DR. ART HISTER'S
Do-it-Yourself
GUIDE TO
GOOD HEALTH

DR. ART HISTER'S
Do-it-Yourself
GUIDE TO
GOOD HEALTH

Random House
Toronto

This book is printed on acid - free paper.

Canadian Cataloguing in Publication Data

Hister, Art
 Dr. Art Hister's do-it-yourself guide to good health

Hardcover ISBN 0-394-22084-6
Quality Paperback ISBN 0-394-22200-8

1. Medicine, Popular.   I. Title.   II. Title: Do-it-yourself guide to good health.

RC81.H58 1990   616.02'4   C90-093176-0

JACKET DESIGN: Andrew Smith
JACKET PHOTOGRAPHS: Robert Karpa
ILLUSTRATIONS: Gary Cody

Printed and bound in Canada.

Contents

Preface		viii
Acknowledgments		xii
Chapter 1	Good Health	1
Chapter 2	Visiting the Doctor	27
Chapter 3	Medical Tests	39
Chapter 4	General Problems	56
Chapter 5	The Eyes, Ears, Nose, Mouth, and Throat	84
Chapter 6	The Respiratory System	105
Chapter 7	The Cardiovascular System	118
Chapter 8	The Gastrointestinal System	147
Chapter 9	The Musculoskeletal System	177
Chapter 10	The Skin	199
Chapter 11	The Female	229
Chapter 12	The Male	262
Chapter 13	Sexually Transmitted Diseases	279
Chapter 14	Contraception	297
Chapter 15	Designer Diseases	326
Epilogue		341
Glossary		342
Index		345

Preface

In which the good, not-so-young doctor reveals why we are about to embark on this journey and advises all those with weak hearts and stomachs to come along anyway

You are often your own best doctor.

Many people disagree with this premise. They argue that just as it takes a mechanic to tell you what is wrong with your car, so it must always take a doctor to tell you what is wrong with your body. Indeed, they will add, it can be dangerous to do otherwise.

But you surely don't take your car into the shop every time the engine misfires or every time you hear a clunk. What you do instead is wait and see if the noise will disappear on its own. Or you ask your friends' advice as to what may be the matter. (Unless you have friends like mine, who don't know one end of a car from another — which doesn't, however, stop them from offering advice gratis.) Or in some situations, you may even get down on your hands and knees and try to diagnose the problem and fix it yourself. (Unless, of course, you are a Jewish male like me and therefore genetically incapable of opening the hood of a car. "Too many parts," Jackie Mason says, and he's right.) Only when you have the feeling that something of major importance or something irreversible is occurring do you go through the bother and expense of taking the car to a mechanic. And then you often cross-examine that poor man (or woman) to make sure that he actually knows what he's doing and is not putting you through needless expense. "What do you mean the muffler needs attention? Can't you just tie it on or something?"

We apply the same approach to most appliances and machines in our lives. But when it comes to our health, we are conditioned to delivering our bodies to our local mechanic every time something goes *ping*. We have developed an entrenched fear that even the slightest delay in diagnosis might result in dire consequences. And when we do show up in our busy doctor's office, we often do not question what is being ordered or prescribed. You may stare at the plumber and pepper him or her with questions, but you will often allow the doctor to order an unpronounceable test without asking why this test is important or how it will change the approach to your problem.

This attitude is wrong. You should not be afraid to use your common sense and knowledge to try to figure out what is happening to that magnificent physical edifice you call your body. And when you do have to visit the medical maven, your family doctor, you should go in armed with enough information that you can intelligently question him or her about your presumed diagnosis and treatment.

There are, of course, many conditions that you cannot — indeed, should not — diagnose yourself. Any time that you do not feel total confidence in your own judgment (or worse, in the diagnoses of your friends, all of whom swear that they have had exactly the same problem for years and therefore know exactly what you should be taking), it is a good idea to get the second opinion of a physician. Often, if you have the kind of practitioner who is comfortable with this approach, you may be able to check out your self-diagnosis over the phone. If there is still doubt, or if the doctor doesn't feel it right to diagnose your particular symptoms that way, then it is always wise to go to the office. It is never a good idea to be left in doubt about your health.

But the simple truth is that most new symptoms that affect a previously healthy fifteen-to-fifty-year-old person are not caused by serious conditions, and there is rarely any need to worry about the consequences of delaying an exact diagnosis for a reasonable length of time. These conditions can best be described as routine, mundane, obvious, and usual. They are very often easily explained and generally do not require fancy tests for confirmation. Furthermore, when you do require the doctor's help, the more informed you are when you go into the office, the more value you will get for the time and effort spent. And finally, if you know why some symptoms occur, then you can often do something on your own to prevent them from recurring.

It is not my purpose in this book to deal with rare or special conditions that you will likely never encounter. Thus, I will not write about Guillain-Barré syndrome or Budd-Chiari syndrome or hepatocellular carcinoma. I will also not deal with those common chronic conditions that do require frequent visits to the doctor, conditions such as diabetes and Crohn's disease. If you happen to be affected by conditions such as these, you should get specialized information that is beyond the scope of this book. These are conditions which can best be addressed by specialists in that particular field, as well as by self-help groups.

This book is written for normal, healthy fifteen-to-fifty-year-olds, those adults who do not have severe, chronic, or unusual illnesses. The book deals with the routine, the usual, the preventable, the treatable, and the recurrent, the problems that account for the overwhelming proportion of visits to the doctor by otherwise normal, healthy adults.

As much as possible, problems are described according to symptoms as you would notice them. But because I am not a particularly consistent person in any aspect of my life, I deviate from this approach whenever I feel I need to.

The first four chapters present general health information. These are followed by chapters dealing with symptoms and problems that occur in each system of the body. The final three chapters discuss sexually transmitted diseases, contraception, and my view of a few contemporary problems, which is bound to make me *persona non grata* in many households. The book ends with a short glossary of commonly used medical terms; you may wish to refer to it as you read the book.

This book is my interpretation of what I have seen over the years and of those conditions I think are common enough to include — the Art Hister Idiosyncratic View of the Medical World. I am sure that I left out some problems that other doctors would have included. In addition, I am certain that I have included conditions that some doctors would argue should always be seen by a physician. No doubt there are also a few errors (although I have attempted to triple-check everything), for which I apologize, and doubtlessly there are several other ways to look at some of the issues. But this is my book, so it is my prerogative to present the information the way I see it. (I used to have a friend who owned the only football in the neighborhood; he set the rules or we lost the use of the ball. This book is my football.)

I hope this information makes you even wiser, healthier, and if possible, more normal.

ACKNOWLEDGMENTS

No book of this type can be written without the help of a lot of friends and advisers. I had plenty of both.

The list of doctors who helped me write this tome is a long and distinguished one. They corrected my errors and reinterpreted some of my information and let me complain about the difficulty of putting all this together. The errors that still managed to elude their sharp eyes are entirely my own fault.

The physicians who read some parts of this text include Elizabeth Whynot, Brad Fritz, Carol Herbert, Jennifer Morwen-Smith, Rob Lloyd-Smith (the hyphenated Smiths are not related), John Hooge, Lorne Kastrukoff, Jack Amar, Laurie Halparin, Craig Beattie, Sam Broome, Andy Chalmers, Neil Longridge, Andy Blokmanis, Jack Rosenblatt, Laurie Lee, Berndt Wittmann, Jon Cope, Lori Kanke, Vera Frinton, Roberta Ongley, Bernard Bendl, Virginia Kilby, Tony Koelink, Bruce Carruthers, John Fleetham, Jeremy Road, Bob Sayson, Vicki Bernstein, David Secombe, Georgia Immega, Bob Rangno, Ray Baker, Pat Rebbeck, Ted Wilkins, and Stephen Sacks.

My friend Dan Pratt offered invaluable advice and helped me focus when I seemed to lose sight of my objective. My wife, Phyllis Simon, read the entire text on a number of occasions (without a gun at her temple) and put life back into me on those many days when I could not see an end to this project. And you have her to thank for eliminating many other examples of my silly brand of humor, much of which still permeates the text. If not for Phyllis, this book would have been twice as long.

My publisher, Ed Carson, never lost hope and offered sage advice and support at the neccessary moments.

My agent, Denise Bukowski, was likewise a long-distance agent of advice and comfort. ("You have to finish it. They paid you an advance.") Thank heaven she has an excellent sense of humor — and an answering machine.

And finally, I have to say a few words about my editor, Nancy Flight (even though she warned me that the acknowledgment section is already twice as long as she wanted). I wrote a book a long time ago that was unfocused and dreadfully long. What you will read now is as much a product of her suggestions and her work as it is of mine. This book would never have been published without her incredible efforts. (It would also be full of many misplaced commas and parentheses.)

DEDICATION

To my family — Looie, Jokie, Timball, and Flossie (the Jericho gang), who put up with my miserable moods and constant complaints, and who nevertheless maintained their great humor and love throughout the last year and a half while I hogged the computer. They have been a constant inspiration for this effort because they make life easier and fun.

CHAPTER 1

Good Health

I am healed (apologies to Dickens)

All of us want to live longer. (At least the people who buy this book
want to.) Even if some of us are sometimes uncertain about how long
we want to survive (because we're afraid that the longer we live, the
greater our risk of acquiring debilitating diseases), we are nevertheless certain that as long as we are alive, we want to be healthy.
Much of my generation, that great demographic blip known as baby
boomers, is convinced that there are secrets to longevity and good
health that can be revealed to us by those who *know* — the "Magic
Formula of Life Theory" — and that those secrets can be learned.
We do not want to grow old and sick the way many of our parents
have, and we believe that even if we can't prevent ill health and death
we can at least postpone them. To that end, we read, watch, listen to
any bit of information that will contribute to our knowledge about
what causes disease and what leads to good health. A quick glance at
the titles in the health section of any bookstore will reveal a plethora
of books about healthful diets, exercise, and other practices that are
unconditionally guaranteed to help us stay young forever. This desire,
I firmly believe, is not a new phenomenon. My theory is that the
second book Gutenberg printed after the Bible was some type of diet
guide for overweight Germans. I am certain that before print every
society was plagued with dietary and nutritional experts standing on
street corners predicting doom for all those who didn't eat their full
portions of taro root or finish their steak behemoth tartare.

In the last fifteen years, health and diet books have become a
growth industry, so much so that I am expecting any day to see a

1

book called *The Berenstain Bears Lower Their Cholesterol*, in which Papa Bear ignores his obnoxious kids' warnings not to consume all that butter and keels over with a heart attack. But despite the generally unprovable claims made in many health and diet books, there really are verifiable bits of advice, nutritional and otherwise, that can help you live a longer, healthier, and better life. You *can* actually prevent many diseases. You can likewise retard the speed with which many chronic diseases affect your health. But none of this information is going to make you immortal or even help you play the piano, for that matter. All we know are general guidelines that seem to contribute to good health. These general rules include avoiding certain "poisons," doing some exercise, eating properly, getting adequate rest, and minimizing stress in your life. This first chapter deals with what we know about these factors and how to follow these guidelines.

These recommendations are best read with a picture in your head of your mother sitting in the room with you and telling you to sit up straight and listen to the wise doctor. Oh, yes, if the information doesn't work for you, there is no money-back guarantee.

AVOID POISONS

I am not one of those people who make hard and fast rules about life (mainly because I can't stick to them any better than you can). So I must recognize that even though the poisons described in this section are bad for your health, I can't simply condemn them with a blanket prohibition. Yes, you should not use these products at all. But if like me, you simply cannot halt your intake of some of these substances, at least make sure that you indulge in them as little as possible. And always plan to stop using them altogether one day.

Tobacco, A Government Cash Crop

I can't tell you how often I've heard it said about someone, often with a sense of awe, that "he was quite a guy — smoked right up to the end." I don't know why it's considered heroic when people keep committing suicide until their last breath.

Smoking is death. There is no better way to put it. If smoking doesn't get you sooner, it will get you later. What's even worse is that you, the smoker, can make me, the shy, quiet, reclusive nonsmoker, sick by forcing me to inhale the secondhand smoke your awful habit produces.

Smoking is responsible for too many diseases to list them all here. But among others, the Smoking Hall of Shame All-Stars includes in its starting lineup lung cancer, bladder cancer, cervical cancer, throat cancer, lip cancer, esophageal cancer, cancer of the larynx, strokes, heart attacks, worsening of angina, emphysema, chronic bronchitis, chronic cough, hoarseness, worsening of asthma, duodenal and gastric ulcers, decreased sensation of taste and smell, increased rate of accidents and fires, and decreased fertility. And please note that that's just the starting team. Then there are the lesser lights, the many other health problems that are also worsened by smoking — the rest of the Alouettes, as it were. (I used to love going to Montreal Alouette games, just to hear the announcer introduce the starting players and, following that, the inevitable announcement that the other players running onto the field were "the rest of the Alouettes." Life is full of the rest of the Alouettes.) What's even worse, therapy for all these problems is much less effective if you continue to smoke.

All smokers could probably quit if they could just find the right therapeutic technique. Every few years a new, "miracle" cure for smoking appears from someone's fertile imagination. In my time, I have seen acupuncture, laser therapy, hypnosis, oral nicotine preparations, relaxation therapy, behavior modification, and several others announced as the answer. They all work to a certain extent on some people (as would being in a comatose state for two weeks — which I am not recommending, by the way). These therapies are most effective for those people who really want to quit this awful habit. But none of these treatments are universally effective.

Despite this somewhat negative assessment, never give up looking for the cure for yourself. If you are a smoking addict, you should try each new therapy to see if it is finally the one that will work for you. Somewhere out there is the perfect method for you, when you are ready. (This is the part of the book where the Hollywood Strings begins to play and a rainbow appears in the background.) The various lung associations in each province usually are an excellent source of information about all the available therapies in your area.

Remember too that it pays to quit at any age under sixty-five. Not only do you save the money that smoking costs you, but for diseases such as strokes and heart attacks, after several years your health risks are about the same as those of nonsmokers.

Secondhand smoke, or passive smoke, has become an important health issue in the last few years, and for good reason. Tobacco smoke is now known to contain over 3800 chemicals, most of which are produced by the unsmoked, unfiltered part of the cigarette or cigar (or pipe, for that matter). We simply do not know the safe blood levels of most of these chemicals, or even if there is such a thing as a safe level for this garbage collection of unwanted substances. But we do know that the rates of diseases such as bronchitis and lung cancer are higher in people forced to inhale passive smoke for long periods of time. Children who live with smokers are known to have higher rates of chest infections, which are directly related to the amount of passive smoke they are exposed to. And most disturbing, the death rates from smoking-related causes are higher in those forced to inhale passive smoke than in those not similarly exposed. So it is not against the rules to tell smokers exactly where you think they ought to put the cigarette they are holding. Do be prepared, however, either to run very fast in the opposite direction or to vigorously defend your point of view.

Recreational Drugs

In one of my favorite anecdotes from the early seventies, a disheveled, hirsute fellow ran breathlessly into the free clinic where I worked and informed the bored staff that he had just experienced the ultimate high from a new, though expensive, drug he had sampled the previous morning. Although he wasn't entirely certain, he thought it was called something like LBJ, and the reaction it produced was "for twenty-four hours, man, you don't feel nothing, you don't hear nothing, you don't see nothing. It's incredible, man." I felt obligated to inform him that for a much lesser expense, the price of a hammer, he could experience the same feeling, if he would just allow me to hit him over the head with it.

People will try anything, so long as it gives them a high that they can't experience without artificial aids. For some reason that I cannot fathom, when drugs are used this way, they are called recreational drugs. What, may I ask you, is recreational about being stoned?

The recreational drugs that I am still commonly asked about include marijuana, hashish (yes, I know that they're basically passé, but some people are still stuck in the seventies), and cocaine.

There really is nothing good to write about recreational drugs except that marijuana may help with severe nausea and glaucoma. Case closed for the affirmative.

There are, however, many negative effects from these substances. Cocaine increases heart rate and increases blood pressure, can cause heart attacks, and most worrisome, in some people it can lead to sudden death from as-yet undetermined factors. Marijuana and hashish can affect the lungs exactly the way cigarettes do, as well as affecting that part of the brain called the hippocampus (a college for the overweight?), where memory seems to be stored. I think it's usually easy to spot all the old potheads at folk festivals and other such events by how spaced out they seem to be and how wonky their memories are. ("Hey, I know you, don't I? Didn't we used to live together or something?") Marijuana can also lead to sperm abnormalities and a lowered sperm count in some males. In large doses, all recreational drugs produce personality changes, an effect that the user is invariably reluctant to acknowledge. ("I am not short-tempered, dammit.")

It is always a source of interest to me that so many people ignore the warnings about drugs because "it won't affect me." Wrong. With apologies to the late Jim Croce, you don't pull on Superman's cape, you don't spit into the wind, you don't pull the mask off the old Lone Ranger, and you don't mess around with drugs. You'll eventually lose and become addicted. (You also shouldn't stand in Ron Hextall's crease without adequate insurance, solicit a contribution from John Turner for a testimonial dinner for Pierre Trudeau, and so on. Life is full of these tough rules, which we must all memorize for our safety.)

What can you do if you are addicted to any of these drugs? The first thing is to admit your addiction. This is the most difficult step.

After you accept that you have a problem, the next place to go for help is to a facility or a physician that is expert at the treatment of addictions. Other family members and friends are not drug counselors; nor should they be put in that position. You may use them for support, but do not rely on them for the intense attention that a drug addiction demands.

And your friendly family physician, me, is often also not the best place to go for help. Although family doctors are generally very knowledgeable about addiction, the ordinary family practice simply doesn't allow the time for the intensive care that an addict requires. Addicts are often charming and manipulative, and they are usually able to pull the proverbial wool over the doctor's eyes, if she or he doesn't have the time and expertise to stay one step ahead of the invariable games an addict will play. It's essential that the addict work with people who can spot these tendencies and prevent them from interfering with the success of the therapy.

Other excellent sources of help are the various self-help groups that deal with addiction and drugs. The people who attend these groups are hard to fool because they've heard it all before. They can also empathize in a way that only people who have similar problems can. And they also often know all the best resources in the community.

Drug addiction is very difficult to beat alone. It generally takes lots of help and lots of time.

Alcohol

Try to explain to a visitor from another planet why we tolerate — even advertise and promote — the use of alcohol, at the same time that we ban a more innocuous drug such as marijuana (although if you are reading this book carefully, as you should, you will know that I don't consider any drug innocuous). The only explanation I can think of is that alcohol was here first, and the government learned to tax its use and subsequently became dependent on the tax. An addiction from addictions, so to speak.

How dangerous is alcohol? Well, let me give you some of the statistics. Alcohol problems are said to affect as many as one in three families in North America. Alcohol is the third leading cause of all deaths on this continent and the leading cause of deaths of adults between twenty-five and forty-five. Alcoholism affects up to 12 percent of the population. Alcohol is involved in 40 percent of all severe burns and 33 percent of all auto accidents. There are many more frightening figures that I can give you, but I think you have enough to get the point.

Alcohol is a toxic substance that injures many body tissues when it is overused. It can damage the liver, producing cirrhosis and liver cancer, and can cause "feminine" changes in some men, such as breast enlargement. Alcohol can increase blood pressure and damage the heart, the nervous system, and the brain. Alcohol produces gastritis, ulcers, and pancreatic damage. It interferes with the production and action of certain hormones, particularly testosterone, and interferes with normal sexual response in both men and women. It can cause birth defects in developing fetuses. When added to other factors, it can increase the risk of some types of cancer. For example, smoking is well known to cause cancer of the larynx. But if you drink excessively as well as smoke, your risk of laryngeal cancer is much higher than if you only smoked. Excessive drinking interferes with normal nutrition and normal sleep. Alcohol interferes with the metabolism of some drugs, particularly drugs that act on the central nervous system, such as tranquilizers. And of course alcohol is directly responsible for many accidents, deaths, and homicides.

So to sum up, if you're a man who drinks to excess, probably you don't eat properly, your breath smells, you can't sleep, you have large breasts and liver spots on your skin, you have small testicles, you stumble around a lot, you can't drive properly, you can't perform in bed, and you may kill your partner and yourself in a drunken rage. Now don't *you* sound attractive! (And just in case the women reading this feel smug, it's not really much different for a woman who drinks to excess, except, perhaps to your chagrin, you probably won't develop larger breasts, and of course your testicles won't shrink.)

In short (to quote the younger Histers), alcohol sucks. In fact, alcohol is so unsafe that if some drug company had just invented alcohol and were trying to get permission from some sober authority for the release of this new product, the company's request would be laughed out of the hearings (unless free samples were given out beforehand).

I must hasten to add, however, that there is something good to say about alcohol. Some studies show that in small to moderate amounts (which is usually defined as the equivalent of one averaged-sized alcoholic drink a day: twelve ounces of beer, five ounces of wine, or one to two ounces of hard liquor) alcohol may protect against coronary heart disease (see chapter 7). There is a lot of controversy about the cardio-protective role of the drink-a-day approach, but results are consistent enough that we have to give them some credence. We do know that at least part of the reason for this beneficial phenomenon is that small amounts of alcohol increase the level of HDL (high-density lipoprotein), the so-called good cholesterol, in your blood-stream. HDL protects your blood vessels from the effects of the bad cholesterol, or LDL (low-density lipoprotein), which in high amounts leads to narrowed coronary arteries and higher rates of heart attacks. So by raising the level of HDL, alcohol may decrease the risk of having a heart attack.

But the problem with promoting a drink a day for the population at large is that along with the obvious increase in alcoholic addiction that would occur, one drink a day may soon turn out to be many drinks a day even for those who do not have addictive tendencies. Far too many people assume that if a little is good for you, a lot must be better. So if one drink every day is good, three must be even better. And then these people run into all the risks of excess alcohol intake.

Until we know a lot more about how alcohol works to protect the heart, and more specifically in whom it works, I believe that we should not encourage anyone to start drinking alcohol to diminish the chances of having a heart attack.

It is not too hard to determine for yourself if you have an alcohol problem. You can obtain a number of questionnaires from books in the library or from various associations concerned with alcoholism that give you a very accurate assessment of whether or not you should seek help. The questions basically ascertain whether you can go without an alcoholic drink for a long time and whether you use alcohol to help you function normally. The truth is that most people already know before they take the questionnaire what the results are going to be.

Now what about the treatment of alcoholism? I hate to disappoint you, but I am not about to reveal any secret recipe for defeating this problem. The only successful treatments I have ever seen occur in those people who have acquired some sort of "religion," something outside of themselves that makes it important that they don't drink anymore. It helps immensely to belong to a group that actively discourages the resumption of drinking. To me, that is why Alcoholics Anonymous is so successful. I am convinced that belonging to any group that cares is the most important factor in curing alcoholism. People who want to use their own willpower, in isolation from any support system, are generally predestined to fail. Alcoholism is an extremely difficult problem to beat alone. The product is too readily available. Our culture glorifies its use. It's too easy to give in.

But even though this is a difficult addiction to beat, if you do have an alcohol problem, it is imperative that you deal with it as soon as you can, preferably today. The longer you put it off, the harder it is to treat. The fact that you have tried to stop drinking before and didn't succeed should not discourage you from trying to stop yet again. But get help. Don't try to do it on your own.

I also am firmly opposed to the idea that people who have a problem with alcohol may eventually drink in moderation. I believe that all alcoholics eventually increase the amounts of alcohol they consume. A person with an alcoholic tendency must assume that alcohol is a substance to be completely avoided.

Caffeine, My Drug of Choice

Having been less than kind to smokers, drinkers, and drug addicts, I want to redeem myself. Caffeine addicts are great people. They are smart, handsome, thoughtful, insightful, and kind to animals and little kids. The fact that I drink about five cappuccinos a day doesn't affect my point of view one bit, although I do tend to rush my words and this tic is driving me nuts and I shake a lot and last night I only slept for four hours and I can't write short sentences. But, hey, all that coffee merely makes me see things more clearly and more quickly. And what I see is that coffee drinkers are real men, even the women.

In truth, caffeine does not seem to be a particularly bad drug to be addicted to. Caffeine is a member of the xanthine family of drugs, which also includes theophylline, an anti-asthmatic medication. The xanthines raise blood pressure, increase pulse rate, cause a general wakefulness and insomnia, and make you jittery (sort of like Robin Williams on a quiet night).

Even though it may sound more like an economic theory from Colombia, caffeinism is in fact the name of the syndrome in which all these symptoms of generally hyper body responses occur when you ingest caffeine (a question on a high school history test: compare communism, capitalism, and caffeinism). By and large, caffeinism occurs most in those people who do not regularly ingest caffeine. If you drink coffee regularly, these effects are not nearly as dramatic. (Tea and soft drinks also contain caffeine, although the caffeine in these drinks is usually not as concentrated as in coffee.)

If you are addicted to caffeine and you have to stop drinking some form of it for a while, you are likely to experience mild withdrawal symptoms, which often include headaches and irritability. Of course a good strong cup of coffee or tea will rid you of these symptoms pretty quickly.

The xanthines weakly (not weekly) constrict arteries, and so some people use coffee to get rid of headaches that they believe are caused by dilated blood vessels to the head, such as mild migraines. Some reports have shown that regular coffee drinkers have fewer asthma attacks than those who don't consume any coffee (regular coffee drinkers are also "regular" visitors to the washroom), presumably because caffeine slightly dilates constricted airways.

Large amounts of coffee, usually defined as more than six cups a day, have also been reported to increase the rate of pancreatic cancer and of birth defects in offspring of mothers who consumed these large amounts while pregnant. These reports have been largely discounted, but I still believe that you should moderate your caffeine intake during pregnancy, on the general rule that you shouldn't go overboard on anything when pregnant. Recently it was reported that women who drank more than one cup of coffee a day had a more difficult time becoming pregnant than women who drank no coffee.

Caffeine does not seem to raise the chances of developing breast cancer, although in some women it tends to make the symptoms of benign breast disease (also known as fibrocystic breast disease) somewhat worse. This is not true for all women with this problem, so the only way to find out what caffeine does to you is to stop ingesting caffeine and see whether the tenderness and swelling in your breasts decreases.

There are conflicting reports on the effects of caffeine on both cholesterol and coronary heart disease, although the general consensus is that large amounts of caffeine minimally increase total blood cholesterol levels and may increase the risk of heart attacks.

For what it's worth, a recent study showed that coffee made with boiled water that comes in contact with the coffee in an unfiltered manner (as, presumably, in a percolator, or horrors! my cappuccino machine) raised cholesterol levels in the blood, whereas coffee made by filtering the coffee through filter paper did not. I suppose someone is working on a study to show that if you drink your coffee from a mug, you are likely to have a higher cholesterol count than if you drink from those awful Styrofoam cups. (Trust me. Even if Styrofoam doesn't raise your cholesterol level, it must do something else that's bad for your insides.)

There are no good coffee substitutes. Nothing really tastes the same. But if you think you are drinking too much tea or coffee, certainly try a substitute, and if you like it, by all means, stick with the substitute. If you can't find a coffee alternative, just cut back on your consumption.

GET LOTS OF EXERCISE

This is one topic that I always feel ashamed to comment on. I believe in exercise, but I don't practice what I preach. You know about lapsed Catholics? Well, I am a lapsed runner, I am a lapsed squash player, and I am a lapsed rower. I am even a lapsed chess player (although I still coach Little League, which merely requires a lot of pleading, cajoling, and standing around). I am proud of one part of my exercise background, though. Just as I used to brag that I was the only person I knew who hadn't seen *Ben Hur* (the movie, which everyone of my generation can recall, along with Bill Haley and the Comets, Patti Page, cars with fins, when Sid Caesar was still funny, and other treasures of that era), I am the only nondisabled, adult professional who has never attended an aerobics class. I realize that

I must be somewhat of a sicko, but somehow the thought of smelling the sweat of two hundred other human beings and being yelled at by an overly pleasant passive-aggressive hellcat in tights for not raising my legs high enough is not my idea of a fun hour.

The trouble is that I believe in the idea of exercise. It's the practice that's hard (which is why exercise and religion are so similar for me). It is so easy to postpone your run for just one more hour or day or week. I am always behind on some aspect of my life, and exercise, which I generally loathe, becomes the easiest part of my schedule to sacrifice (as if it's ever a sacrifice).

Exercise is good for you. Really. Because you burn off excess calories, exercise is the most effective way to lose weight and to keep the weight off once you've lost it. (You lose anything else, you never get it back. Weight, however, like the cat in the song, never stays away.) Exercise improves muscle tone and flexibility. Specific types of exercises can improve muscle strength and endurance. Exercise is beneficial in raising HDL, the "good" cholesterol. Exercise may help in preventing osteoporosis, the disease in which bones "soften" as we age. Exercise lessens fatigue caused by daily stress. There is some recent evidence that exercise may prolong life by retarding the deterioration of certain body functions, and it may improve the quality of life in old age by retarding the deterioration of some brain functions. There is some proof that some tumors, such as bowel cancer and breast cancer, and certain diseases, such as rheumatoid arthritis and diabetes, are either less frequent or less severe in people who follow a regular exercise regime. Moderate amounts of exercise seem to increase immunity and lessen the frequency of infections. Interestingly, though, excessive endurance exercise seems to lessen immunity, leading to the not-unusual complaint of frequent colds and flus in long-distance runners. (I think they all secretly like to be sick so that they don't have to keep training.)

But beyond the obvious physical benefits, exercise is extremely beneficial for psychic health. There is the obvious benefit of feeling good *after* you finish. I never feel good while I'm exercising, but boy do I feel better after. There is the benefit of sticking to something you clearly have to work hard at, the benefit of sticking to a schedule, the benefit of having some sort of discipline in your life, the benefit of bragging to your friends that you are doing something most of them aren't.

Aerobic versus Anaerobic Exercise

About twenty years ago, exercise became categorized into the subgroups of aerobic and anaerobic. It had become clear that like everything else, not all exercise is created equal. Aerobic exercise refers to exercise that promotes efficient oxygen use by the body, meaning that you can do the exercise for several minutes without getting short of breath. This type of exercise must be steady and uninterrupted. Examples of good aerobic exercise include jogging, brisk walking, rowing, cycling, and swimming.

Sporting activities that do not promote the same efficient, steady use of oxygen are called anaerobic sports. Tennis, squash, and basketball are examples of start-and-stop exercises that do keep you in shape but tend to be more anaerobic (although when they are played at a very competitive level, I am certain that these sports are quite aerobic).

To protect against heart disease, aerobic exercise is considerably more beneficial than anaerobic exercise. So if you are mostly interested in the cardiac benefits, the general consensus is that you need to exercise aerobically for twenty to thirty minutes three to five times a week. If you want to increase muscle tone and flexibility, obviously the more exercise you do for the muscles that concern you, the greater the benefit. If you are interested in preventing osteoporosis, it is clear that you need some exercise, but just how much of what type still remains a mystery. Remember, we really had no idea of the benefits of exercise until relatively recently, so we just haven't had enough time to effectively compare longevity and eventual quality of life between the couch potatoes, the daily walkers, the placid joggers who stop to smell the flowers, and the messianic runners.

How to Start an Exercise Regime

When starting out on a new exercise regime, it is absolutely essential that you proceed in a cautious and sensible manner. This is especially important once you hit the big four-oh. If you have spent a lifetime doing no more than eating chips, swilling beer, and flipping channels, it is quite normal to take several months to get over this state of semihibernation, and if you try to produce a new, healthy body in four weeks, you run a great risk of developing some type of injury, or even of getting a heart attack. I also recommend that if you are over forty, or if you have a family history of premature heart disease, you should discuss your exercise plans with a doctor.

After you have decided that this blimp you see every morning in the bathroom mirror has to be replaced by the svelte bod that has been hiding inside you for lo these many years, there are a number of steps that you must go through.

1. Most important, decide what you like to do. Be honest. You may live beside an Olympic-sized pool, but if you hate getting wet, as I do, you will likely stop going at the first conceivable excuse.

2. Next, you must evaluate your present physical state for risk factors and possible disabilities. This evaluation is extremely important because each sport has specific requirements that may disqualify you, even if you are dying to participate in it. For instance, if you have a bad knee from previous trauma, it is unlikely that running should be your sport. If you have a chronically draining ear, then swimming or diving should not be high on your list of possibilities.

3. Now comes the hardest part, where you pass from the cerebral to the physical. Set the time aside and start. I know, I know — it's hard to set the time aside. You're busy saving lives or making beds or being pleasant to an unappreciative public or family. But honestly, who can't find thirty minutes a day, if that is the number-one priority? I have used every excuse in the book (there is a book of excuses, you know, a copy of which can be obtained from any teenager) so I know how easily you can fool yourself. But that's exactly what you're doing — fooling yourself. If you make it a priority, the time will materialize. (My favorite cartoon is of a man sitting down to finally write his great novel, and having found that all the necessary preconditions for writing are perfect, he then turns around and leaves the desk and his writing for that day because the conditions seem too perfect. It doesn't take much

of an excuse to abandon an exercise when you really don't want to do it.)

4. Start by doing the chosen activity twice a week for a few minutes at a time (although you can probably start with more than a few minutes if you choose an activity such as swimming or walking).

5. Always remember to do an adequate warm-up and to warm down (which, contrary to folklore, is not done with an alcoholic beverage). Warming up properly means doing several minutes of stretching and gradually increasing the intensity of your activity. Each type of exercise and each exerciser requires a unique stretching regime. Read a book on stretching, figure out for yourself what kind of stretches you require, and then, hardest of all, spend the time doing this relatively boring preparation. Then you should take several minutes at least to hit the maximum intensity of your workout.

6. While exercising, "listen" to your body and don't try to do more than you are capable of. If you develop a pain in your knee while running, for example, unless the pain quickly disappears, stop running and consult a doctor to ascertain the cause of the pain. Just because you are capable of continuing your exercise despite the discomfort doesn't mean that you should continue. You may be doing yourself some long-term damage.

7. After the exercise, warm down by slowly returning to complete rest and by doing a few stretches.

Once you've started, you will probably become heady with self-congratulation. Each time around the block, or each extra lap of the pool, will lead to a delusion that next time you will do it faster, better, longer (even for me, who usually considers each new milestone to be one more station of the cross that has been passed). This is precisely how most people develop problems. They overtrain. What's the rush? You've spent the last thirty years on a couch in a fetal position. Why not take six months, rather than two weeks, to get to your prescribed goal? Of course you can push your body, but the cost is likely to be an overuse injury. Only an idiot or a weight lifter (yes, I know, there are some normal weight lifters) would try to lift 300 pounds just a day or two after he had finally lifted 250 pounds. But you would be amazed at how many idiots there are who try to run five miles several days after they have struggled to do four. These people are begging for an injury.

Remember that a chain is only as strong as its weakest link. For those pushing forty — and especially those who have opened the door to forty and are charging in to the next decade — remember that the weakest link can be your cardiovascular system. You should not exceed a certain heart rate in training. To get this magic number, first subtract your age from 220. Then take 70 percent of that figure. That, dear reader, is your theoretical target heart rate in aerobic exercise. So for the slower ones out there, if your age is forty, your target heart rate should be about 70 percent of 180 (220 − 40 = 180), which is 126.

A Cautionary Note

Are there any drawbacks to exercise? First, as already mentioned, there is the risk of injury, especially if you don't train properly.

Second, in some men, intense exercise decreases the production of testosterone. It can also decrease the sex drive in some overzealous athletes (so if your spouse starts suggesting that you run 20 k every day, you might just question the reason for this gratuitous advice).

Third, a recent article described a syndrome that the author called hypergymnasia. People who suffer from this syndrome, usually young women, are so addicted to exercise that they absolutely have to work out very intensely every day. Many of these women have previously had eating disorders and have merely replaced one type of psychiatric illness with another. Me? I guess that you could say I suffer from hyperrestonia.

For me, the biggest hazard of intense exercise is the boring personalities that too many overachieving athletes develop. There was a time, happily somewhat passed now, when every second jerk seemed to want to discuss personal record times and 10 k times. Stocks and real estate and how to prepare pasta are considerably more interesting topics, don't you think?

GET YOUR SHUT-EYE

I lost great gobs of sleep while writing this book. As a result, I was often a miserable something-or-other, which means that I made life miserable for those nearest me. Sound familiar? People vary in the amount of sleep they need to function properly. There really are folks who can manage on four hours of sleep a night. But for most of us, eight to nine hours is more like what we need, although we all tend to cheat, of course.

Once we pass into middle age, the need for adequate sleep increases. So, yes, when I was an intern (my kids usually leave the room whenever I start a sentence like this), I often got less than seven hours' sleep a weekend (pity the poor patients), and yet I was still able to function in the hospital (which tells you a lot about how hospitals work). At the ripe age of forty-three, I know I could never do that again. I would fall asleep on my feet, probably on the first night shift.

If we don't get enough sleep, we lose our ability to reason as well, we lose our facility with certain mental functions, and we become irritable. One study showed that 35 percent of interns reported falling asleep during a phone conversation while on duty at night (even in conversations in which they were not speaking to their spouses or in-laws).

Lack of sleep should always be treated by first trying to eliminate the reasons for the insomnia. It is obviously more beneficial to decrease the stress in your life, if that is the cause of the insomnia, than it is to start to treat the lack of sleep, which is really only a symptom. Don't drink stimulants such as coffee or soft drinks that contain caffeine at night. If your work agitates you, don't do any in the evening. Any relaxation technique you can find or follow — warm milk and honey, yoga, biofeedback, exercise, sexual (not verbal) intercourse (used here for purely therapeutic reasons, of course) — may help you relax enough to drift off to dreamland. Naps during the day are very effective for some people, minimizing their need to sleep as long at night (but try not to nap during office hours, unless the boss is napping as well).

Never force yourself to try to sleep by lying in bed, tossing and turning for hours on end. If you haven't reached slumberland in twenty to thirty minutes, get out of bed and do something. Any quiet activity will probably do, but one of the best is reading some boring book (not this one, goodness knows, which will instead keep you up for hours; try any publication on the GST instead). After a few minutes of this activity, quietly return to your bed (although your partner will probably make some rude comment about the idiot who has just woken her up) and try to sleep again.

If the insomnia lasts for more than two weeks, however, you should visit your family physician to see what can be done. Some new research shows that sudden onset of profound insomnia is often associated with significant psychological problems, such as major depression. In those cases, the depression needs to be treated (either with psychotherapy or with antidepressant medication) or else the insomnia itself will eventually lead to more severe psychological problems.

Lack of sleep should rarely be treated with sleeping pills, but unfortunately that's exactly what most people do far too often. Sleeping pills, also called hypnotics, all have two effects that should make everyone cautious of their use. First, they can have a carryover effect, resulting in fatigue the next day. Second, they are addictive, often resulting in a strong rebound insomnia when their use is discontinued. In addition, there have been occasional reports that some of these medications can produce profound psychological changes, such as hallucinations and psychotic episodes, when they are used continuously for any length of time.

Hypnotics should be used only once in a while — for example, that night you have to get a good night's sleep and you know you are too anxious to fall asleep on your own. The only other valid use of sleeping pills is when you have not gotten a good night's sleep for a few nights in a row and you need to break the pattern. In those situations, using sleeping pills for one or perhaps two nights is acceptable, but never use them for more than that.

EAT PROPERLY

I am ashamed to admit this, but when I was in medical school, the total lecture time spent on nutrition was, as I recall it (and the older

I get, the less I recall), several hours. What's worse, we treated nutrition as a subject akin to voodoo, and many of us skipped the lectures, including me.

Please forgive me. I was young. And besides, nutrition wasn't the only lecture I skipped, and to use that famous Second World War excuse, I wasn't the only one. I knew of one student who refused to attend lectures on the kidney because she claimed the topic was incomprehensible, an observation that given our lecturers, was not far from the truth. Rumor had it she couldn't recognize a kidney if one bit her, something she probably thinks that kidneys do.

It was entirely possible to graduate as a doctor from McGill University in 1970 knowing next to nothing about such a vital topic. It wasn't only possible, it actually occurred — witness Dr. Hister.

Nutrition is very difficult to study objectively, except in people living in very deprived circumstances, or in extremely ill patients who cannot absorb certain products from their gastrointestinal tracts. Because it is unethical to eliminate something that you know people must have in their diet just to study the effects of a lack of this product on their system, nutrition has never lent itself well to the classic double-blind studies that doctors accept as the most valid research method. In the double-blind method, which is not quite the same as the blind leading the blind, neither the researcher nor the subject can distinguish the product under study from a placebo, or from some other product. Is it tape or is it Memorex?

The lack of precise information on this vital topic leaves an informational void into which many nonmedical theories and fads are inserted. These fads and theories have a great appeal for the nonmedical world because people generally prefer to find answers and cures that are under their own control. They want to help themselves, much more than they want to depend on the medical edifice. And what could be more alluring than the thought that we can control our own health destinies simply by eating properly?

I do believe that we can control certain aspects of our health by following some basic nutritional guidelines. If you follow most of these recommendations, you will likely live a healthier life, and you may live longer. But there are no guarantees.

In general, you need to eat protein, carbohydrates, fats, vitamins, minerals, and trace elements, and you need to drink plenty of liquids.

The recommended daily requirements for these substances allow for a large excess of all you need. (I will not print a table of these recommendations, but they are readily available from any health unit and from most doctors' offices.)

Having given you the motherhood statement on nutrition, I will now reveal Hister's Vague Rules on Eating. These rules must be taken with a grain of salt (although you must, of course, be careful of your salt intake). I do not expect that you will actually go out and weigh your portions of food or compulsively measure the exact number of calories in one teaspoonful of olive oil. So when I say, for example, that you should cut your total fat intake from 40 percent to 30 percent, the easiest way to do this is simply to replace several fried dishes a week with poached or boiled or baked dishes. You don't actually have to measure anything. These are general rules and are meant to be applied with a broad interpretation. (I live in perpetual fear of the measuring police, who come into your life from time to time with a weight scale, measuring cups, or calorie and cholesterol counters. There must be an island, near Antarctica, I hope, where we can send them all.)

Eat Moderately

Most of us eat too much. The first rule of good nutrition is to maintain a total caloric intake that keeps your weight at a level that is desirable for your height and age. (Weight tables are available from your doctor or in most diet books.) You and your twin sister may need different amounts of calories to maintain your weight. (It's sad but true that my wife can pig out — and she does — and maintain her weight, whereas I only have to look at a plate of food and I am already two pounds heavier. Of course I seldom merely look, but that's beside the point.)

Decrease Your Intake of Fats, Especially Saturated Fats

Many of us now get more than 40 or 50 percent of our calories from fats. To minimize your risk of premature coronary heart disease, reduce fats to no more than 30 percent of your daily caloric intake and try not to get more than 10 percent of your total intake from saturated fats (which come mostly from animal products but also include such important sources as palm oil and coconut oil). For most of us, this means cutting back on our consumption of dairy products, as well as fried foods, marbled meats, thickened sauces, and prepared foods and fast foods, which are often saturated with saturated fats. Use only skim-milk cheeses, drink only 1 percent milk (which you can still use for making frothy milk for cappuccinos), and, cut out butter (which I do not believe that you should replace with margarine, something I cannot conceive of as being a food). Cook with mono-unsaturated or polyunsaturated fats (if you have to use oil at all when you cook), and remove the skin from chicken before you cook it.

For years, people assumed that if you just replaced saturated fats with polyunsaturated or mono-unsaturated fats (such as safflower oil and olive oil), then you could take in as much fat as you wanted. (Doesn't the thought of eating fat turn your stomach?) This assumption is wrong. Fats yield nine calories per gram, as opposed to four calories for carbohydrates and four for proteins. So if you don't cut down on fats, you will get fatter (or stay fat). High fat intake has been correlated with increased rates of several cancers, including cancer of the bowel, the rectum, and the breast. Also, most successful low-cholesterol diets only succeed if the *total* fat intake is decreased, not just the saturated fats.

Eat More Carbohydrates

To replace the eliminated fat, eat more carbohydrates, such as pastas and whole grains. This rule is one that most people have no trouble following. The recommended percentage of carbohydrates is about 55 to 60 percent of your diet.

Eat Less Protein

You probably don't need as much protein as you are now getting. Protein should represent 15 percent of your calorie intake. Most of us get considerably more protein than this in our diets because we've always been told that protein is good for us. This is true, but the excess protein is simply not needed. Better to take in more fiber and carbohydrates. Don't tell my mother I said this, but you don't need to eat meat or fish every day to be healthy. You can cut your meat and fish intake down to two or three times a week and still get more than enough protein.

Eat Your Veggies

Try to eat five or six servings of fruits and vegetables every day. If you really want to be a food fetishist, you can try to balance your intake of yellow and green vegetables. This is guaranteed to drive your kids nuts, or out of the house. (Nuts are good foods too.)

There is some pretty good evidence that beta carotene, present in vegetables like carrots and broccoli, can decrease the rates of certain cancers, even lung cancer in smokers. Citrus fruit peels (a real favorite for a main course in our house, as I am sure it is in yours) contain something called terpenes, which have caused tumors to shrink in animals. (I'm sure that the prospect of eating only citrus fruit peels may have had something to do with the animals' improvement.) My favorites, garlic and onions (the national dishes of my homeland, Poland), are also thought to decrease tumorous changes in some types of tissue. The ellagic acid in strawberries and raspberries and some nuts has been found to protect against tumors.

Get Plenty of Vitamins, Trace Elements, and Minerals

We need vitamins to help with certain metabolic processes. A normal, well-balanced, North American diet gives us enough of every vitamin that we need, although certain people, like vegetarians or people with chronic bowel inflammation, do require more of certain vitamins than a normal diet provides. Vitamins in very large doses, however, can be dangerous. This is especially true for those vitamins stored in fat tissue in the body (A, D, E, K), particularly vitamins A and D.

We also need minerals. The most written-about mineral these days is calcium, which is of course found primarily in dairy products but is also present in green, leafy vegetables. There is some good evidence that the rate of osteoporosis, a disease in which the bones soften, is lower in postmenopausal women who take 1000 to 1500 milligrams of calcium daily *before* menopause (although anyone prone to kidney stones should be careful about this level of calcium intake). There have also been some reports that calcium may be effective in preventing bowel tumors.

Iron is necessary for the transport of oxygen to your tissues by means of the red blood cells. A low iron intake results in an iron-deficiency anemia. Endurance athletes, pregnant women, and women with heavy periods require extra iron in their diets. Good sources of iron include meats, eggs, spinach, and milk.

We really don't know too much about the required doses of the other minerals, like magnesium and aluminum. Some researchers have identified aluminum as a potential agent in the development of Alzheimer's disease, meaning that you shouldn't eat the tabs on aluminum beer and pop cans, I guess.

If you are a vegetarian, God bless you, but in case He or She forgets, make sure to take in foods with adequate amounts of iron and vitamin B_{12} such as dairy products. If you don't eat dairy products, you should be on vitamin B_{12} supplements. And remember that the best sources of complete proteins, those containing all the essential amino acids we require, are animal products. So as a vegetarian, you must learn to combine different protein foods to get all your amino acids. And always remember that you are not a better person just because you don't eat meat. You're just more likely to be anemic.

Potassium-rich foods like bananas, citrus fruits, and nuts may protect against developing high blood pressure. And there are some reports that high potassium intake decreases the rate of strokes.

Trace elements like selenium and zinc are probably the next great source of wonder in the field of nutrition. We simply don't know how important they are, so make up a theory, find three friends to test it, and write a book. I guarantee it will sell some copies.

That's Not All

Try to eat as few smoked foods and cured meats as you can, because the nitrites in these foods increase the risk of bowel cancer. (This food rule hurts me the most. I live for the taste of hot smoked meat from Schwartz's in Montreal, which I can unfortunately get only once a year.)

Fiber is currently a favorite son. Fiber is the indigestible part of plants. We certainly don't eat enough fiber in North America. We don't really know exactly how much fiber we need, but it is quite obvious from studies of other cultures that when significantly greater amounts of fiber are taken in, the rates of certain tumors, like bowel and rectal cancer, decrease. Fiber also seems to lessen the rates of other bowel disorders, like appendicitis, irritable bowel syndrome, and diverticulosis, and perhaps of other diseases, like diabetes.

The way you get more fiber is to replace refined foods with the unrefined equivalents. Eat whole-grain breads and baked goods, more whole-grain cereal, more bran, and more veggies and fruits. You do not, however, have to eat bran at every meal (such as bran chicken or bran soup). Eating too much bran can lead to stomach cramps, gas, and bloating (as well as loss of friends for dinner).

If you have high blood pressure or kidney disease, don't eat too much salt.

And then there is the whole area of pesticides and additives. As anyone who reads and has an IQ greater than 70 knows, there is a good deal of debate about the hazards of certain chemicals added to foods. Consumer advocates are ready to blame any food additive or pesticide for all of humanity's ills, whereas the chemical industry, which is of course composed of only fine, upstanding people who only want the best for humanity and are not in the least interested in profits, defends itself by saying that anything less than instant death immediately upon ingestion of their products means that whatever the industry is doing must be safe. We are caught in between. You must make up your own mind about whether or not specific pesticides and preservatives and hormones and antibiotics added to the foods that you eat can do you much harm. They don't sound good, but does that mean they are necessarily harmful? Life is so complicated.

Finally, there is overnutrition. Many of us are simply too fat, and we go on frequent diets. What can I say about weight-loss diets that you can't read in much greater detail in books written specifically on that topic? The answer is not very much, which will not stop me from saying something.

I work in an area of Vancouver in which people are extremely well read and well fed and willing to try just about anything to improve their health. So I think that I have heard of every conceivable diet plan ever devised by any health maven wanting to make a quick buck.

Practically all diet plans have three things in common. They all work for a while, and they are rarely unsafe. Those two common factors make each new diet that comes along worth trying and make all diet books best-sellers. But the other factor that links most diets is that few of them are effective in the long term for most people.

If you have heard that a new diet based on eating as many apple cores (with the seeds) as you like is guaranteed to make you thin and wealthy, then as long as you have no health problems, go ahead and try it. If you develop any symptom (dizziness, excessive fatigue, headaches, an aversion to anything that looks like an apple, and so on) after starting on one of these regimes, see a doctor about the symptom, just to be certain that it doesn't stem from the diet. But remember, no matter how dramatic your weight loss is in the first few weeks, the rate of loss will eventually slow down or plateau. And unless you are prepared to permanently change the way you eat, and unless you are prepared to finally start on an exercise regime, that same exercise program that you have been avoiding for lo these many moons, I can assure you that you will regain all your lost poundage, and many of you will actually end up fatter in the long term.

The only way to keep off lost pounds (or kilograms, and even grams) is to change the way you eat and exercise. All else is likely to fail.

AVOID TOO MUCH STRESS

Finally, we come to stress.

I have left it for last mainly because I believe that for most of us, stress is just not that bad (and also because I do not have much to tell you about how to avoid it).

Stress in life is normal. We fool ourselves when we think that more primitive cultures than ours are stress-free. Other cultures may have less stress, but none are completely free from some types of anxieties, which often appear unpredictably and probably have much the same physical and emotional effects as stressful events do in our lives.

It is only when stress starts interfering with our ability to function normally that I believe it needs to be looked at. If you get a headache every day when you have to go to work, if each school day is accompanied by a stomachache, if you are beginning to act differently at home or at work because of the constant pressure, if you find you need a drink every night to unwind, then you need to do something to alleviate the situation. Stress-related symptoms are as varied as the people who get them. Some people (especially men) get chest pain, some develop rashes or headaches, and many have mood or personality changes. The list indeed is endless.

There is no current proof that stress alone can produce illnesses such as cancer and heart disease. Excess stress is probably not good for you, but by itself, without other factors, it probably doesn't produce severe disease.

What can you do if stress is interfering with your ability to function normally? For the relief of general stress-related symptoms, there are the motherhood treatments of relaxation techniques. These include various relaxation methods (see *The Relaxation Response* by Herbert Benson), as well as exercise, dance, music, prayer, stamp collecting, massage therapy, watching television, talking — in short, anything but drugs, alcohol, and overeating. You must find what you like to do that relaxes you, and then you must do it regularly.

If a specific situation produces your feelings of stress, there are only two solutions. You can either learn to tolerate it, or you can get away from it. Never assume that the situation will change just because you are unhappy with it. A spouse who drinks will not suddenly stop drinking because it's driving you nuts. A boss who is a tyrant will continue to be one, despite your daily headaches and persistent skin rash.

So you should learn to develop the general ways of relieving stress already mentioned above. You should also try to find ways out of the situation. And you should perhaps look into some type of therapy that can help you find ways to cope better with a situation that may not change for a long time.

CHAPTER 2

Visiting the Doctor

In which the good young doctor argues that the only reason
that the good die young is that they just don't get quality
medical care

Now that I've told you all those things you could do to make yourself healthier, it's time to recognize that you may still need to visit the doctor from time to time, if only to check that you are following all my advice properly.

When you go, there are some simple rules to follow that will make your visit more fruitful. These rules are based on certain preconceptions. First, you have a right to the doctor's time and advice. You are, after all, paying for the privilege of occupying a seat in the waiting room for sixty minutes. Second, you can argue with the doctor. You can even interrupt while he or she is explaining something to you if you don't understand what's being said. (In contrast to my own invasive style, most patients seem too polite to interrupt while I am monologuing them. I often only know that I'm droning on when I see their eyes cloud over or wander to a minute inspection of the articles on my desk.) Third, the more you know and the more you ask, the better the medical care you will receive. If the health provider is insulted or threatened by your questions, you should find another person to help you. We all learn best from questions we can't answer.

Remember that good health care is a right in this country, not a privilege. Your right to health care comes not because of the kindness of strangers (although it's true that doctors frequently don't introduce themselves when bursting into your hospital room, generally searching for the person who occupies the bed next to yours but who has been ensconced in the communal bathroom for the last hour) but because you live here.

We are privileged to have one of the best health care systems in the world, in that practically everybody in this country has access to the same uniformly high level of medical care. (Some people, mostly politicians and doctors, argue that it is simply *the* best, but I don't know how you rank systems numerically. Let's just give it a 9.3 out of 10, which would qualify it for a bronze medal, since Canada rarely seems to win the gold.) The great majority of people who choose to serve in this system are caring, kind, and thoughtful and willingly offer you the best care that they can.

As in most empires, however, some of the people who work in the health care system lose sight of their original objective. Thus, the patient often becomes a number in a clinic, a sort of commodity of trade. The patient's story becomes an accumulation of statistics and entries in a file. The person, the human being, is lost in a mass of details about that person. Doctors, nurses, physiotherapists, administrators, and cleaners can become arrogant, unfeeling, thoughtless.

As a patient, always remember that the system is there to serve you. It is not there as a sinecure for the health care workers or the health care bureaucracy. You pay handsomely for this service. You deserve the best care available.

HOW TO PICK A DOCTOR

Choosing a new doctor is always a problem, but it seems to be particularly acute for people moving to a new city or a different part of town. I am not certain how you can invariably find a doctor who is right for you, but I definitely know how you can *not* find a doctor who is right for you. You should not go through the phone book or call the College of Physicians. You shouldn't search for a contractor for your house by flipping through the Yellow Pages for the one nearest you (the telephone company will disagree); nor should you select a physician that way. The College of Physicians merely gives you what the phone book gives you — the two or three doctors closest to your home, usually in alphabetical order. (Why should a doctor whose last name begins with A be more to your liking than one whose last name begins with Z?)

The best way to find a new doctor is the same way you would find a plumber, a dentist, or a hair stylist. Ask your friends. Chances are your friends, if they have a lifestyle similar to yours, will be seeing a physician whom you will also like.

The most important factor in choosing a doctor is the style of the doctor, how comfortable you feel in her office. If a physician makes you uncomfortable, if you can't relax in her presence, then it's unlikely that she is the right doctor for you, no matter how highly recommended she may be. Medical knowledge may seem like a more important factor than comfort, but I honestly believe that most doctors offer virtually the same degree of knowledge. (My mother disagrees, insisting that I am the world's smartest doctor, although the dumbest son.) Doctors do differ in their areas of interest. Some doctors are more comfortable with teenagers than other doctors are. Some of us enjoy counseling; some don't. But the type of knowledge doctors have is often very similar. It is how we dispense the information, how we deal with you, the patient, that is probably our most important distinguishing feature.

There are other considerations. You should consider the age of the physician. Some people only trust older doctors because they have more experience. Others feel that only young physicians are up to date on the latest treatments and diagnostic tools. (That's what ages a doctor prematurely. Twenty years ago, I was too young for some; now, alas, I'm too old.)

The sex of the doctor matters to a lot of patients. For example, a lot of men will not let a female doctor examine them. Many women, however, feel much more at ease with a female physician.

Some other factors to take into account include the proximity of the doctor's office to your work or home, the office hours, the telephone access to that office (I know all doctors have phones, but do they answer them?), and similar logistical concerns. A small aside. Patient advisories often warn you to ask to which hospital the doctor admits his patients and where he graduated from (University Hospital at UBC, and McGill, in case you have to know). But the medical school from which the physician graduated matters little in the development of his skills because much, if not most, of the information doctors use in practice is picked up after graduation. Doctors learn a great deal, perhaps the bulk of their skills, on the job.

Nor should you worry too much about the hospital to which your family doctor admits her patients, because as an average healthy adult, you should rarely need this service before old age. Even if your doctor doesn't admit her patients to a certain institution, she can often arrange for temporary privileges for herself if it's important enough. Or she can find you an equally sympathetic physician in the institution more convenient for you.

There are other issues that might matter to you, but make sure that they are really of importance. These issues may include whether or not that doctor delivers (babies, not pizzas), encourages or scoffs at holistic or alternate therapies, pays house calls, offers advice and referrals on the phone, solicits second opinions when you ask, and so on. Most of these matters are related to the issue of style I mentioned earlier. If you are comfortable with the physician, chances are that most of these issues will be resolved in a manner acceptable to you.

One area that is always of concern to patients is telephone access to the physician. Can you get through to the doctor when you want? Are you put on hold, to die of your condition before the receptionist returns to your line? Does the doctor return your phone calls? The same day, or once a month? Will she or he inform you of normal results over the phone?

In our (inefficient) office, the phone is a constant source of complaints, and we have been trying to solve the problem for the last five years. To me, this has become a Sisyphean task. (I'm certain that Camus had his doctor's phone lines in mind when he wrote *The Myth of Sisyphus*.) Telephone lines are like bridges. New lines are overused as soon as they are opened. I'm sure that some new lines are connected with a busy signal. If someone has a good suggestion for improving our system, please let me know. But don't phone, because you won't get through. Write me instead.

YOUR RIGHTS AS A PATIENT

If you are unhappy with the medical service you receive, you can shop around for better service. You *can* visit a second doctor for the same complaint, although every system limits this type of visit somewhat. You can, and should, find another doctor if the first doctor is not treating you with the respect and consideration you believe is your due. Doctors all have different personalities, and they all hit it off with different kinds of patients. There are some patients who adore me. (My kids don't believe this.) There are other people who would rather endure an hour of listening to fingernails scratching a blackboard than visit me again. (I doubt that many of them will buy this book.)

You can, you should, go back to see your physician if the treatment isn't working. You should always ask how quickly the prescribed treatment is meant to take effect. If you don't, you may be in for some surprises. One man once called me an hour after he took his first antibiotic capsule to inform me that he was still coughing. I referred him to his mother.

You are completely entitled to second opinions if you are not happy. If the doctor perceives this as a threat, then you should probably not be seeing that doctor anyway. In complicated or uncertain situations, the doctor also is usually only too happy to have the unbiased opinion of a colleague.

HOW TO VISIT THE DOCTOR

A visit to the doctor should be like a visit to Safeway when you are shopping for a special meal. Bring a list.

Most doctors are very busy, and we often rush the patient. So it's best to come prepared with details and questions. If both Aunt Ida and Uncle George had a similar problem, make a note. You are likely to forget Aunt Ida's traumatic time with her abdomen when you are confronted with the harried physician. Write down a history of the symptoms *as you have felt them.* Think about the circumstances of the symptom. Is the pain intense, does it come and go, is the pain accompanied by other sensations, such as nausea and fullness, was there a fever, when did the pain start, is it relieved by food (for my son, everything is relieved by food), and so on. I realize that the doctor should ask all these questions, but what if he or she forgets? Your note is a quiet reminder of what matters to you.

In the hall, ushering the patient from my office, I frequently hear something like, "Art, I need to ask you something, but I've forgotten what it is." Don't trust your faulty memory. Write it down.

If a test has been ordered, ask what it is for, how safe it is, how reliable it is, and when the results will be available. Once the proposed diagnosis and treatment have been explained to you, make absolutely certain that you fully understand what was said. If the word "tumor" was used, for example, it may mean something completely different to you than it does to your physician. Ask if there are other possibilities to consider or other treatments that might work. Ask if you need to come back, and why. What will be gained from another visit? Your time is valuable. If you are returning simply to hear that all the test results were normal, there may be (there definitely is) a better way to spend an afternoon.

Medicine is still as much an art as it is a science. There are frequently several approaches to a problem. Doctors often disagree about a treatment or an investigative tool. Ask. Argue. Don't be obnoxious, but be assertive and questioning. You will be a better patient and make your physician a better doctor. Always end by asking what you can do for yourself, either as a treatment or to prevent the condition from recurring.

RULES FOR TREATMENT

When you do require a medication, there are a great many questions you should ask about each prescription. You can usually get what you need to know if you are polite and direct. You will often not get it if you are shy and unquestioning. The information is important and can occasionally save your life. Like most doctors, I have prescribed penicillin for a patient who didn't tell me she was allergic to it. I have written a prescription for a beta blocker (a drug for high blood pressure) for a person who has asthma (beta blockers have been known to set off severe asthmatic attacks). Just remember that doctors make mistakes, and you don't want to be one of them.

Here are the main questions you should ask:

1. When getting a drug, you should always ask your doctor why she is choosing the particular one whose name she has just illegibly scribbled on a prescription sheet.
2. Ask about the cost of the drug. Because I have worked in areas

with many poor patients, I am aware of the price of many medications. Frequently I obtain this information because of a loud complaint from a patient that some doctor who filled in on our call system has prescribed a forty-dollar prescription. Often the condition could have been treated just as successfully with a ten-dollar prescription.

3. Ask about side effects. Which side effects are common? Which are rare? Which are merely a nuisance? Which are potentially life-threatening? Take the birth control pill, for example. The absence of periods on the low-dose pill is a common side effect that is of no real concern. The development of sudden sharp leg pain can indicate a clot in a vein that can lead to a stroke. This type of pain needs to be promptly evaluated. Yes, of course you should read the packet of information that comes with the prescription. But you should also ask your doctor what to watch for before starting on this potent medication.

4. Ask how often you should take the medication. If a drug needs to be taken four times a day, does that mean you have to wake up at night to take a pill, or can you safely spread out the pills during your waking hours? If you miss one pill, as all of us often do, should you take two to compensate?

5. Ask if there are prohibitions on this particular medication. Can you take it with milk? Can you take it with other foods? Can you drink alcohol when you are taking this drug? One drink only, or can you party?

6. Ask how this drug affects other drugs you are taking. Many medications interact with other drugs, resulting in potential complications. As an example, cimetidine (Tagamet), commonly used for ulcer therapy, shouldn't be mixed with tranquilizers, which are also often used in the same patients.

7. Ask how long you need to take the pills. Should you come back to see the doctor when the prescription runs out? How long can you take these pills without expecting long-term complications? How soon should you expect to be feeling better? Do you have to take the entire prescription? What if the symptoms disappear in one day and you have a ten-day prescription? Is there a shorter course of a different therapy that might work as well, although it may cost more?

8. What else can you do for yourself? Are there dietary modifications that you can make? Should you exercise? Must you stay home? In bed? Can you watch "Geraldo"? Do you have to?
9. Always report all suspected adverse reactions to the doctor. If your hair starts turning green shortly after you start a new medication, always phone to ask if the green hair is an expected side effect. If it is, perhaps you should switch drugs.

The doctor should never feel challenged by this line of questioning, although if he is terribly busy, he may feel rushed in giving you the information. My detractors call me hyper, but I have learned to give much of this information in a rapid manner, often while I am busily scribbling the prescription.

WHEN TO GET A ROUTINE CHECKUP

Every doctor seems to have his or her own rules concerning the need for an annual physical examination (in the interests of brevity, and my editor's sanity, this will be referred to simply as a physical from now on). What follows, then, are my guidelines. Other doctors will no doubt disagree. Let them write their own books.

All women between fifteen and forty should have the following:

1. *An annual pelvic examination and Pap smear*
    I believe that all women who are sexually active should have an annual pelvic examination. This category includes all sexually active young teenagers and the newly celibate, if they have had several sexual partners in the past. (The newly celibate are like all converts. They are more religious than the true believers for a while, but in time . . .)
2. *An annual breast examination*
    Every woman should also have an annual breast examination. She should also be shown how to do breast self-examination and should be actively encouraged to do it every month.
3. *An annual blood pressure reading*
4. *Special examinations in the presence of certain risk factors*
    If there are certain family risk factors (such as premature death

from heart disease or excessive cases of bowel cancer) or personal risk factors (such as excessive use of alcohol or a history of severe sunburns in childhood), a more thorough physical should be done periodically, and certain additional tests should be conducted. If you have symptoms at the time of the routine visit, then obviously the source of the symptoms should be pursued with more aggressive investigation.

Between the ages of fifteen and forty, no more is required. When a woman reaches age forty, I recommend a full and thorough physical with a complete cholesterol count, a urinalysis, and a blood test for hemoglobin. This is called a base-line examination and is used for future reference.

All women between forty and fifty should have the following:

1. An annual pelvic examination and Pap smear
2. An annual breast examination
3. An annual blood pressure reading
4. Special examinations, if necessary

In that decade, more attention needs to be focused on possible bowel tumors, glaucoma, and potential cardiovascular problems. Some authorities have also advised all women in this decade to have yearly mammograms, but this is still a contentious and unsettled issue. At all times when you visit the doctor, you should discuss issues that may matter to you, such as contraception, osteoporosis, menopause, exercise, and diet.

For men, unless you have symptoms of disease or are at risk for some problem because of family history or poor health habits, there is rarely a need to see a physician before the age of thirty.

At thirty (or thereabouts) all men should have:

1. A blood pressure reading
2. A cholesterol count

Note that a physical is not required or necessary at that time.

Over the next decade, the average male (I know that no male thinks of himself as average) should be encouraged to have a blood pressure reading periodically, perhaps every three years. While he is seeing the doctor for this, they can also discuss factors for cardiovascular disease (see chapter 7 if you want to know why men are more affected than women) such as lack of exercise, poor diet, and smoking.

At age forty, men should have:

1. A full physical examination with particular emphasis on the cardiovascular system
2. A cholesterol count
3. A urinalysis
4. Special examinations, if necessary

If there is any reason to suspect glaucoma, it should be checked for.

Everyone seems to still recommend annual rectal examinations for prostate and rectal tumors beginning at this age, but I am not so sure that annual examination is necessary. There is no doubt that *some* prostate tumors can be felt through a rectal examination, but many of these tumors have spread by the time they can be felt. In addition, although a tumor can be diagnosed in this manner, there is some doubt as to whether anything can be done to prolong that patient's life. As for rectal cancers, about 10 percent can be felt with a rectal exam, but this type of tumor is still quite rare among men under the age of fifty.

So if we are not doing the forty-year-old male much of a favor by invading his rectum, why bother? Perhaps it is wiser to start rectal examinations as a routine at a later age, say forty-five or fifty, when men don't seem to mind this intrusion on their dignity quite as much. Most men make more willing patients if you can delete the rectal from the rest of the examination.

Between forty and fifty, there is still no need to do an annual examination in the absence of symptoms. Periodic reassessment, perhaps every three years, is probably not overkill (a great word to use for a medical procedure, wot?) and does nicely for everybody's reassurance. In this decade, emphasis is put on finding high blood pressure, cardiovascular disease, and rectal, prostate, and bowel cancers.

So these are my ivory-tower recommendations. The real world is, of course, another matter entirely. Many people, particularly men, are addicted to an annual *complete* physical. Not doing one is sure to bring on signs of withdrawal (manifested by increasing signs of hypochondriasis) or to send them to another doctor's office in search of that holy grail of medicine — perpetual life. The male world has become convinced of the urgency of annual medical exams by some variation of the ultimate male horror story in which a man suddenly collapses while jogging or making love or raking leaves (not as pleasant a prelude to sudden death as making love) and dies without warning at the age of thirty-eight. And every man believes with all his heart that this would never have happened had this poor chap had an annual physical exam. Which is a load of rot.

Assuming there were no previous symptoms or undue risk factors, chances are quite good that this man could have had *daily* physicals and the outcome would have been the same.

There are other arguments one can make in favor of annual physicals. For instance, the need for an exam brings the patient to the office, where he can discuss medical issues that matter — diet, smoking, exercise. This is true, but why pretend that the physical part of the visit matters?

Then there is the argument that the patient sleeps better at night having the reassurance of a normal examination. (And the doctor sleeps better at night because physicals pay a lot.) This is also true, but it just shows how much the public has bought the false hope implicit in a normal examination. Better to reeducate the members of the public about this false reassurance so that they can better take care of their own lives and we can instead spend health care dollars where they are really needed.

Let me reemphasize that these recommendations are based on two preconditions. First, the patient has no symptoms. And second, the patient has no risk factors to worry about. If both of these conditions are met, you can safely leave an annual visit to the doctor for a physical off your calendar. Visit Disney World instead. I don't think they do rectals there.

HOME TESTING

I am sure that within thirty years you will be able to sit down in your parlor and attach yourself to some type of gizmo with multiple knobs, arms, bells, and sirens, and depending on the printout, you will be able to determine whether or not you need extra vitamin C that day, or whether or not the pain you have in your side requires any medical help. Medicine is definitely moving in the direction of home testing and home monitoring.

Currently, good home-testing kits are available for giving blood pressure readings, measuring glucose levels in the blood, identifying ovulation peaks in women, detecting hidden, or occult, blood in the stool, and determining pregnancy. Also on the drawing boards are cheap machines to measure your own cholesterol level, home kits to culture for strep throats, and self-testing for allergies.

As always, it's buyer beware. Some machines are more efficient than others. More important, it is sadly true that a little knowledge can be dangerous. A machine cannot provide you with perspective. Just because a reading does not fall into the normal parameters does not mean that you have to do anything about it. Many problems (many vaginal infections, for example) self-correct without intervention. More important, many people have slightly abnormal results in certain measurements without having any disease. For example, many people have a level of bilirubin (a breakdown product of red blood cells) in the blood that is above the commonly accepted "normal" level, yet there is nothing wrong with these people. This normal "abnormally" high bilirubin level does not require any treatment or investigation. So it is with many test results. A white blood count of 10,400 may be normal or may be an important sign of infection. Perspective, perspective, perspective.

CHAPTER 3

Medical Tests

*In which the author discusses all the things
that may be done to your wonderful body*

Nothing seems to shake people as much as being told that they have to be sent for "some tests." Me? Tests? Why me? What's wrong? Does the doctor really think I have cancer and doesn't know how to tell me? *What are the tests for?*

Most medical tests are done for the reassurance of either the physician or the patient. "How can you tell, doc, that my bleeding doesn't represent a tumor?" "Frankly, George, unless we do some tests, you'll just have to take my word for it." "In that case I want to be tested, doc." And another probably negative test is ordered.

Many medical tests are ordered for what we call the rule-it-out reason. Practicing by the rule-it-out method means ordering tests just to eliminate or to rule out certain possibilities, many of which are fairly remote. For example, in a person with persistent abdominal pain, barium X rays are frequently ordered just to rule out a malignancy, even though the history and physical examination indicate that the condition is very likely benign. These tests do have a use, in that negative results take a lot of worry away, and the patient can then more confidently follow the originally recommended treatment plan.

But this kind of overtesting has significant drawbacks, not the least of which is the cost to the health care system. A lot of money is spent to confirm what was readily apparent in the preliminary examination. There is also the cost to the patient's long-term health. Obviously a few extra blood tests over the course of your life are not going to harm you in any way. But how many barium X rays can the average patient have without increasing his or her risk of cancer?

39

FALSE POSITIVES AND FALSE NEGATIVES

There is one other aspect to random testing that I must address. Frequently I am asked by a nervous (usually male) patient to be tested for "everything." Everything? "Yeah, you know. Cancer and heart disease and all the things that can go wrong." This kind of patient needs a lot of time.

We cannot, nor should we, test for everything. That is because medical tests produce a significant amount of false positive and false negative results.

If you test enough patients, you will find that a small number of test results are abnormal, or what in our perverse logic we call positive, even though the person tested really doesn't have any medical problem. This is called a false positive result and usually is no more than a confusing nuisance for the doctor. But certain false positives can present real problems to the patient. As an example, a false positive in an X ray for breast cancer usually results in breast surgery, with the attendant risks inherent in any surgical procedure no matter how minor.

A false negative is a test in which the results are negative when the person actually has the disease that is being tested for. Blood tests for rheumatoid arthritis, for example, are negative in a substantial proportion of people who actually have arthritis. Likewise, if you have a breast lump that is growing, never assume you don't have a breast tumor just because the breast X ray, or mammogram is negative. As any mammogram report will stress, these X rays are not perfect at distinguishing a benign lump from a cancerous one. If there is any question about a cancer, the lump should be removed no matter how reassuring the mammogram report is.

Random testing of everyone for everything would result in a lot of needless apprehension and a lot of useless investigations in many people, and a lot of false reassurance in others. Tests should be reserved for specific reasons and risks.

WHAT TO ASK

If you are going to have a test, no matter how innocuous it seems, there are some questions you should always ask:

1. Why am I going for this particular test? Is it necessary?
2. Why do you suspect that I have the condition that you are testing me for?
3. Is the test innocuous, or are there potential side effects and complications? If so, what are they?
4. What is the likelihood that the test result will determine the future course of action for my problem? In other words, am I just wasting my time if there is no treatment anyway?
5. How reliable is this test? Or to put it in the words you learned above, what are the false positive and false negative rates for this test? Are you really going to make up your mind as to what I have on the basis of these results?
6. What should I be careful of before I have the test? Should I eat? Exercise? Fast? Drink alcohol? Have sex? None for six months? No, thank you.

If you ask all these questions, you may assume that the doctor will only have time to see two patients a day. But much like the information about medications that you are prescribed, this information about tests is necessary to have, and it can be dispensed relatively quickly, often in conjunction with other aspects of the problem that brought you into the office.

I have been dissuaded on numerous occasions from ordering tests by patients who protested that they didn't want those particular tests for some reason or other. It is your body. Do not allow it to be invaded without knowing exactly what is happening and why. (This stance will be easier if you just think of doctors as Visigoths, or better yet, as the "brain specialists" in Monty Python skits. "Are you the brain specialist?" "No, no, no! Yes, yes! I am the brain specialist. Yes." "My brain hurts." "It will have to come out." "Out of me head?" "All the little bits of it.")

Always remember that tests are meant to help elucidate a solution to a problem. They are not an end in themselves. There is an old medical joke in which a surgeon says to a colleague, "The operation was a success. But the patient died." We treat people, not test results. If the tests are negative and your symptoms continue, press the doctor to reassess the situation. Reassess once, twice, as often as necessary, until the situation either stabilizes or defines itself more clearly.

The tests described on the following pages are the more common ones that are ordered.

BLOOD TESTS

There are thousands of blood tests. And they are becoming more sophisticated every day. You can probably find someone, in California no doubt, who can measure the level of boredom that David Letterman or Donahue produces.

But there are only a few tests that are used for the common problems. The other blood tests are reserved for more esoteric conditions or for more difficult situations.

ART Test

I just had to list this one first.

I will leave all ridiculous comments up to you, my readers.

ART is the screening test used for syphilis. If it's positive, it should always be followed by more specific syphilis tests. ARTs (automated reagin tests) can be falsely positive, and they can stay positive for many years.

Tests for Blood Levels of Medications

We can now measure many medications in your bloodstream. Dilantin, theophylline, digitalis, and lithium are just four commonly prescribed drugs that should be periodically monitored with blood tests.

There are several reasons that we may want to know a drug level in your blood. First, most drugs are not effective unless you absorb a specific amount from the pills you swallow, and everyone absorbs different amounts of the same pill. Theophylline, commonly used for asthma, is a perfect example of a medication that differs widely in how much each person absorbs.

Second, many drugs become toxic if too much is absorbed. Testing levels of the drug in your blood helps determine a safe level for you.

Finally, there is the occasional situation where someone has taken far too much of a medication, either accidentally or on purpose. Testing the blood level of the drug at that time helps determine the emergency treatment to be administered.

Tests for Blood Urea Nitrogen (BUN), Creatinine

Why would anyone want to have the amount of buns in their blood measured? Actually, these tests are used to measure kidney function, although you have to lose a significant degree of function before these tests become positive.

Tests for Calcium, Protein, Phosphates

These are frequently thrown in as a part of other routine tests. Even when they are abnormal, they are very, very, very seldom correlated with significant disease, unless the patient has significant metabolic problems — for example, from starvation or parathyroid hormone disease. A normal blood level of calcium does not mean that your bones have enough calcium. There is no correlation between the calcification of your bones and the level of calcium in your blood; thus, this is not a useful test for osteoporosis.

Cholesterol Count

Despite other surprises you may find in this book, the serum cholesterol count actually does measure the cholesterol level of your blood. Several subfractions of your cholesterol count are important. Thus, in the usual complete cholesterol count you can measure the levels of total cholesterol, the level of high-density lipoprotein (HDL), the level of low-density lipoprotein (LDL), and the amount of triglycerides in your blood (see chapter 7). This complete screening test should be done only after a twelve-hour fast (nothing to eat after the evening meal) and with no alcohol intake for seventy-two hours.

Complete Blood Count (CBC)

This does not refer to a measure of how the mother corporation is getting on your nerves. Nor is it really a complete blood count, because it is anything but complete. The CBC is used to measure certain properties of your red blood cells and includes a white blood cell count (see below).

Early Pregnancy Test (EPT)

This is not a test that is done at 6:00 A.M. to see if you're pregnant. Rather, it's a blood test for pregnancy that should be positive for both a normal pregnancy and an ectopic pregnancy (an abnormal pregnancy that is growing in the fallopian tubes instead of in the uterus). The test measures the amount of a product called beta HCG, which is produced in increasing amounts by all pregnancies, not just the normal ones.

Electrolytes Test

Most people hear of electrolytes when they develop vomiting and diarrhea and are told that replacing the water that they have lost is not good enough; they should also replace their lost electrolytes. The major electrolytes are potassium, sodium, and chloride. The easiest way to think of these is as salt ions, which you lose in urine, sweat, and bowel movements. They must be continuously replaced or else you may suffer cardiac and metabolic complications. Patients who are on diuretics — drugs that make you urinate more — can develop electrolyte abnormalities because many diuretics also allow your kidneys to filter out more electrolytes, especially potassium, along with the excess urine. Eat lots of bananas, dried fruits, and peanut butter if you've been put on those diuretics that don't conserve potassium, like furosemide (Lasix) and hydrochlorothiazide (Dyazide).

Erythrocyte Sedimentation Rate (ESR)

The ESR is a nonspecific test that measures how heavy your red blood cells are. The ESR is measured by determining how fast red cells settle to the bottom of a tube when the tube is allowed to sit. In some chronic illnesses, especially the arthritides, the ESR goes up, often quite dramatically. By monitoring the ESR, you can measure how well the treatment is progressing.

Ferritin Test

The ferritin test measures the amount of iron you have stored in your body. You draw on these iron stores in times of physical stress. Ferritin levels can be very low in female endurance athletes, as well as in some male runners. A low ferritin level can interfere with physical performance and can leave you tired even in normal circumstances.

FSH and LH Tests

Testing for the follicle-stimulating hormone (FSH) and the luteinizing hormone (LH) can help determine the hormonal status of women — for example, whether or not menopause has occurred — and can diagnose certain causes of infertility.

Glucose Tests

If the glucose level in your blood is consistently above a certain level, you have diabetes. There are several different ways to measure the blood glucose level, including, most commonly, to measure the fasting level (done after an eight-hour fast). The fasting glucose test is often supplemented by other tests done one and two hours after breaking the fast (which does not mean breakfasting but rather ingesting a glucose mixture).

A glucose tolerance test is considerably more complicated. To do this test right, the pancreas must be "primed" for several days beforehand. You do this by eating lots of carbohydrates, usually for three days before the test, which is one pretest preparation that nobody seems to mind. You then fast overnight, show up at the lab with your morning urine in hand (preferably in a container), and your veins are tapped every hour until you either cry "enough!" or the test has run its course after four or five hours (paranoid people who think "they" are out to get them should not volunteer for this test). Only a masochist, or a health nut, volunteers for a six-hour glucose tolerance test. This test determines whether or not you have hypoglycemia, an abnormally low blood glucose level (see chapter 15).

Hemoglobin Test

Hemoglobin is the part of the red cell that transports oxygen to your tissues. When your hemoglobin is low, you are anemic. There are many causes of anemia, the most common being iron deficiency.

Hepatitis Test

We are able to measure antibody response to the hepatitis B virus, the cause of the liver infection that used to be called serum hepatitis but is now called hepatitis B. This test should be done on anyone who may be acutely ill with this infection, anyone who once had hepatitis but is not sure which type it was, and anyone who may be a carrier of hepatitis B.

HI Titer

It is crucial that you not confuse this test with the HIV test (see below). The HI titer determines whether or not you've been exposed to rubella, or German measles.

HIV Test

This test measures antibodies to the human immunodeficiency virus (HIV), the virus that causes AIDS (Acquired Immune Deficiency Syndrome). A positive test indicates that you have been exposed to the virus. It does not mean that you will get AIDS. Currently we do not know what percentage of people who are HIV positive will get AIDS, although as time goes by it seems that the percentage is getting higher and higher.

Immunoglobulin (Antibody) Test

The serum immunoglobulin test measures antibody levels in your blood. People like to have this test done when they feel their "immunity" is low, having identified themselves as those special ones in the community who always seem to come down with any cold or flu that is passing through. But the truth is that we don't know why most of these people get sick more often than others, and when we do measure their antibody levels, they are nearly always found to be normal.

Liver Function Tests

These tests, of which there are at least five, do exactly what their name implies. They measure how well your liver is working. Occasionally the levels of some liver enzymes can be raised for no apparent reason, so unless you really are suspicious that the liver is misbehavin', don't go chasin' an isolated slightly raised liver function test.

Bilirubin is a substance produced when your body recycles the red cells of your bloodstream by breaking them down. When the liver can't function properly, the bilirubin level goes up because the body can't handle this normal recycling function. This rise in the blood bilirubin level may cause your skin to become jaundiced, or turn yellow.

The bilirubin level is frequently raised in otherwise normal people who have absolutely nothing wrong with their livers. This is called

Gilbert's syndrome. (This syndrome is not named after the Gilbert of Gilbert and Sullivan — the G is soft in Gilbert's syndrome.)

Platelet Test

Platelets are blood cells that are important in the blood's ability to clot. The platelet count establishes how many platelets are circulating in your bloodstream.

Rheumatoid Factor Test

The rheumatoid factor test is the blood test used to help diagnose rheumatoid arthritis. But a large proportion of people with arthritis never have a positive rheumatoid factor test, and a lot of people with a positive test do not actually have arthritis (and you wonder sometimes what drives doctors crazy).

Spot Mono Test

This is not a test to find the best place to get mono but a test to actually diagnose an acute bout of infectious mononucleosis. Although it's often done for this reason, the mono test is useless if you are looking for that syndrome called chronic mono, which is not at all chronic mono (see chapter 15).

T_4, TSH Tests

The T_4 test measures the amount of thyroid hormone circulating in your bloodstream. The thyroid is the gland situated in the front of your neck that is intimately associated with the metabolic functions of your body. The thyroid is a very complex gland, and the T_4 is, at best, only a somewhat accurate measure of thyroid function. Although this isn't always true, a good rule to remember is that if your T_4 is low, you are likely to be hypothyroid (low in thyroid function); if your

T_4 is normal, you are likely to be euthyroid (normal for thyroid function); and if your T_4 is high, you are likely to be hyperthyroid (a free copy of this book to the first person who guesses what this means).

Another useful thyroid test measures the level of TSH (thyroid-stimulating hormone) in your bloodstream.

Testosterone Test

Testosterone is the main male hormone, but women produce testosterone as well. It should be measured in women who have an excess of body hair or certain other malelike physical features (with the exception of male braggadocio). Testosterone has gained prominence in the last few years because weight lifters (and other athletes, I hasten to add) have been injecting themselves with huge amounts of testosterone derivatives (anabolic steroids) to build muscles.

Uric Acid Test

Uric acid levels go up under certain conditions, most prominently in gout, a disease in which the excess uric acid is deposited in various body parts, particularly the joints and the kidneys. But you can get gout even with a normal uric acid, and you can have a very high uric acid and not have gout. (Don't even ask.)

Vitamin B_{12} and Folate Tests

These tests are administered when a vitamin B_{12} or a folic acid anemia is suspected. Any vegetarian, especially a strict one who avoids even fish and eggs, who has the symptom of fatigue should have these tests done.

White Blood Count

The white cells in your blood are responsible for fighting off foreign invaders such as bacteria and viruses.

Several different types of white cells are lumped together in the white count, and each has a different significance. The total white count goes up in acute bacterial infections like appendicitis. The white count tends to go down in prolonged viral infections. The percentage of different white cells that are present also helps with diagnosis. Thus, in an acute viral infection like infectious mononucleosis, there tends to be a preponderance of cells that used to be called lymphocytes (but are now called large white cells), and they look abnormal. (As soon as a generation of new doctors is comfortable with a new nomenclature, the renaming police reactivate themselves and change all the familiar titles to newer ones, which all of us have trouble remembering.) In leukemia, faulty white cells are greatly overproduced.

URINALYSIS

Everyone seems to get a urinalysis done periodically, but hands up all those who know what is being tested for.

There are three parts to a urinalysis (although you, of course, only take part in one part). In the first, a stick of different-colored reagents is put into your urine and the doctor watches the colors change on the stick. (Be serious, now. What else is there to do in a lab?) In this way we can tell if your urine has too much glucose or protein or white cells or hemoglobin. This is a rapid and useful screen for diabetes, kidney and bladder disease, and some prenatal problems.

In the second part, the specific gravity of your urine is measured to determine how concentrated your urine is.

The third part of a urinalysis is to rapidly spin the urine in a test tube and examine the sediment that settles to the bottom of the tube. We look for red and white cells, which are more numerous in infections and tumors, and for something called casts, which are a sort of construction of cells that shouldn't be there. Certain casts indicate specific kidney problems (or problems for the producer).

X RAYS

X rays are very helpful in diagnosing certain problems. But every X ray that you have means that you are exposing your body to extra radiation. It is true that we are exposed to much background radiation already — from radon, for example — so in the scheme of things, you are really adding very little extra radiation to yourself by having an X ray. But this is *excess* radiation that you are exposing yourself to, so if you have a decent alternative to the test, why not use it? A perfect example is the use of skin tests for TB instead of chest X rays.

Most body parts can be X-rayed, but some areas show up better than others.

CT SCANS

Plain X rays have several limitations. Because they are two-dimensional pictures, they cannot show depth very well. Plain X rays are very useful when it comes to "hard" tissue like bone, which always shows up well on X ray films. But they are not useful for picking up injuries to soft tissue areas, such as the brain or cartilage.

CT scans (the letters stand for computerized axial tomography — CAT or CT) are computerized films that can show up some soft tissues, as well as give a measure of depth to the picture. CT scans have revolutionized the diagnosis, and consequently the treatment of many problems, including especially brain and skull injuries and diseases, certain abdominal problems, disc disease of the spine, inner ear disorders, and a host of other conditions.

BIOPSIES

Biopsies are tests in which a piece of tissue is removed for further analysis, often to determine whether or not cancer is present. Simple biopsies from the skin can often be done by shaving some cells from the lesion, but biopsies that are taken from the inside of the body, or even biopsies from more complicated skin lesions, require the use of some type of anesthetic.

It seems that a biopsy result should be foolproof, but like anything else in this business, it's buyer beware. On at least two occasions, I have been very surprised at a certain biopsy result. I subsequently asked a second pathologist to review the specimen — anonymously, of course. On both occasions, the second pathologist disagreed with the original report and issued a far more reassuring report, which eventually proved to be correct. In addition, a biopsy may occasionally not remove enough of the tissue you are concerned about. If the result doesn't make sense, it's worth reviewing the case.

CULTURES

A culture is a test in which we try to grow the little culprits that are invading a part of your body by concentrating colonies of these rascals on specific culture media that allow easy growth of pathogens. You can have cultures taken from any body part. I discovered just how many parts can be cultured while I was still in medical school, when a surgeon who didn't have all his oars in the water decided that I was causing all the infections on his ward. In a sensitive and caring moment, he ordered me to go to the lab to be "completely cultured" (and I don't believe he wanted me to listen to Mozart or read Shakespeare). Like the fool that I can be (especially when confronted with a madman holding a scalpel), I went. You would be amazed at just how many tests they were able to do. Luckily, I passed. Turned out that he was growing *Staphylococcus* in his nose and was probably responsible for his own infections.

With the technology we currently possess, it is relatively easy to grow bacteria but very difficult to culture viruses outside a specialized lab. The areas that are commonly cultured include the throat, the lung (sputum), the bladder (urine cultures), the skin, the vagina, the cervix, and the rectum.

ELECTROCARDIOGRAM (ECG)

The ECG is a great example of a test in which a little knowledge often leads to no good. The ECG is a tracing that measures the electrical activity of the heart. The resting ECG is done by strapping a patient into electrodes attached to the arms, legs, and chest while the patient lies quietly on the examining table (scared half to death and utterly convinced that she will be the first person ever to be electrocuted by her doctor). The resting ECG is very useful, indeed crucial, for checking on the rhythm disturbances that can occur in the heart or for determining if heart damage has already occurred during or following a heart attack. But what most people want from an ECG they simply can't get, and that is the reassurance that their heart is "sound" or that the particular bout of pain they are having is not the prelude to a heart attack. Unfortunately, many is the intern who sent a Mr. Cohen home to his bed with the reassurance that all was okay for the night because the ECG was normal, only to have Mr. Cohen return hours later with a full-fledged heart attack. In short, resting ECGs have limited use for the normal, healthy adult, because they are simply not sensitive predicting tools.

Of more value when used properly is a stress ECG. In this variant, the patient is strapped into the electrodes and then exercised, usually on a treadmill. Although also a rather imperfect tool, the stress ECG is somewhat more likely to pick up hidden heart disease than a resting ECG because the heart is being worked hard.

In the last few years, a twenty-four-hour ECG tracing called Holter monitoring has become a more important test in those people at high risk for "silent heart disease," since it monitors the heart continuously, presumably including those silent attacks of decreased blood flow to the heart (see chapter 7).

ENDOSCOPY

In the last ten years, excellent instruments have been developed that permit us to look directly into organs and spaces that a few years ago were beyond our ability to invade easily. Thus, we can look directly into the stomach (gastroscopy) at the stomach lining, meaning that fewer barium X rays need to be done. We can look directly into a knee or shoulder (arthroscopy) and even do a lot of the surgery on these joints with arthroscopic tools. And laparoscopies (see chapter

11) have revolutionized the diagnosis and treatment of many gynecological problems.

NUCLEAR MEDICINE TESTS

In nuclear medicine tests, an infinitesimally small amount of radioactive material is injected into your blood, and depending on which
radioactive substance is used, it will concentrate in different organs
or in bones. This concentration of nuclear material then produces a
type of picture of the organ when it is scanned (on top of which the
U.S. Navy will use you as a beacon in foreign harbors). Nuclear scans
are quite helpful in sports injuries because they are the only accurate
method of diagnosing an overuse or stress fracture in a bone, and for
many thyroid disorders.

TESTS FOR OVA AND PARASITES

Anyone who experiences prolonged or severe diarrhea, especially
after traveling to a foreign country, should be tested for ova and
parasites. This totally unglamorous test involves collecting a stool
sample (I know half the population doesn't know what stool is, but
it's hard to write a book discussing poo or number two, so stool it is)
in a container. The sample should be brought to the lab as soon as
possible (don't collect it Friday night and leave it in your fridge until
Monday — yes, Virginia, there are people who have done that),
preferably to a lab that specializes in finding these little critters. The
test may have to be repeated several times until the organisms are
found.

SKIN TESTS

Skin tests are invaluable in detecting allergies. A small amount of
the material you may be allergic to is injected under your skin and
any reaction is measured.

Another common skin test is for the presence of reaction to a TB protein. The test is positive when you get a reaction that is red, raised, and over one centimeter in diameter.

ULTRASOUND

Ultrasound in medicine works in much the same way that ships send sonar waves into the deep to find lurking submarines. The same is done to the body, although it's rare to find a submarine in anyone's abdomen. High-frequency sound waves are beamed onto certain tissues. The tissues return these waves, producing a picture on a screen. Ultrasound is particularly useful for pelvic, abdominal, thyroid, and heart valve problems, as well as in pregnancy. For gallbladder stones, ultrasound has virtually eliminated the need to do gallbladder X rays.

An ultrasound examination of the heart, by the way, is called an echocardiogram.

I will close this chapter by simply restating that all tests can have problems associated with them. Always think about whether what you will learn from the test is worth the cost.

CHAPTER 4

General Problems

In which the good doctor expresses the feeling that life is not fair, because there are no easy answers — or questions, for that matter

This chapter covers the common problems that drive patients and doctors batty. These complaints may or may not be difficult to diagnose, but they are either hard to treat or tend to recur. They take up a good deal of office time, yet they do not lend themselves to easy solutions. These problems often send patients doctor shopping (doesn't doctor shopping conjure up the image of a supermarket with a lot of little specialists on the shelves?) in an attempt to find a better answer than the one their original doctor gave them. This chapter presents information about these conditions that may help you make fewer visits to your doctor.

SOME GENERAL SYMPTOMS

Pain

Pain hurts. (I doubt that this insight will earn me a Nobel Prize, but if Henry Kissinger can win one for peace, who knows?) Most humans don't like pain. We want to get rid of it as quickly as possible.

Pain is a symptom. When the symptom is overbearing or when it interferes with our ability to function normally, the symptom often needs to be treated on its own. But generally most pain needs to be monitored only because it indicates some problem in the body.

Pain is best classified as chronic or acute. Chronic pain refers to pain that is present for a long time. It may wax and wane, but it usually does not worsen much with time. In many cases, chronic pain is a very difficult medical problem to understand unless there is an obvious cause, such as a form of arthritis. Even though there is often no evident pathology to explain the pain, the person with this problem complains of persistent bouts of discomfort. The pain is real; it is not imagined. But for many people, there are few explanations for why it persists.

There are many therapeutic regimens for chronic, unexplained pain, including TENS (transcutaneous nerve stimulation) machines, physical therapies, acupuncture, biofeedback, behavior therapy, hypnotherapy, antidepressant medication, psychotherapy, yoga, and others. All of these treatments are worth a try because even though they may not work, they are not going to make you worse, so you have little to lose by trying them (although a patient on medication must be carefully monitored when a drug is used for a long time).

In my experience, though, very few people with chronic unexplained pain show great improvement on any of these therapeutic regimens. Each new therapy works somewhat for a while, but the pain soon seems to adapt to this new intervention and resumes its chronic course. That is why most people with chronic pain use analgesic medications as their primary method of pain relief. These people must monitor their use of analgesics very carefully because most of them will become addicted to whatever analgesic they use regularly. With time, the body adjusts to every medication, and the chronic pain sufferer needs higher and higher doses of the medication just to get the same amount of pain relief.

Acute pain comes on suddenly and may be mild or intense. There may be an obvious explanation, such as a fall, for example, or the reason may not be apparent. Depending on the severity of the pain, whether or not it is abating quickly, which body system is affected, and what other symptoms (such as fever) accompany the pain, it may be important to find the cause for the pain and not just treat the symptom.

How can you tell when to actually worry about a new pain or when to simply monitor it for a while? Most of us are smart enough not to run off to the doctor with each new ache. We use certain clues to help distinguish the significant pain from the insubstantial. Doctors too use their own criteria to help them decide whether a patient's pain needs close monitoring. What follows, then, are Dr. Hister's Clues to Monitoring Pain in Adults. (It's different for kids. Diagnosing the source of pain in kids is frequently akin to veterinary work. And teenagers are of course another story altogether. The grunt that I often get for an answer from a teen is no different from the woof my husky uses to communicate with me.)

The first criterion is the presence of other symptoms associated with the pain, especially fever and vomiting. The second is the intensity of the pain, particularly if the intensity is increasing. The third is the presence of tenderness. Tenderness means the area hurts more when you touch it. And the last criterion is the duration of the pain.

If your abdomen begins to hurt and you have a rise in temperature, that pain should be observed. If tenderness accompanies the pain, then you should see a doctor relatively soon. If the pain is getting worse, it should be promptly evaluated. Even if the pain is not increasing but is persistently intense, then you should probably be seen by a doctor. If the pain is abating and the fever is decreasing, then that pain can be safely observed for a while. Any pain that is prolonged — that is, going on longer than makes sense — should be evaluated by a doctor as well.

Headaches, of course, are not associated with tenderness, but otherwise the same criteria apply. A headache that is accompanied by vomiting and fever needs to be evaluated by a doctor, whereas most other headaches that are not caused by trauma, even though they can be intense, can be safely observed for the development of other accompanying symptoms.

On the skin or in a joint, pain accompanied by redness of the surrounding tissue or by tenderness should be evaluated for the presence of an infection or other inflammation that may require treatment.

For chest pain, we have to use other clues, including the apprehension level of the patient, the description of the type of pain, the risk profile of the patient, and other accompanying symptoms. In most adults, chest pain is not usually due to serious disease, but it's very important not to err with this symptom.

Remember that these are general rules for previously healthy adults. When in doubt, call your doctor. Also remember that very few conditions in the previously healthy fifteen-to-fifty-year-old must be seen instantly or sooner. One can usually wait a few hours and see what develops. (I have learned over the years that generally the patient who wants me to call back ASAP — that is, *now* — merely wants the urgent phone call because he is going to play golf in an hour and would like his question answered before then.)

When dealing with a new acute pain, you should not take pain-relieving medication until you have diagnosed the source of the pain and the probable outcome of the problem. With abdominal pain produced by an inflamed appendix, for example, the use of enough analgesic may alleviate the pain, but the analgesic merely hides the severity of the condition, increasing the risk of eventual complications. Likewise, with a blow to the head resulting in a headache, the drowsiness produced by a strong analgesic may mask the drowsiness produced by a brain injury.

Once you have established that the pain does not come from a problem that may require other treatments, such as hospitalization or surgery, then you can relieve the pain with an appropriate over-the-counter (OTC) analgesic. Most OTC analgesics are either in the ASA family or in the acetaminophen family.

ASA has been around for generations, and its benefits and risks are well known. It is an effective painkiller, as well as a potent fever reducer and anti-inflammatory. In high doses, ASA can produce gastric upsets, nausea, and ringing in the ears. In high doses over a long period of time, it produces gastric irritation, resulting in gastric ulcers that bleed and may even rupture, as well as kidney damage.

Acetaminophen likewise is a good painkiller and fever reducer. It does not produce gastric irritation, but in chronically high doses it produces severe kidney damage.

The Canadian government has recently allowed ibuprofen (Advil), a nonsteroidal anti-inflammatory drug, or NSAID, to be sold over the counter for pain relief. NSAIDs should be used very cautiously because there is a high risk of gastric ulcers with long-term use of this class of drugs.

When stronger analgesics are needed, the ASA or the acetaminophen is usually combined with codeine (292s, Tylenol 3 and 4). Besides producing the uncomfortable side effect of constipation, codeine also causes drowsiness and fatigue. Long-term use produces addiction.

Two good rules to remember are first, anything that you take for pain relief will have have some side effect that you should learn about, and second, if you use the medication regularly for a chronic condition, you will become addicted to it, no matter what reassurance you get to the contrary.

Fatigue

The single most frustrating complaint one hears in a typical medical office that caters to fifteen-to-fifty-year-olds is the complaint of fatigue.

Fatigue is universal (see chapter 15). We work too hard, we play too hard, we are under constant stress, and we don't rest or relax enough. Every thinking adult knows this, but occasionally some of us stop believing that this is a sufficient explanation for our tiredness. So we go trooping to the doctor, expecting a battery of tests to determine a physical cause for this symptom.

After eighteen years in practice, I can safely say that in the absence of other distinct physical symptoms, fatigue is rarely due to a defined physical cause. Sure, you may be anemic or hypothyroid or have mono. But if so, you are likely to have other symptoms that help define the problem more clearly. If you don't, a visit to the doctor is likely to be a waste of time.

Fever and All That

A Canadian question. If fever is so bad for you, why did God invent it, eh?

Fever has become a frightening prospect for many people. Perhaps it's because we are inundated with television ads telling us we can, indeed we must, control all our symptoms, particularly fever. The ads make it look as if the fever was the *cause* of our problem rather than the result of some inflammation.

Fever is a *symptom* of a problem. In an adult, fever by itself is not a hazard, unless the temperature rises to the range where it can begin to be destructive to tissue (41°C, or 106°F).

How do you deal with fever? First, buy a thermometer. About twice a week someone calls me and tells me she has a temperature. (I should hope so!) I inform her that what she means is that she has a fever, and I then ask her to tell me what her temperature is. Two out of three of these people then mumble a reply that they don't actually have a thermometer, but they feel hot, and after all, they know what a fever feels like. I am a patient man. I tell them to go and invest in a thermometer and call me back. They rarely do.

Feeling hot is not the same as having a fever. If your internal "thermostat" tries to reset itself, you will feel hot. Yet often you will not develop any rise in temperature. Drink lots of liquids, call your mom for sympathy, relax, and wait. It is likely that you will soon recover. Or else you will develop more obvious symptoms to show where the problem lies.

If you experience a rise in temperature, the fever is merely an indication that your body is dealing with a problem, which you should try to localize. Are you coughing? Does your throat hurt? Are you having abdominal pain? Does your head hurt? Is your back sore? Are you urinating more frequently?

It is these other symptoms that will determine whether or not you need medical therapy. A sore throat, even a severe one, in an adult with a fever is usually caused by a viral infection and usually does not require any antibiotics. Abdominal pain accompanied by a rise in temperature should always be checked by a doctor. If you're not sure, a phone call to your doctor for advice will help you determine your course of action.

If the fever is making you uncomfortable, or if it is climbing too high (and every doctor has a different idea of what too high means; for me, a fever over 39.5°C, or 103°F, in an adult is too high), use cool or room-temperature (not cold) baths or compresses to the forehead to reduce it. This treatment is often sufficient by itself. If the cool baths do not work, you can use either ASA or acetaminophen. But never give ASA to a child who may have a viral infection, as it may cause Reye's syndrome, which can be fatal. And as I am constantly reminded by incautious parents, even though teenagers under sixteen think of themselves as apprentice adults, they are still children.

HEADACHES

I hate my headaches. A headache, any headache at all, makes me feel powerless. Although I usually understand why I have one, I still can't control it. I can always feel a headache coming on, I know what's producing it, I know that if I can relax or change the circumstance I am in, the headache will go, and yet I am usually incapable of avoiding it. A headache also frustrates me because I occasionally have to take medication to make it go away. I hate taking medication for the sole purpose of symptom relief, so I too often allow the headache to become unbearable before I take a pill. Sometimes this attitude is the proper one; often it is not. (There really is no one keeping score and awarding martyr points.)

Headaches are extremely common. They are the leading cause of time lost from work for fully employed adults.

We have all at one time or another had a headache in which we wanted to separate our body at the neck and park the upper portion on someones else's torso, preferably our boss's or a hated enemy's. Usually enough OTC medication works. Medication is the appropriate treatment if the headache is an occasional event and you only have to use pills once in a while. But if your headaches are very severe or fairly recurrent, then it is important to identify specific causes and to learn other methods of pain relief, such as biofeedback therapy or relaxation techniques.

Tension Headaches

Tension headaches are by far the most common variety of headache. They are called tension headaches because they generally seem to be produced by tension and because there is no doubt that the muscles of the skull or neck are tense, or in spasm, when you have these headaches. Tension headaches can occur anywhere over the head, and the pain often extends into the muscles of the neck.

The pain of a tension headache is often quite mild, a pain-in-the-ass type of pain in the head. But tension headaches can also produce severe pain and nausea, sometimes lasting several days and often necessitating the use of extra-strong analgesic medication. Tension headaches can last all day and frequently do not disappear with sleep.

Tension headaches would seem to be easily amenable to treatment. But just speak to anybody who has frequent or severe headaches of this type, and you will quickly learn just how debilitating and how resistant to treatment they can be. It seems obvious to tell people to avoid the situations that produce the headaches and to relax more. Make sure to tell them at the same time to honor their parents and to donate to charity and to eat everything on their plates. Most of the time, for that kind of person the tension is largely unavoidable. All of us worry, work hard, sleep too little. We either have too little money or sex, or too much. (Yes, too much sex can be a problem. Why do you think so many spouses seem to have a constant post–8:00 P.M. headache?)

For most of us, if we didn't worry about one thing, it would be another. It's comforting advice to relax, but who is going to pick up your children from their endless lessons, pay your bills, prepare the meals, do the shopping, fight with the staff or the boss, and perform a million other daily necessities, each of which may be altered, but the sum total of which cannot be changed.

Anyone willing to do all these things for me and my family is more than welcome to come and take over our household. Of course I will then have to worry about how to pay you and whether you are doing a good enough job and whether my kids like you, and this will eventually lead to even more headaches for me.

Certainly if you are prone to tension headaches, you should try to minimize stress in your life. You should also learn techniques that can abort a tense situation before the pain builds. Thus, after a tense conference or confrontation, you may want to exercise briefly. You may want to pray. You may want to call your spouse. You may want to meditate. (I tried meditating once, but I couldn't relax because I kept thinking about what else I would rather be doing.) You may want to breathe deeply several times or chant.

We are all different. What works for me (eating, alas) may not, probably does not, work for you. Every noninjurious method of relaxation therapy is worth a try, if you have the patience.

There are clinics that teach biofeedback and relaxation techniques to minimize headaches. In these clinics, you learn to identify your body's signals, such as the first signs of pain or which muscles tense up before the headache appears. You then learn techniques such as how to change your breathing pattern or how to gradually relax your muscles so that you can abort this symptom. There are thousands of (expensive) stress management books, clinics, gurus. Depending on your wealth and your health, these may be of benefit, and I would certainly encourage anyone with significant headaches to give these a try.

Despite the proliferation of nonpharmaceutical interventions, medications are still the main treatment for tension headaches. Several general groups of drugs are used. These include analgesics, anti-inflammatories, tranquilizers, antidepressants, and muscle relaxants. Some of these are available without prescription, but I would caution all those who have to use pills regularly to discuss their use of these pills with a physician from time to time. All medications for tension headaches should be used with extreme caution. Many of these medications are potentially addictive. When you are going to treat a condition that is unlikely to disappear in your lifetime, this addictive potential should be very carefully weighed.

If nonpharmaceutical approaches do not work and you have to take a pill, always use the least amount of medication necessary, and in the lowest dose. If one pain tablet works, use only one. If you have to increase the strength of the medication for a particular headache, do it the one time only. If you find that you are gradually increasing the dose of medication, seek the advice of a doctor, preferably someone accepting of nonpharmaceutical therapies. Never repeat a prescription for narcotic analgesics without consulting the physician.

If you are prescribed tranquilizers for headaches, remember that they are highly addictive. Tranquilizers are useful medications for occasional use only. Occasional means once in a while, seldom, every so often. If you do become dependent on tranquilizers, the addiction to the medication will eventually present more problems for you than will the stress.

A unique type of headache occurs when an analgesic is suddenly stopped for whatever reason, usually because the sufferer decides to try to see if he can get along without his pills that day. Anyone taking regular analgesics for headaches will get more severe headaches if the medication is discontinued temporarily. This is called a rebound phenomenon. It is very hard to recognize rebound headaches, because the headache sufferer will still probably be under the same stress as usual and will simply ascribe the headache to more tension. He will then take the same analgesic as before, which will no doubt work, and start the cycle over.

If you are on a steady dose of painkillers for headaches and you want to discontinue taking them, just prepare yourself for the fact that your headaches will be more severe for a while. Ultimately, though, you will be much better off if you stop.

When a tension headache is particularly severe for a few days, or when the headaches suddenly become more frequent, patients often arrive at the office frightened to death that they must have finally developed a brain tumor. This phenomenon of "brain tumor until proven otherwise" is especially prevalent in men. (Remember Woody Allen in *Hannah and Her Sisters?*) Women seem to put up with headaches longer than men do, perhaps because men cause more headaches in women than vice versa. (You can dispute this observation by writing my editor.)

How *do* you know that the new headache you are experiencing is not the first sign of a brain tumor? To play to your paranoia, you can never be absolutely certain. But there are some reassuring clues that can allay your fears. In the fifteen-to-fifty-year-old age group, brain tumors are extremely rare, whereas tension headaches are practically mandatory, a badge of success. Unlike innocent headaches, brain tumors generally do not appear with a sudden severe pain when there is no previous history of other appropriate symptoms. Tumors usually present with pain that gradually worsens with time, and the pain is often accompanied by neurological or ophthamological signs, like double vision, difficulty with memory or speech, convulsions, and so on.

Certainly anyone with a prolonged, severe, or unusual pain in the head ought to see a doctor. But once the doctor has seen you and has reassured you that a tumor or meningitis is unlikely according to the presentation of your symptoms, you should relax and accept this analysis. Do not stay awake at night fearing missed diagnoses and wondering who will come to your funeral.

Migraines

Migraines are not just severe headaches. Rather they are headaches that are associated with an increase of blood flow to the brain, which is why they are often described as pounding. The increased blood flow is caused by an expansion of the blood vessels to the brain, which is the result of an imbalance in a hormone called serotonin.

Migraines are divided into two rough categories — classical and common. (Who would want a common migraine when you could own a classical one instead?)

Classical migraines are often described as pounding, occur on one side of the head, are associated with a strong family history of migraines, are more common in women, are common in kids, often disappear with age, and often have accompanying neurological symptoms, like visual disturbances. A classical migraine is often preceded by a sensation that it is going to occur, called an aura. The aura usually consists of visual symptoms, such as double vision or flashing lights.

Common migraines, which really are more common, are all those migraines that do not include classical features (surprise), especially ones that don't have neurological symptoms.

When a migraine strikes, it can be associated with severe nausea and vomiting; an aversion to daylight, noise, or smells; ringing in the ears; and neurological, speech, or visual disturbances.

Although most migraines do not seem to be triggered by specific events, in some people some migraines are associated with specific causes, primarily dietary. Chocolate, cheeses, red wine and beer, coffee, cola drinks, and citrus fruits are especially well known to cause these headaches, but any food can be responsible in the sensitive individual. Stress, tobacco, medications, odors, menstruation, hormonal changes, noises, bright lights, fatigue, even atmospheric changes can be other contributing factors. Some people only get migraines on the weekend. (These people must be a joy to live with. All week long you don't see them, because they're too busy, and on the weekend they're sick.) In fact, migraine patients should carefully analyze any factor they think is responsible and try to avoid that trigger.

If you have symptoms warning you of an impending migraine, sometimes you can treat it before it actually strikes by lying down in a dark room or by taking some analgesic or an ergotamine preparation, which is available by prescription only. Ergotamine works by constricting arteries but probably has other antimigraine properties as well. It is only effective if it's taken at the first hint that the migraine is starting. Ergotamine compounds are not painkillers — they either short-circuit the pain or they don't. If they don't work in the prescribed dose, taking more of them will not help and can cause serious side effects.

As with all recurrent headaches, relaxation techniques may minimize the pain of migraines. When they are full-blown, however, migraines often require very strong analgesics.

Some prescription medications can prevent migraines. The one most often used is propranalol, a type of high blood pressure medication known as a beta blocker. It was discovered, by serendipity (I love that word), that some people had less frequent migraines while taking propranalol for their high blood pressure.

A number of beta blockers work equally well. They are effective in some migraine sufferers, but not all. They usually do not have to be given in the same high doses that are used for high blood pressure.

Other prescription drugs that can be useful for preventing migraines include antidepressants, pizotyline (Sandomigran), calcium-channel blockers like nifedipine (Adalat), and anti-inflammatories like naproxen (Naprosyn).

Cluster headaches are very severe migrainelike headaches that occur in clusters. Even I can remember that definition. They are most common in young and middle-aged males, are one sided, and are usually centered on the eyes. They are often associated with tearing and redness of the eye on the same side as the headache, as well as clogging of the nasal passages on that side. They are extremely severe headaches that occur daily for several days or weeks at a time and frequently require narcotic analgesics for pain relief, even though they may only last for thirty minutes to an hour. Cluster headaches are also considered vascular headaches, and the best treatment is to begin preventive medication at the very onset of the cluster.

Vascular Headaches

Two interesting types of headache due to increased blood flow to the brain include exertional headaches, which occur during heavy labor or exercise, and benign orgasmic headaches, pounding headaches that accompany intercourse. (Maybe those are the people who think the earth has moved.) Sadly, one of the proposed treatment approaches is to avoid the initiating trigger. Better to take medication as a preventive, I think.

Headaches from Trauma

Obviously, getting hit in the head can result in a headache. Every hit to the head results in a jolting of the brain. The brain floats in fluid that cushions the impact, but there is still some transmission of force to the soft brain tissue.

A concussion is an injury in which there is a temporary impairment of consciousness, what football players call having your bell rung. Impairment of consciousness doesn't mean loss of consciousness, so you don't have to be knocked out to suffer a concussion. The degree of impairment determines the grade, from one to three, of your concussion. More important, if you participate in contact sports, the grade of the concussion often determines when you can play the sport again.

The headache following a concussion, called a postconcussion headache, can last for several weeks, even months, and can be accompanied by nausea, dizziness, and a dazed sensation. Generally, the only treatment for a postconcussion headache is observation. As the headache clears, the person can return to normal activity.

Head trauma can result in serious problems. If there is bleeding into the skull cavity from a blood vessel that doesn't clot, there is nowhere for that blood to go. The result can be pressure on the brain, either immediately after the trauma, if there is a lot of bleeding, or weeks later, if there is a slow leak. If you have been hit in the head and the headache is getting worse rather than better, or if you have visual or neurological disturbances, you should see a doctor.

Miscellaneous Headaches

Sinus headaches are usually severe headaches that localize on the face, often on the forehead or around the eye sockets. They are produced by infections of the sinus cavities, so this type of headache should have other signs of a sinus infection, such as a thick nasal discharge or a postnasal drip. The headache will only go away when the infection is adequately treated.

TMJ syndrome (or as some wanted to call it, TMJ disease) refers to pain in the area around the joint where the upper and lower jaws meet, the temperomandibular joint (TMJ). Early in the 1980s, TMJ syndrome threatened to become a designer disease (see chapter 15) because it became fashionable to blame this problem for every headache for which another cause couldn't be found. Methods of diagnosis of this condition vary greatly, so it is possible to argue that just about anyone with pain in the area of the jaw may have this condition.

TMJ syndrome is said to occur mainly in thirty-to-fifty-year-olds as a daily ache on the side of the head, which can spread all over the skull. The pain is aggravated by most excessive uses of the jaw, especially (alas) eating. In all TMJ syndrome patients, stress, or what some doctors refer to as psychological overlay, greatly contributes to the pain.

Treatment is geared to reducing use of the facial muscles. (Don't eat and don't talk — eliminating my favorite pastimes.) There are all sorts of (expensive) dental techniques to change how you bite or chew, but weigh the potential benefits carefully against the costs of these bothersome treatments.

ALLERGIES

This may come as a surprise to all wheezers, snifflers, coughers, nose wipers, eye wipers, and scratchers, but there are lots of people who believe that allergies are nothing more than a sign of neurosis. According to these insightful souls, there is no physical problem that accounts for allergy symptoms, but the allergy sufferer is so neurotic that he has somehow managed to make his nose run and his airways wheeze. Obviously, these theories are always held by people who don't have allergies. I am living proof of how wrong these heartless people are. I have lots of allergies, and I am not in the least bit neurotic — I am a doctor, after all.

Allergies are an overreaction of the body's defense system to some foreign insult. This does not mean that you "throw a hairy spaz" (in my son's immortal description) or suffer a convulsion when a foreigner calls you a pig. What it does mean is that certain factors, often external to your body, can send your body into an overreaction to protect you from those factors. This overreaction results in too much mucus, wheezing, a skin rash, or diarrhea, depending on which body system is affected.

A factor or substance that causes an allergic reaction is known as an allergen. Different allergens act on different systems. The common systems and organs affected by allergic reactions include the nose (reaction: a runny, stuffed nose, called rhinitis), the eyes (reaction: red, itchy, runny eyes, called conjunctivitis), the bronchi (reaction: coughing or wheezing, known as allergic asthma), the skin (reaction: hives and itchy, irritated skin patches, known as atopic dermatitis), or the bowel (reaction: gas, bloating, cramps, or diarrhea.)

Common allergens include molds, the tiny mites present in dust (it still bothers me that there are things, no matter how tiny, that actually live in dust; in our house they must be so plentiful that we should charge them rent), trees, grasses, weeds, animal dander, feathers, metals (which does not mean that you can be allergic to a bridge), insect venoms, medications, and foods.

Allergies often develop over time. I find that one of the hardest things to do in this business is convince a thirty-year-old patient that the sniffles he has had for thirteen weeks are not really due to a cold that didn't go away but are much more likely to be a sign of an allergy. If I then tell him that he may be allergic to old, gentle, moribund Flossie, whom he has had since the Great Flood, I recognize that he will demand a second opinion. (And if he doesn't, Flossie should, if she could only move.)

Allergies are best diagnosed by tests in which a small quantity of the allergen is injected into the skin, and the reaction is then measured. An allergy to the injection results in a red, itchy bump.

Some allergens lend themselves much better to skin testing than others. Grasses, trees, weeds, animal danders, insect venoms, and dust are easy to test; foods and drugs are not. Foods do not lend themselves to verifiable, repeated skin tests for two reasons. First, they can produce an allergic reaction in other ways from that measured in skin tests. Second, foods also produce many false positive reactions. Drugs such as penicillin do not lend themselves to skin tests because even a small amount of injected material can result in overwhelming allergic reactions in some people. Just as confusing is the fact that some people who are allergic to penicillin do not show positive reactions to the skin test.

The best way to treat an allergy is to avoid the allergen in the first place. This is easy to do if you are allergic to the feathers of the Norwegian Blue Parrot. It is not that easy to avoid dust. In fact, I think it's impossible to live as dust-free an existence as an allergist would like. Nor is it easy to get rid of a favorite cat. Or dog. (They just don't stay away.) But you should, if you develop allergies to them. Anyone with repeated coughing or sniffles or throat clearing who also has a dog or cat is likely to be allergic to that animal. Sorry, but that's how it is.

If avoiding the allergen doesn't work, then it's time to reach into the medicine cabinet. Allergic reactions in the upper respiratory tract and nasal passages (that is, runny noses and sniffles) occur when an inhaled allergen binds to the surface of certain blood cells known as mast cells and basophils. A reaction is produced in which the cell wall is disrupted. The cell then releases several chemicals, most notably histamine, which are responsible for those symptoms that we identify with allergic reactions. Now do you see where we are going with all this technical jargon? Antihistamines are the mainstays of relieving allergic nasal congestion. They work by counteracting the effect of histamine, but they are most effective if taken before an anticipated exposure to an allergen.

Antihistamines, like rock and roll hits, can be divided into two categories, old and new. The old antihistamines, most notably chlorpheniramine (Chlor-Tripolon), are notorious for producing drowsiness as a side effect (unlike the old rock hits) because these drugs pass into the brain from the bloodstream. They work, but you should not drive or operate heavy machinery (such as a tractor) if you are not used to taking them. The older antihistamines have one added benefit in that they also block other body chemicals besides just histamine. They can therefore be useful in other conditions that cause congestion but are not real allergies, like vasomotor rhinitis (see chapter 5). The newer antihistamines, including astemizole (Hismanal) and terfenadine (Seldane) are heavily promoted as being non-sedating, so you can still operate your tractor if you wish. But they are considerably more expensive.

For nasal allergy symptoms, you can also use steroid (cortisone) sprays. The best known are beclomethasone dipropionate (Beconase) and flunisolide (Rhinalar). Taken in recommended doses, these drugs do not seem to be absorbed into the bloodstream in sufficient quantities to produce any of the well-known problems associated with long-term steroid use. (Nor will you end up running like Ben Johnson if you use a steroid nasal spray. Different types of steroids, I'm afraid.)

In some people, a spray of a drug called sodium cromoglycate (Rynacrom) can be used to prevent allergic reactions. But it doesn't work in a lot of people, it has to be taken every four hours, and it costs a lot.

In addition to nasal congestion, an inhaled allergen can also cause an asthmatic attack (see chapter 6). This type of reaction is caused by the release of other chemicals, not histamine, so needless to say (but I will say it anyway, as all people who use that phrase are wont to do), antihistamines don't work in an asthmatic attack, and in some people they can even worsen the asthmatic reaction. To treat allergic asthma, you have to use anti-asthma medication.

For runny eyes (allergic conjunctivitis), there are eye drops, like cromoglycate (Opticrom), that can minimize the symptoms, although the most effective treatment is to avoid the allergen in the first place.

For certain allergies, most notably to dust, weeds, grasses, and trees, you can take shots that will decrease your allergic response. In a shot program, a series of progressively increasing doses of the specific allergen responsible for the symptoms is injected under the skin. These injections fool your body into producing different types of antibodies from those that lead to allergic symptoms. These different "blocking" antibodies then prevent an allergic response when you are exposed to the allergen. This type of therapy is called desensitization therapy, or immunotherapy.

Not everybody can take desensitization shots. People on certain high blood pressure medications, people with certain heart rhythm problems, and those with migraine headaches should not get desensitization shots.

Anaphylactic Reactions

Every year you read about someone who ate fish at a party (who goes to a party where they serve fish?) or a cake with nuts or took penicillin when he or she shouldn't have and collapsed and died virtually instantly. These people had an anaphylactic reaction. An anaphylactic reaction is an overwhelming allergic reaction in which hives and skin swelling occur. These symptoms can be followed by marked congestion in the breathing passages. The allergic reaction in the airways can then result in shock, heart stoppage, and death.

The most common allergens that produce anaphylactic reactions are the penicillins, with venom from the stings of such insects as bees, wasps, hornets, and yellow jackets being a distant second. Less common causes include many other medications and such foods as shellfish, other fish, nuts, seeds, egg whites, and peanuts.

Anaphylactic reactions never occur the first time you are exposed to the allergen. On this first occasion, if you are a person capable of being allergic to shellfish, for example, your body develops antibodies to the shellfish. This is called a sensitizing reaction. Once you've been sensitized, future exposure to the same allergen, even in small amounts, can result in an anaphylactic response because there are lots of antibodies waiting to pounce.

People who have severe allergic reactions in response to any allergen, especially insect stings, should be instructed to carry anti-allergic kits (Epipen or Anakit) with them. These kits contain adrenalin and an antihistamine. Adrenalin can stop an anaphylactic reaction if given quickly enough in adequate doses. Always remember to carry the kits into situations that may expose you to the allergen. If you are allergic to insect stings, for example, you should take a kit with you on camping trips, when you go hiking, or on joyful trysts in those fields of grass that represent eternal youth and hope. It would also, of course, be inadvisable to keep a wasp as a pet. Once a year check to see that the adrenalin hasn't become outdated.

Reactions to Medications

Probably the most overdiagnosed allergy to medication is an allergy to penicillin. Studies show that 10 percent of North American adults think they may be allergic to penicillin. The reason that there are so many people who think they are allergic is that it is not unusual to get a rash when one is ill, particularly with a virus. If you happen to be on penicillin at the same time, there is a great tendency to diagnose the rash as being of allergic origin.

Remember that an allergy to penicillin means an allergy to all the drugs in the penicillin group. This includes cloxacillin, ampicillin, amoxicillin, and others. There is also a cross-reactivity with the cephalosporin group of antibiotics that include common drugs like cephalexin (Keflex).

Be aware that even perfect doctors like me occasionally forget to ask if you're allergic to any medication before writing an antibiotic prescription. Don't be shy. If you think you're allergic to penicillin, ask if the antibiotic you are about to take is in the penicillin family. If you need an antibiotic and you can't take penicillin, there are always good alternatives. Another antibiotic family that many people become allergic to is the sulfa group of drugs. This includes sulfamethoxazole-trimethoprim (Bactrim, Septra), sulfisoxazole (Gantrisin), and others, which are frequently used for bladder infections. Neomycin, used in certain skin antibiotic creams and ear drops, is also commonly the source of allergic reactions.

Any time you are on a medication and you develop a new symptom, like a skin rash, you should run this past a physician before you take the next pill. It is unlikely that you will suffer a severe, life-threatening reaction merely by ingesting the next pill, but why take the chance?

Humidifiers

Home humidifiers are a not-uncommon source of airborne particles that can cause allergic symptoms. Humidifiers are often advised for children with croup, especially for those living in that type of domicile that most Canadians are addicted to, the overheated house (this structure is usually found with other variants, often including the overwatered lawn). Humidifiers are rarely completely emptied or cleaned, and the water reservoir serves as a breeding ground for molds and bacteria, which are then released into the air when the machine is turned on. Don't be lazy. Empty the humidifiers daily, use new water, and clean them.

COMMON VIRAL INFECTIONS

Like opinions, viruses are ubiquitous. You cannot completely avoid them.

When they invade your body, they enter your cells. To kill the virus, medications must either enter your cells and only selectively kill the virus or prevent it from multiplying while leaving your cells alone, or the drugs must prevent your cells from taking up the viral cells in the first place. And of course the medication must also be relatively nontoxic, meaning that the person receiving the drug is not made too sick from taking it.

Unlike bacterial infections, which are usually easily treated with antibiotics, there are no effective antiviral drugs on the market that are selective for the virus and not toxic to your own cells (with the exception of a few specific antiviral drugs such as acyclovir for herpes simplex infections).

Since we can't cure a viral infection with medication, it becomes obvious that a visit to the doctor when you have such an infection is usually a waste of time. A visit to your mother would probably do you far more good, if you could stand the lecture you would receive at the same time. (Mothers, unlike doctors, only see one patient at a time, which is why their advice can be so prolonged.) Drink plenty of fluids, rest, take good care of yourself, and wait — the treatment that's been called tincture of time (not thyme, which a friend of mine adds to every awful dish he cooks).

Because of this difficulty with treatment, it's especially important to avoid acquiring a viral infection in the first place. I strongly believe that any preventive strategy includes good health practices. Listen to your mother. Don't get too run down, get enough sleep, eat well-balanced meals, and get some exercise. If you believe that extra vitamins or other food supplements (such as garlic, which is really not a supplement but a staple to me) help your resistance, by all means take in extra quantities at the time you are exposed to the virus (as long as those quantities are not in the toxic range).

Likewise, I am certain that a poor mood contributes to one's propensity to become sick. So don't get depressed, silly. Some viruses are also avoidable by immunizations. These include German measles (rubella), measles, mumps, hepatitis B, influenza, and polio.

You can avoid exposure to some viruses, but it is virtually impossible to avoid others. Thus, hepatitis B and the human immunodeficiency virus (which causes AIDS) are easily avoided by not participating in high-risk behavior (see chapter 13). In contrast, colds, which are also caused by viruses, are virtually impossible to avoid, and that is why you will likely come down with one or two colds a year.

Influenza

Every year the annual flu epidemic kills a few people in every community. Usually flu kills the very young or the very old or those with preexisting heart or lung problems. But it can and does strike anyone at all, and if you're unlucky enough to get a complication such as pneumonia, flu can kill you too, even if you were previously quite healthy.

Influenza is caused by one of the viruses in the influenza family of viruses. Flu is not just a severe cold; it is an illness of your whole body that causes more severe symptoms than a cold. These symptoms include cough, sore throat, fever, headache, achey muscles and joints, digestive system upsets such as diarrhea, and depression. Despite what your mother may have told you, flu is not easier to get if your hair is wet or if you go out in the cold. Flu *is* spread by direct contact, such as by touching doorknobs that infected people have touched before you, and by airborne spread of the virus through coughing and sneezing (which is why people with the flu should be sent home when they develop symptoms).

You can prevent the flu. Just get a shot every year. It is successful in about 80 percent of people who get it. But make sure that you get immunized at least two weeks before flu season because it takes that long to build up adequate antibodies. You must also get a new vaccination every year, since the influenza viruses are wily characters that mutate somewhat every year. There is one medication, amantadine HCL (Symmetrel), that can prevent influenza caused by type A strains of the flu, although it doesn't work on type B strains.

Colds

A cold is not the flu (I had to say that again because many people use the terms interchangeably). Colds are caused by nearly two hundred different viruses, most notably the rhinoviruses, which is why it's so hard to develop an effective vaccine. Colds are usually confined to the respiratory tract, even though many of us complain loud and long about how bad we feel all over when we have a cold.

Colds are common in the summer because many of us experience a drop in immunity in the summer, probably through an effect of the sun. Colds are also common in the winter, when we spend more time indoors and are exposed to more sick people. Colds too are spread through direct contact and through the air.

Fluids are important in the treatment of colds and flu because the more dehydrated you are, the worse the symptoms. I take vitamin C at the first hint of either a cold or the flu. It's probably more of a placebo effect than anything else, but I am convinced that for me, large doses (up to six grams a day) make the infection milder and make it disappear more quickly. I did recommend this treatment for everyone in my practice for several years, only to find out that it didn't seem to benefit most people the way it benefited me. Not everyone is an advanced specimen, I suppose.

Stomach Flu

Most of us on occasion develop diarrhea and stomach cramps of sudden onset and say that we have had stomach flu. Strictly speaking, there is no such thing as stomach flu. Although it is true that these symptoms are often caused by a viral infection, it is also true that they are rarely due to one of the influenza viruses. But who cares what we call it? We still treat it with fluids and patience.

Acute Mononucleosis

Acute mononucleosis, aka mono, is a viral infection caused by the newly famous Epstein-Barr virus, a member of the herpes family of viruses (these families of viruses remind me of the Mafia, which of course doesn't exist). Most people are exposed to the E-B virus while very young and usually develop few or no symptoms from the infection.

In its symptomatic form, the disease we call infectious mononucleosis, the E-B virus is generally most prevalent in adolescents and young adults. Although I haven't heard this term in many a moon, mono used to be called the kissing disease, implying, of course, that close exposure to an infected person is what gives you infectious mono. But remember that most people who develop an acute infection are rarely aware of who passed the virus on to them.

The most common symptom of an acute infection is overwhelming fatigue of recent onset. This is invariably accompanied by a sore throat. Other common symptoms include skin rash, swollen glands, depression, and headache. It is also not unusual to get a type of hepatitis (liver inflammation) with acute mononucleosis. There is no known treatment except the usual rest, preferably in bed and alone. Most people recover in two to three weeks; some remain ill for as long as three months.

Hepatitis

Strictly speaking, I should not discuss hepatitis at any length because hepatitis is definitely a problem that should be monitored with regular visits to the doctor. However, this is also a disease that is often preventable, so I believe there is much you can learn to help you avoid it.

The term "hepatitis" means an inflammation of the liver. There are many reasons that this can occur, but the most common forms of hepatitis in young adults are due to viruses. These include hepatitis A (which used to be known as infectious hepatitis), hepatitis B (which used to be known as serum hepatitis), and (surprise, surprise) non-A, non-B hepatitis (NANB). There are others, but these three account for most significant infections. Hepatitis A and NANB hepatitis (less commonly) can be passed through direct household exposure. All forms of hepatitis can also be transmitted through sexual contact or the exchange of blood products, such as by sharing needles for intravenous drug use or blood transfusion. (These are the only ways that hepatitis B can be passed on; blood transmission accounts for the majority of cases of NANB hepatitis.)

When the liver is inflamed, several symptoms occur. These include jaundice (usually) due to a rise in the bilirubin (I knew a guy once called Billy Rubin — do you suppose his parents knew, and is he now known as William Rubin?) level in the blood, itching, lack of appetite, fatigue, decreased urge to smoke, abdominal discomfort, and depression. The best place to spot jaundice is in the whites of the eye, which generally turn a sickly lemon yellow color, as does the skin. In addition, the urine generally becomes very dark (Coca Cola colored), and the stools can become quite pale or colorless (you have to look).

Hepatitis A invariably causes a mild, benign, three-week illness. NANB hepatitis and hepatitis B are likewise generally short, mild infections, although they can occasionally be much more severe. Both hepatitis B and NANB hepatitis can also develop into a chronic relapsing form of the disease that can come back periodically. About 5 to 10 percent of the patients who develop hepatitis B are left as chronic carriers of the disease who can transmit the infection for the rest of their lives to sexual partners or by donating blood. Similarly, about 40 percent of people who develop NANB hepatitis are left as chronic carriers. Hepatitis B and NANB hepatitis both also increase the risk of a type of cancer of the liver called hepatocellular carcinoma.

There are vaccines against both hepatitis A and B (and it is likely that there will soon be a vaccine against one of the likely causes of type NANB). The serum that can be given for hepatitis A only provides protection for a few months at most but should be given to those traveling to parts of the Third World or to other areas where there is a high risk of infection, and to close household contacts of infected persons.

The vaccine against hepatitis B does not offer protection to those who have already been exposed. It is given as a preventive to high-risk persons. Its major drawback is that currently it costs about one hundred dollars. Certainly for high-risk people, especially for the sexual contacts of type B carriers and for medical personnel, this cost seems a small price to pay for preventing a serious disease.

The only treatment for an active case of hepatitis is rest. It's also a good idea to avoid substances, like alcohol, that can tax your liver, although it's doubtful that you need to avoid these products for any length of time once you have recovered. Some medications (such as the birth control pill) should likewise be avoided by a person with hepatitis.

People who may have had hepatitis B in the past, when there were no reliable tests to differentiate the various forms of hepatitis, should be rechecked to see if they have antibodies to the hepatitis B virus and if they are chronic carriers.

ANEMIA

Anemia is a disease in which there are deficiencies in the red cells of the blood, those cells that carry the oxygen to your tissues. Either there are too few red cells or they don't work properly. Hemoglobin, which contains iron, is that part of the red cell that carries the oxygen to your tissues, and most anemias are diagnosed by finding a low hemoglobin count.

Iron-deficiency anemia is by far the most common anemia in young adults. It is fairly common in women who menstruate heavily (for example, those with IUDs) simply through the mechanism of excess blood loss. It is also especially common in athletes, particularly women, who train hard, partly because of the excess destruction of red cells caused by the heavy pounding of running, partly because of microscopic blood loss in the gut, partly because of the restrictive diets that many women athletes follow, and partly for unknown reasons. The treatment is obvious. Correct the correctable, and take in extra iron, either by eating iron-rich foods or by taking iron pills.

Whenever an iron-deficiency anemia cannot be readily explained, it behooves you to have stool tests and a urinalysis to see if you are losing microscopic amounts of blood in the stool or urine.

Vitamin B_{12} deficiency anemia occurs fairly often in vegetarians, especially the strict vegans — those who eat no animal products at all. B_{12} is most easily obtained from meat, but it is also present in eggs, milk, and fish. If a vegetarian refuses to eat these foods, the next best way of getting this necessary vitamin is by regular B_{12} supplementation.

Anemia also accompanies many chronic conditions, such as rheumatoid arthritis. The more successfully the chronic condition is treated, the greater the chance the anemia will disappear.

MISCELLANEOUS PROBLEMS

Carpal Tunnel Syndrome

The carpal tunnel is the area in the middle of the wrist through which a large nerve, called the median nerve, passes on its way to innervating some of the fingers.

In some people, the median nerve becomes compressed in the carpal tunnel, leading to numbness and pain in the digits, especially in the thumb, middle and index fingers. This condition is known as carpal tunnel syndrome. It is best diagnosed by tests that measure nerve conduction. There is usually no obvious cause, although the condition is more common in those occupations that involve repeated unusual use of the wrists, such as drywall plastering, typing, or playing the violin.

Resting the wrist, especially with splints at night, tends to alleviate the symptoms. But if you continue to do the work that produced the problem in the first place, the symptoms gradually worsen. In those cases, an operation to relieve the pressure may cure the problem.

Raynaud's Disease

Raynaud's disease is a reaction in which the small arteries of the extremities go into spasm when exposed to cold. This reaction is most common in the fingers but can also occur in the toes and the nose. It is also much more common in women than men. When a Raynaud's reaction accompanies other diseases, it is known as Raynaud's phenomenon.

My wife has a particularly obvious case. When she exposes herself (this is an odd choice of words, because she rarely ventures out without clothes on) to cold, her fingers turn white and start to hurt. This can even happen on a spring day when she is out on a long run. (I keep telling her that she wouldn't get Raynaud's if she stayed home more. She tells me to get stuffed, by which she is not talking about my allergies.)

The only good immediate treatment I know is to immerse the digits in warm water right away. Calcium-channel blockers like nifedipine (Adalat) can prevent Raynaud's, but they must be taken before going into the cold.

Never treat Raynaud's lightly. There have been instances where the arteries did not come out of spasm and a finger had to be amputated. Again, this is very unusual, but it is a good idea to stop the spasm as quickly as possible.

The best treatment for Raynaud's is to prevent the reaction in the first place. Keep your tootsies (and your fingers) warm.

Night Sweats

In the first three years that I did my television show (a subtle plug for my ego), we asked people to write in with questions that their family doctor couldn't answer. After snoring and impotence, the problem that seemed to provoke the most questions was night sweating. Interestingly, it was seldom the person who sweated that wrote in. More often it was the spouse who wrote because she (usually) was tired of waking in drenched sheets.

Night sweats are common. They are more prevalent in overweight, heavy-sleeping males, especially when they have a tendency to drink too much alcohol. There is seldom a definable physical cause, but this symptom has been described as a part of other diseases such as TB, hyperthyroidism, anemias, and AIDS. Obviously, if there is a risk of one of these other problems, that should be evaluated, but the great proportion of people with this symptom will have nothing else wrong with them.

I hope you haven't read this far expecting to find a miracle cure. I don't have one.

Night Leg Cramps

This symptom is also often called restless leg syndrome. Some people develop cramps when lying down, especially at night. The cramps are invariably most prevalent in the calf muscles. Many treatments have been proposed, including elevating the foot of the bed, putting various concoctions under the bed, and taking calcium supplements, magnesium, dolomite, quinine, and various other medications such as calcium-channel blockers (Verapamil). They're all worth a try, especially the quinine, but don't be surprised at how stubborn a problem this can be.

CHAPTER 5

The Eyes, Ears, Nose, Mouth, and Throat

*In which the good young doctor explains that he had to
put the eyes into the same chapter as the ears
because there is simply not enough information
on the eyes to give them their own chapter*

This brings me to my favorite anecdote from medical school, which
occurred in a class ahead of mine. The class members were studying
X rays and had been discussing the skull, although they had not yet
seen any films of it. The lecturer, out of some perverse logic that
seems only too common in medical lecturers, then put an X ray of the
pelvis up for review. When he asked if someone in the class could
discuss the film, up shot the hand of Hershhorn (not his real name —
I have always wanted to say that), who began by saying, "It's a film
of a skull, sir," and I am told on good authority, proceeded to describe
how he could distinguish the ears and other features of the cranium
on this X ray. After a stunned silence, the lecturer responded. "Congratulations, Hershhorn," he said. "You've finally figured out what's
wrong with this poor chap. He's got his brains in his ass."

When the head is included (as it generally ought to be), the organs
described in this chapter are collectively known as the HEENT
(which I believe is not pronounced as one word). The HEENT is the
source of many visits to the doctor, many of which are not necessary.
Read on.

THE EYE

A brief description of the structures of the eye will help make what
follows more comprehensible (I hope).

The visible part of the eye consists of a central pupil; the iris, which

84

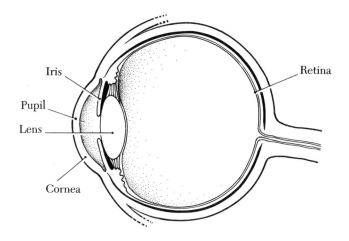

Iris

Pupil

Lens

Cornea

Retina

THE EYE

is the muscle that opens and closes the pupil; and the white of the eye, known as the sclera. The pupil and the iris are covered by a transparent coat called the cornea. The sclera is covered by a lining known as the conjunctiva.

Behind the visible eye, the lens, the disc that changes shape to allow near and far vision, sits in a fluid-filled chamber. The shape of the lens is controlled by a ring of muscle around its edge. Behind the lens sits the retina, which receives the image formed by the lens. From the retina the signals pass to the brain.

That's as clear as I can make it. I hope you see that.

Red Eye

Most red eyes in the fifteen-to-fifty-year-old are due to an infection of the conjunctiva. In viral conjunctivitis, which is more common in the spring and fall than at other times, a watery discharge is produced, especially overnight, so the person with the infection wakes up with her eyes caked shut. Although the discharge from the eye may be profuse, viral conjunctivitis will clear without antibiotics. A useful treatment is to apply warm compresses, such as towels soaked in warm water, to the affected eye. It is a very easy infection to transmit to others, so the patient should wash her hands frequently and use her own towels.

Bacterial conjunctivitis usually produces a thicker, more purulent (made of pus) discharge. This condition responds rapidly to the appropriate antibiotic drops.

Two other causes of red eye, which are not as common, need to be treated totally differently.

If a red eye is accompanied by pain, especially if there is aching and excessive sensitivity to light, then it is likely that the red eye is caused by an inflammation of the iris, called iritis. Iritis should always be seen by a doctor, since it often requires steroids for complete resolution.

Glaucoma, which is rare under the age of forty, can also present with a sudden onset of a red eye and is often accompanied by pain. Glaucoma is due to the buildup of pressure in the chamber that houses the lens of the eye. If untreated, it can lead to blindness. Glaucoma is often silent, so a check for glaucoma should be done periodically as a part of routine checkups in all those over forty.

Blood in the White of the Eye

Subconjunctival hematoma is a fancy name for a collection of blood under the conjunctiva. It usually shows up as a red spot several millimeters in diameter located in the white of the eye. It is often caused by bleeding in fragile blood vessels in the eye and is often noticed upon waking in the morning. (After your shock wears off, you will of course believe that the angels, or your spouse, tried to gouge your eyes out while you were sleeping. And you may be right.)

The other not-uncommon cause of a subconjunctival hematoma is some kind of trauma to the eye, such as a poke in the face from an altercation (although every single person who has ever shown up in my office with one has invariably told me that he walked into a wall, a feat so many patients seem able to do but something I, a total klutz who trips over nonexistent barriers on the sidewalk, have never managed to do). A subconjunctival hematoma does not require treatment, and much like a black eye, it will disappear in fourteen days.

Inflammation around the Eyelid

Blepharitis is an inflammation of the margins of the lid. The symptoms of blepharitis are lid margins that are red and scaly, accompanied by an itchy or irritated sensation. The treatment consists of lid scrubs, in which the lid margin is washed carefully (if you use soap, very carefully) three or four times a day. Very rarely, a topical antibiotic cream may be useful.

Styes

A stye is an infected gland in the eyelid. I don't know why, but most people who get them swear that the stye is associated with increased stress in their lives, although ophthamologists will tell you that styes are much more commonly associated with chronic blepharitis.

Styes should be treated with warm compresses and antibiotics. When a stye is recurrent, or when it results in a permanent lump, it is frequently removed surgically for cosmetic reasons.

Herpes

You should never allow a doctor to prescribe cortisone for an eye infection unless he or she can guarantee you that you don't have a corneal ulcer, also called a dendritic ulcer, which is caused by the herpes simplex virus. Cortisone cream or solution, which is an excellent treatment for certain types of iritis, can worsen a herpetic eye infection and in a worst-case scenario can lead to blindness.

If you have a herpetic sore on your lip or at the corner of your mouth, don't rub your eyes with the back of your hand after wiping your mouth with the same hand. You should know better than that, silly.

Thickening in the Lining of the Eye

A pterygium is a thickening at the side of the cornea nearest the nose and is caused by the heaping up of a layer of the conjunctiva at that point. It can be left alone unless it is encroaching too far onto the cornea, when it needs to be surgically removed.

Corneal Abrasions

Corneal abrasions, which are cuts on the surface of the cornea, hurt like hell, and often the patient is very sensitive to light, a symptom known as photophobia. (Photophobia does not mean that you're afraid to have your picture taken. That's called Greta Garbo disease.) The eye should be patched and reexamined for signs of infection every twenty-four hours until the cornea has healed.

Some corneal abrasions, especially those due to cuts from an organic source like a tree branch, tend to recur. What happens is that many months or years later the eye in which the abrasion originally occurred suddenly starts to hurt for no apparent reason, and a new abrasion can be detected. These recurrent abrasions should be treated in the same way as the original.

Floaters

Boy, do these things drive people nuts. Floaters are objects that one notices floating across the field of vision. These are usually tiny, ill-defined objects, though I suppose if you keep seeing a fridge in all visual fields, there may be something seriously wrong with you. They are due to thickenings in the jelly that surrounds the lens and fills the inside of the eye. They are totally harmless and should be ignored, which is much easier said than done.

THE EAR

The part of the ear that you can see is called the pinna. Leading from the pinna to the inside is the external ear canal, home to that sticky stuff known as ear wax. The canal ends at a thin membrane or drum. Behind the drum is the middle ear cavity, which contains three little bones that transmit sound waves to another membrane farther in. Also emptying into this middle ear is the eustachian tube, which connects the middle ear to the throat. The purpose of this tube, as any flyer will tell you, is to relieve pressure that builds up in the middle ear cavity. The inner ear is home to two major structures — the hearing organ, called the cochlea, and the organs of balance, the semicircular canals.

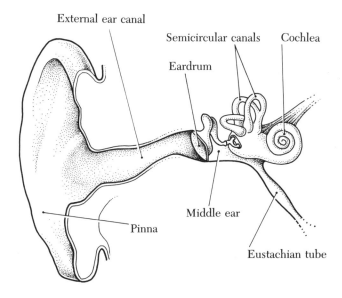

Ear Wax

Ears are either self-cleaning or they're not. For many people, Q-tips merely push the wax in farther. (I believe that Q-tips were invented by a doctor who stumbled on an easy way to supplement his income by cleaning plugged ears.) Unless your ears are plugging up, they do not need to be cleaned. A few drops of warm oil, such as mineral oil or vegetable oil, help loosen the wax from the sides of the ear canal. Warm does *not* mean hot. Of course if the oil that you put in the right ear begins to run out the left, you have a bit of an extra problem to deal with.

Ringing (Tinnitus)

The symptom known as tinnitus is a sensation of noise in the ears or head. The noise is frequently described as a ringing or a buzzing sensation. Tinnitus (which is not the same as a tin ear) can be present in only one ear or both (such as when you have a phone attached to both ears), or it may sound like it's located in the middle of the head. Tinnitus is one of those symptoms that drives people nuts. It can accompany any ear problem, but is most often idiopathic, which means we don't know the cause. Tinnitus also frequently accompanies hearing loss as we age.

All new cases of prolonged tinnitus should be investigated for correctable causes, such as fluid in the ears or tumors (which are rare). There are many proposed treatments for tinnitus, including devices that mask the sound. But most tinnitus patients will tell you that little works, except learning to live with the symptom.

Decreased Hearing

Decreased hearing in people under fifty is often due simply to poor concentration. When they are tested, their hearing turns out to be normal. These are often the people who come in to ask for a hearing test by saying, "My wife (or husband) says I don't hear well."

Other common causes of temporary hearing loss include excess wax in the ears, allergies that plug up the eustachian tube, and middle ear infections. These are easily cured by attending to the main problem.

Real hearing loss in adults is often due to damage to the hearing nerve from exposure to excess noise at work or from exposure to excess noise years ago. This damage is often uncorrectable. It is advisable — it should be compulsory — to wear earplugs if you are exposed to a great deal of noise at work.

Aging is the most common cause of hearing loss, but I am not too thrilled with the only known solution to this problem.

Ear Infections

The most common ear infection in young children is of the middle ear cavity. This infection is called an acute otitis media and is invariably due to an infection that has spread to the middle ear cavity along the eustachian tube from the throat. The reason otitis media is so common in young children is that the eustachian tube runs a more horizontal course in children between the ages of two and five, resulting in poorer drainage from the ear, and because they generally suffer more colds and upper respiratory infections than adults. Otitis media is not nearly as common in adults, who have a much more vertical eustachian tube and better immunity.

A cold or flu causes swelling of the tissues of the back of the throat, with consequent swelling of the opening of the eustachian tube in the throat. This swelling allows bacteria to settle in the middle ear cavity, leading to infection.

The usual symptoms of otitis media are sudden onset of pain in the ear, along with a decrease in hearing on that side.

Otitis media is treated with antibiotics. If the infection is left untreated, the fluid that builds up in the middle ear cavity often bursts through the eardrum. This relieves the pressure, and consequently the pain, although the infection can then enter a relatively silent chronic phase. The drum usually heals well after a rupture, and there is rarely a resultant hearing loss after only one untreated case of otitis media. If, however, otitis media becomes chronic, with the production of a sticky gluelike fluid, there is often associated hearing loss. This condition needs to be treated with tubes that are inserted into the middle ear and allow the fluid to drain into the outer ear.

Otitis externa is an infection of the outer ear. The symptoms include pain, discharge, and itching. In the chronic form it is often known as swimmer's ear because it is usually caused by repeated wetness in the outer ear canal. It can also be the result of excess trauma to the canal from Q-tips. The best treatment is to use appropriate antibiotics and keep the ear as dry as possible. Some people claim that a dilute vinegar solution, applied into the affected ear in the form of drops once or twice a week, can lessen the frequency of acute flare-ups.

Ear Pressure

If you have a cold or an allergy and you have to fly, it is advisable to take a decongestant about half an hour before going up in the plane, but especially half an hour before descending. The decongestant may help prevent severe pain and a burst eardrum from poor function of the eustachian tube.

THE MOUTH

The mouth is not the primary source of a lot of visits to a doctor's office. Most people are able to deal with their oral problems by themselves. Or else there simply are not that many things that go wrong in the oral cavity that require a doctor's attention. Many oral lesions are actually skin diseases, so they are dealt with in the chapter on the skin (chapter 10).

Halitosis

Bad breath is never the primary reason for visiting a doctor, but often patients will sneak in a question about halitosis, usually towards the end of a visit. They generally begin by referring to an imaginary friend or relative. It's usually something like, "You know, Art, my sister's breath is awful. I'm so embarrassed for her. What should I tell her to do?" The thought often strikes me how odd it is that halitosis seems to run in that family.

Halitosis is in the eyes (the nose?) of the beholder. It can be caused by any process that changes the bacteria in the mouth, or very occasionally, the gut. Often the source is the obvious — poor dental hygiene, infections, or mouth breathing. Treatment should be geared to the appropriate cause. If no cause is easily detected, try eliminating certain food groups (always start with dairy products) for a few weeks to see if that works, but don't hold your breath (although that may diminish the complaints from your family).

Cankers

Canker sores are shallow irritations or ulcers on the tongue, lips, gums, or palate. Although many are probably due to viruses and some may be transmittable, they are not caused by the herpes simplex virus.

Like herpes, though, canker sores recur, often with a prodrome, or warning sensation, for twenty-four hours before. Once you have one canker sore, you can have others for the rest of your life. Stress and other infections are notorious precipitating events. Canker sores are also occasionally associated with Crohn's disease.

Canker sores hurt. There are no universally effective treatments, although tetracycline swished around the mouth for two or three minutes occasionally works. Various OTC medications are available, but if they have any effect, it is probably a placebo effect. Many home remedies are available for cankers, including my previously mentioned favorite appetizer, main course, and dessert — namely, garlic. They can all be tried, and if they work for you, by all means, continue to use them. (Even if garlic doesn't get rid of the sore, no one else will allow you close enough to risk passing it on.)

There is one other aspect of canker sores that bears emphasizing. They can last for a long time. We frequently tell patients that the sores will last for several days, up to two weeks, and they should then disappear. But the sad fact is that for many people, the sores can last considerably longer.

Herpangina is the name given to a specific viral infection, more common in children, especially in the summer and autumn, that is associated with shallow ulcers on the palate. Symptoms include the usual bag of viral symptoms — fever, sore throat, headache, fatigue. Wait four or five days, and this too shall pass.

Swellings on the Lips

Mucous cysts are small, pearly, circular swellings, usually on the lips. They are benign and often disappear on their own. They should only be treated when they interfere with chewing or when they keep getting bitten. The only effective treatment is to remove them surgically. Unfortunately, unless the incision is both wide and deep enough, they tend to come right back, leaving a less than happy patient.

THE NOSE

As a wise lady once pointed out, a nose is a nose is a nose. (She didn't quite say that, but that's what she meant to say.) Each nose is different, although many are eventually shaped by plastic surgeons into clones of the current version of the perfect proboscis. These days the perfect nasal shape seems to have absolutely no ridges, no bumps, and no character, alas.

Noses collect oxygen. They also warm the air we breathe, trap foreign particles, and play an important role in the immunological system of the body.

The nose is also essential for the sense of smell, the least-understood sensation in the body. Smell is something that we rarely worry about, because in contrast to animals, this sense is not important to our survival (although when I watch my husky smelling the backside of every mutt she meets, I admit I am somewhat puzzled by what all this nose-to-the-rear-end stuff has to do with survival). When the sense of smell is absent, however, it greatly diminishes our quality of life.

This sense disappears far more commonly than most people think. I have seen a report that 15 percent of significant head injuries result in some loss of smell, much of it permanent. Unfortunately, we know little as yet about how to restore this sense once it's gone. (If my husky ever lost her sense of smell, I am sure she would commit doggie suicide. She would eat herself to death.)

Nasal Congestion

Doctors seem to like nasal congestion (in others, not in themselves, of course) because nasal congestion provides a great deal of income to most physicians.

Everybody gets at least one or two bouts of a stuffy nose every year, which are most often due to the colds that we all come down with. Many people, however, walk around with a constant "cold." Dese people talk like dis. They are also commonly asking to borrow a Kleenex. (Why do people "borrow" Kleenexes? Does anyone ever return a used Kleenex?)

There are three common reasons for chronic nasal congestion. Very frequently this symptom is due to an unrecognized allergy (see chapter 4). If the allergy is treated properly, the patient is generally able to get rid of the symptom.

A second common reason for frequent, recurrent bouts of nasal congestion is a condition called nonallergic rhinitis, or vasomotor rhinitis. Rhinitis means your nose is running (but not trying to get in shape). Vasomotor rhinitis is the term used for every congested nose in the absence of allergies or other well-established physical reasons. One theory for this problem is that people with vasomotor rhinitis have noses that are overly sensitive to certain everyday irritants like smoke and pollution. Although your nose or my nose may not like polluted air, we'll politely cough once or twice, or sniff, or not react at all, and proceed with our business. The noses of the people with vasomotor rhinitis, however, react physically to these same irritants by overproducing mucus. There is no good way of diagnosing this problem except by eliminating allergies as a cause.

The best treatment for this problem, as for allergies, is to recognize the factors that produce the symptoms and to avoid those factors as much as possible. This is not terribly easy to do if the rhinitis is produced by normal environmental pollutants. For the same reason, there are not many home remedies that relieve the continuous flow of mucus in this condition. The most effective treatment for this condition is to regularly use some type of cortisone nasal spray.

A word about self-treatment. There are several OTC noncortisone nasal sprays available for the treatment of rhinitis. These medications work as nasal decongestants by decreasing the blood flow to the nasal lining, and they are quite effective at relieving a stuffy nose. But for every benefit in this business, there's a price to pay, and the price for these medications is that they are highly addictive. By addictive, I do not mean that you can get high by sniffing these products. Rather, what happens is that your nose becomes reliant on these medications after steady use. (Steady use may be as little as several days in a row.) When the nose doesn't get its regular hit, it produces a more severe discharge than the one for which you took the medication in the first place. This is another example of a rebound effect. Rebound rhinitis obviously responds well to more medication, and the circle can go around and around, until you forcefully withdraw from taking the medication for several very stuffy nights. So listen to your worried doctor. Never take OTC nasal sprays for more than three days in a row. Instead, save them for an especially bad day, or more commonly, bad night.

A third reason for recurrent nasal congestion is a deviated nasal septum. The nasal septum is that tissue that separates one nostril from the other. Instead of running straight up and down, it can deviate, pushing more to one side than the other. This condition can occur from a blow to the nose, or you can be born with it. Deviated septa that cause problems are operated on.

Nosebleeds

Nosebleeds are a bother. They are seldom very serious, though in rare circumstances people have died from them. Nosebleeds are often recurrent, for up to several weeks at a time.

Nosebleeds are usually caused by a blow to the nose, nose picking, or the drying out of the lining of the nose. This latter effect is more noticeable in the winter, when the air inside our houses is very dry as a result of the Great Canadian Tendency to overheat our homes and buildings. Nosebleeds can also be due to general bleeding problems, but they are rarely the only manifestation of these diseases.

Don't lie down with a nosebleed. You don't want to swallow the blood or choke on it, so always lean forward, even though you are probably bleeding all over someone's best couch. Apply pressure to the probable bleeding area by pinching the soft part of the nose for several minutes. This is often sufficient for the acute bleed. If the bleeding keeps recurring, depending on the source of the bleeding and how heavy it is, you must either have the bleeding area cauterized (a type of chemical burning) or have the nose packed with gauze, neither of which elicits screams of joy from the bleeder.

Don't pick your nose, and never overheat your house — two good rules to live by.

Snoring

When I was younger, I took a tour through Europe one summer, staying mainly in youth hostels. I remember the one in Lausanne, Switzerland, best of all, partly because the hostel was located in a particularly lovely setting. But mostly I remember Lausanne because along with 118 other men, I had to share a huge dormitory with a man who snored so loudly he kept that entire room awake all night. This was accomplished despite several less-than-pleasant attempts to wake him, none of which succeeded.

Statistics vary for this problem because snoring is to a large extent in the ears of the listener, and our ability to tolerate snoring in our bed partner varies tremendously. Some studies show that up to 75 percent of males and, not to be sexist, over 50 percent of females snore (although women will always deny that they snore, just as they always deny sweating). Let's just say that snoring is a significant problem of grand dimensions, and much like the stories about the ones that got away, often the subject of much exaggeration.

People snore because the manner in which they breathe while asleep sets up a noisy airflow through the mouth and throat and down to the larynx. Simple enough. But a cure for this breathing pattern is another matter.

There are probably as many home cures for snoring as there are for herpes, which means that there are many. As with any other home remedy you hear of for any other condition, you should always try each of these treatments as long as it causes no harm, but remember that if any of these treatments were universally effective, the person recommending it to you would probably have already retired on the profits of the book he or she would have written.

Many people will tell you that if you change your sleeping position, snoring will diminish, especially if you stop sleeping on your back. To keep off your back whilst you are dead to the world, you are supposed to sleep with a tennis ball sewn into the back of your pajama top, assuming, of course, that you wear one. It's worth a try (for best results, try a Slazenger), but don't hold your breath. (Holding your breath doesn't work either.) Drinking alcohol at night worsens the symptoms for some people. Curing allergies and nasal congestion is occasionally effective in others. Taking out adenoids also works sometimes, especially in kids. Losing weight also can't hurt, because there is some proof that overweight people snore more.

There has been a recent spurt of interest in an operation that changes the shape of the palate, presumably allowing a smoother flow of air in the back of the throat. This operation clearly works for a few, but it is not a universal cure, despite the impassioned protests of some of the surgeons.

The best treatment for snoring is to train your partner not to listen.

Sleep Apnea

Apnea means a stoppage in breathing. People with sleep apnea are loud snorers who repeatedly stop breathing for various periods of time while they are asleep. They usually stop breathing for only a few seconds, but it can be considerably longer — up to a minute and a half. The reason that they start breathing again after an apneic period is that apnea luckily produces changes in the blood chemistry that lead to an automatic restart of breathing.

The most common symptom of this abnormal sleep pattern is daytime drowsiness. Most people with sleep apnea do not sleep well, and they wake up more tired than when they went to bed. More important, sleep apnea taxes the heart and leads to a greater risk of heart attacks during sleep.

The best way to diagnose sleep apnea is to be tested in a sleep disorders clinic, where they literally watch you sleep and monitor your breathing. (Yes, you're right. It's as exciting as watching the grass grow.)

Significant sleep apnea is treated with gadgets that supply the snorer with oxygen while he sleeps, or with surgery.

Sinus Congestion

Sinuses are air pockets in the skull bones. There are four pairs of them, four on each side of the face.

We are still not sure what the sinuses do. They are probably most important in helping the head deal with air pressure on the bones of the skull.

The sinuses have a lining, and this lining can become infected, either as an acute infection or as a chronic problem. Because the opening from a sinus is very narrow, the sinus quickly fills with inflammatory fluid when it is infected. The pressure from the fluid causes the sinus to ache. This pain is usually located in the front of the face, either above or below the eyes, depending on which sinus is involved. A thick, yellowish discharge from the nose is also often present. An infected sinus usually hurts if you tap the area of the skull immediately over it. An X ray can confirm that the sinus is blocked, but it is frequently not necessary for accurate diagnosis.

Acute sinusitis is treated with antibiotics and any other measure that helps the sinuses drain, such as breathing in steam or nasal decongestants. A sinus infection that gets out of control can abscess or spread (it is not that far from the sinuses to the brain).

The sinuses can also become chronically inflamed. When this happens, the sinuses constantly drain some discharge and feel plugged. People who have chronically inflamed sinuses are miserable, and they complain of constant headaches and pain in the face. They must learn to recognize the irritants that make the sinuses more plugged (such as smoke, allergies, occupational chemicals and fumes) and avoid these irritants at all cost. They also require regular vaporizing treatment for their congestion, and they often become dependent on medications that help the sinuses dry up. These people look for, and deserve, your sympathy. When all else fails, the sinuses are drained surgically.

THE THROAT

Basically, the throat is a chamber that connects the nose to the airways and the mouth to the esophagus. You can think of the throat as an atrium, a collecting room. But, unlike the *grands salons* of Paris, the throat is not a simple receiving room. It is a very important part of the immune system of the body and contains stacks of lymph tissue — say hello to the tonsils and to the adenoids. The tonsils sit on either side of the back of the throat. The adenoids are located at the top of the throat, where the nose connects to the back of the throat.

Lymph tissue is a vital cog in the body's ability to fight off infection. It is where the body tends to concentrate the white blood cells and antibodies that fight off the invaders that constantly try to penetrate the body's defenses. Even when the tonsils and the adenoids are removed, the throat lining still contains huge amounts of anti-invader material, explaining why doctors have always believed that (with some exceptions) you are not any more prone to infections when your tonsils are removed.

Tonsillitis

A doctor's version of a bedtime story.

When I was a lot younger, Emily, doctors were meanies who took little boys and girls off to a big hospital to have their tonsils taken out. These unsuspecting children were lured there with promises of Jell-O and ice cream, and their parents were bribed with promises the children would have fewer throat infections once their tonsils were removed. Kids who were mouth breathers or kids who snored were promised that these symptoms would also disappear.

Those were mean times for kids, Emily. Many of those who were operated on still got frequent sore throats. Some kids did snore less when the adenoids were removed because there was less blockage of the passage from the nose to the airways. But many mouth breathers did not improve; nor did many snorers. Close your eyes, dear.

Things are different now, sweetheart. Tonsillectomies are done much more infrequently. We recognize that there are some people, not just children, who do have faulty tonsils. In these people, the tonsil tissue swells and hurts each time there is an infection in the throat. These folks have to use a lot of antibiotics because the tonsils are usually infected with bacteria. But these people are the exception, not the rule. If someone is missing a significant amount of time from school or work because of repeated tonsillar infections, it may pay them to have their tonsils out. But we can't promise that these people will be any better off after the operation. The infections may simply move to other areas of the throat and occur just as often.

Always remember that a tonsillectomy is not a minor operation. It has all the potential complications of any operation requiring anesthetic, as well as a potential for excessive bleeding.

In adults, adenoids are rarely the reason for mouth breathing or snoring, and removing them usually doesn't help solve the problem.

Go to sleep now and remember not to grind your teeth.

Strep Throat

Patients often come into the office with the self-diagnosis of strep throat. They are usually wrong.

Most people think that strep throat is automatically the diagnosis if they are suffering from a severe sore throat or if fever accompanies the sore throat. They have come to believe that all such sore throats are due to an organism called group A beta-hemolytic streptococcus, or strep for short. (Actually, the patients have no idea what the organism is called. They just know that the condition is called strep throat and that they have to have an antibiotic to cure it.) This is not so.

The great majority of sore throats are caused by viruses. These sore throats do not require antibiotics.

Generally, strep throats occur in younger patients (those under thirty), are quite painful, and are accompanied by a fever and swollen glands. However, the only way to know for certain if your sore throat is caused by strep bacteria is for the doctor to take a swab from the back of the throat to try to isolate the offending organism. (Whenever I use the term "offending organism," you can picture a leering bacterium or virus that not only is snarky and talks back but also is not in the least bit remorseful or afraid of you — sort of like Sean Penn.) In study after study, it has been reliably shown that doctors cannot accurately distinguish viral sore throats from strep sore throats purely from the patient's symptoms. Unlike the little engine that could, doctors cannot diagnose this condition just because they think they can.

Throat swabs are about 90 percent accurate at finding the responsible bacteria. If the test does not indicate any strep growing in your throat, it's unlikely that you require antibiotics. If you are given antibiotics for a viral sore throat, you will no doubt get better while on the penicillin or erythromycin. But your improvement is simply coincident with your taking of the antibiotic, because you would have improved anyway whether you were taking medication or not. But because most people improve while on the antibiotic, they tend to (erroneously) give credit to the medication for their improvement.

The result of a throat culture can be obtained, in most large centers, within twenty-four hours. Newer tests promise even quicker results. If there is strep growing in your throat, a delay of one day in instituting treatment will not have any effect on long-term healing. (Just to confuse you some more, it must be pointed out that some people carry strep bacteria in the throat silently, and a positive throat swab in such people does not necessarily mean that the organism is the cause of their infection. But it's easier to understand all this if you just ignore that I said that.)

Why, oh why should we not give everyone antibiotics right away, pending the culture report? One day of unnecessary medication surely wouldn't hurt. Why, oh why, oh why?

Because antibiotics can cause serious complications such as allergic reactions, because antibiotics cost money, because antibiotics produce side effects like diarrhea and vaginal yeast infections, and because overuse of antibiotics has led to all sorts of bacteria that are now resistant to these antibiotics. That's why.

If left untreated, the strep bacteria can spread from the throat to other parts of the body, particularly to the heart valves, where they cause rheumatic fever, a condition that can lead to progressive heart damage. When I was in medical school, I served part of my training in a poorer part of Montreal. A large number of the adults in that community had had rheumatic fever, presumably because as kids they had not used antibiotics to treat strep infections. But we did not see nearly as much rheumatic fever in their children, because those kids had better access to antibiotics.

In the last few years, however, sporadic cases of rheumatic fever (as well as scarlet fever, which is caused by the same organism) have again begun to reappear all over the continent. Perhaps doctors are not prescribing as much antibiotic as they did a few years ago. Perhaps the bacteria have changed. Or perhaps antibiotics are not the sole reason why strep organisms do not spread to the heart valves from the throat. There may have been another still-undetermined factor at work over the last few decades that along with the use of antibiotics prevented this complication, and maybe that other factor is no longer as active.

It still remains prudent to treat all proven group A streptococcus infections of the throat with penicillin or its alternatives. But if you visit the doctor with a sore throat, I urge you to always ask for a throat swab and to only take antibiotics if the results of the swab are positive for bacteria. Strep does spread to other members of the family, and it may not be symptomatic in everyone. If you have a positive culture result more than once in a short period of time, you should probably get the other members of the family tested.

Oh, yes, the family pet too may harbor strep organisms. For recurrent strep throat, it may pay to get Fido cultured (which doesn't, of course, mean getting him tickets to the symphony). One other cause of sore throats bears mentioning. Infectious mononucleosis (see chapter 4) has been responsible for some of the worst sore throats that I have ever seen. Anybody who complains of excessive fatigue and has a severe-looking sore throat with pus should have a mono test.

Chronic Sore Throats

Many people complain of sore throats that linger long after an infection is gone. This phenomenon is more common in the winter than other seasons. The sore throat is frequently described as worst on rising in the morning and improving somewhat as the day wears on, only to reappear in full flower the next day. This symptom is caused to a large extent by the Great Canadian Tendency (see above). The dry atmosphere inside an overheated house, combined with no intake of fluids at night, leads to a dried-out throat lining that hurts. The pain diminishes as the day progresses because sufferers lubricate their throats by drinking liquids. If you have a persistent waxing and waning sore throat after a throat infection, try sleeping with the window open (heaven forbid!) and turning the heat down. Of course you must convince your partner that the doctor ordered you to freeze your tootsies.

Hoarseness

Sudden onset of hoarseness is nearly always due to an infection of the larynx, or the voice box (unless you've been yelling at the ref in a soccer game). Laryngitis generally accompanies or follows a cold or other condition of the upper respiratory tract. Because it is most often caused by a virus, antibiotics are rarely necessary. The only known treatments are to rest your voice (which does not mean whispering; this may actually tax your larynx more than talking), to humidify your respiratory tract with the use of steam and vaporizers, and to drink lots of liquids. Although it usually disappears in about a week, laryngitis may last up to two weeks, a complication that seems to happen more to actors, singers, and radio personalities than to the general public.

Chronic hoarseness, which really means hoarseness that persists more than two weeks, should be investigated for other potential causes, which can include nodes and polyps on the vocal cords and cancer (especially in smokers).

CHAPTER 6

The Respiratory System

In which the author wheezes his way into your hearts

When I was growing up, my mother's harshest admonition to me was
that if I didn't dry my hair completely or put more clothes on when
I went outside, I would surely catch pneumonia. This warning was
invariably hollered in my direction as I left the house with still-wet
hair following one of my semiannual baths, or else it was screamed at
me while I was running around outside on a typically frigid Montreal
morning, clad in just a T-shirt and pants after she had carefully
dressed me in a snowsuit, scarf, and mittens. (How can you possibly
play ball hockey in a snow suit?) I had absolutely no idea what
pneumonia was, but I lived in perpetual fear of catching it (although
not enough fear to follow her advice, of course).

I did know that coughing was one symptom that accompanies
pneumonia, because every time I coughed, or even cleared my throat
loudly after one of those semi-naked ball hockey games, my mother,
in her usual subtle, guilt-provoking manner, would natter, "See?
What did I tell you? It's starting. Your pneumonia is starting."
(According to my mother, you own every disease that affects you.)
Every break after a goal, especially if one of us Jean Beliveaus
happened to cough, allowed me a moment's pause to feel guilty.
Luckily, play always resumed quickly, and I was able to forget her
dire prediction. And I never did get pneumonia (nor did I ever get
to play at the Forum, where ball hockey, after all, is not what the
patrons pay for.) But I did get asthma as an adult, so in a way my
mother's predictions of respiratory problems for her elder son did
turn out to be true.

HOW THE SYSTEM WORKS

The respiratory tract is a simple system to understand anatomically. The nose collects air. You need this air because it contains oxygen, the gas that fuels the energy cycles of the body. The air is warmed in the nose and sent down the back of the throat — the pharynx — to the main breathing tube — the trachea. The trachea in turn divides into two major air tubes called the main stem bronchi, one for each lung. The main bronchi divide into smaller bronchi, and those divide into even smaller bronchi called bronchioles. The smallest bronchioles end in millions of tiny air sacs called alveoli. The lung is a spongey kind of organ composed of these tiny alveoli.

It is at the level of the alveoli that the fascinating work of the lung takes place. The alveoli are extremely thin. This extreme thinness allows oxygen to pass through the alveolar walls and enter the tiny arteries that run throughout the lung tissue. That's how you get the oxygen into the blood stream. Carbon dioxide, a waste product of various body processes, passes the other way, from the tiny blood vessels back into the alveoli and up the air passages.

This whole process is called gas exchange. (I bet you thought that gas exchange occurred in a different area of the body. And between at least two people.) Interfering with gas exchange for only several minutes can result in permanent severe damage to many organs, especially the brain.

How do the lungs manage to expand to draw air into them? Think about it for a minute. A balloon doesn't just fill with air if it's left lying around. You have to work at blowing the balloon up. But the work involved in taking a breath is relatively minimal. You clearly don't work hard enough to blow up the lungs with each breath. So how do the lungs fill with air?

The answer is rather ingenious. The lungs are located between the shoulders and the abdomen in the part of the body called the thoracic cavity. The thoracic cavity has negative pressure, meaning that the pressure within the cavity is less than air pressure outside the cavity. As a result, air rushes into the lungs to even out the pressure. So it takes very little effort to draw air into the lungs with each breath. Any hole in the system (such as one produced by trauma to the chest cavity), however, will even out the pressure between the thoracic

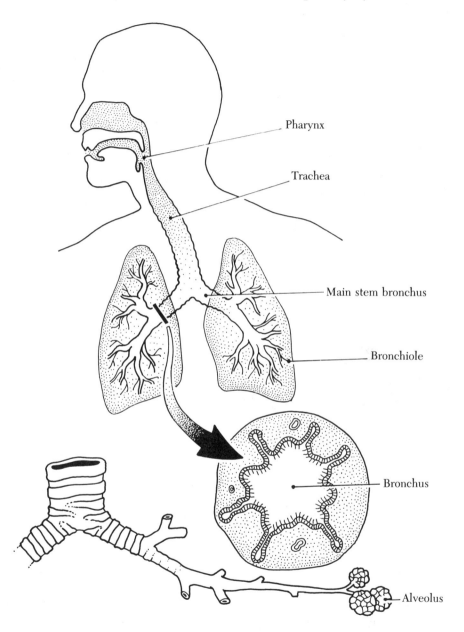

THE RESPIRATORY SYSTEM

cavity and the outside world, resulting in collapse of the lung on that side (much like a balloon collapses when it's punctured) and preventing proper breathing.

Although gas exchange is the most important work that this system does, the respiratory tract performs several other very vital functions. The respiratory tract is also a filter system. The whole passage is lined with little hairs called cilia, which trap tiny particles that we breathe in and send them back up to be expelled from the body.

The respiratory tract is also a very important cog in the body's continuous battle against foreign invaders. Through the use of coughing, mucus, lymph tissue, cilia, scavenger cells known as macrophages, and antibodies, the respiratory system helps the body deal with the relentless assault of bacteria, viruses, fungi, and other zealous invaders that are only too ready, like little children, to invade your private space.

COUGHING

Nobody likes coughing. Actually, that's not exactly true. My son has his seat in class next to another kid who coughs continuously and happily, mainly (I think) because my son can't stand it whenever this second boy coughs.

This latter boy notwithstanding, most of us feel that coughing, much like pain, is a symptom we could definitely live without. But coughing does have a useful purpose. When you cough, you clear the respiratory tract of whatever is irritating it.

Coughing can be caused by mucus (or other fluids, such as blood) draining down the back of the throat from either the nose or the sinuses, or from fluids produced in the bronchi or in the lung tissue.

Coughing Produced by Colds

When coughing is produced by a postnasal discharge, or by irritation of other tissues in the upper respiratory tract, the cough will clear when the primary condition (either a cold or some other infection) clears up. These infections are usually viral in origin (see chapter 4) and rarely require treatment beyond the usual rest and fluids.

Coughing Produced by Bronchial Irritation

If you visit the doctor with a productive cough (that's a cough that produces mucus), you are often told that you have acute bronchitis, a diagnosis that immediately strikes fear in the heart of every adult Canadian. It is true that the bronchi are usually inflamed in such cases, but this certainly doesn't mean that you are very ill. Nor does it mean that you automatically require an antibiotic. Most cases of bronchitis are caused by viruses and respond to the usual measures of rest and fluids. To see if you do need an antibiotic, get a sputum culture.

Cough suppressants, either those prescribed by the doctor or those purchased OTC, are often taken for bronchitis. But cough suppressants should be used only after a couple of questions have been answered. Is the cough really interfering with your ability to function normally? And what do you think is going to happen to the mucus that you don't cough up when you're on the medication? Much like diarrhea or fever, coughing is a mechanism the body uses to help itself fight an inflammatory condition. A productive cough is helping rid your respiratory tract of mucus produced by the inflammation in the bronchi. This is important because mucus that collects without being cleared properly can be a focus of new infection and can also interfere with proper breathing and lung function. So a cough should be suppressed only when it interferes with your ability to function normally during the day or when it interferes with your sleep (and your partner's).

The most effective cough suppressants contain codeine, so they can usually be obtained only by prescription. Dextromethorphan, the DM you often see on the bottles of cough medication on drugstore shelves, is also a cough suppressant, though not as effective as codeine.

There are medications, known as expectorants, that claim they help you cough up the mucus that is collecting in your airways. I am not convinced that any of these medications do that. To me, the most effective expectorant has always been some hot liquid drunk in great big dollops (and yes, chicken soup is at least as effective as anything else I know of and tastes considerably better than most other liquids).

Pneumonia, that disease most dreaded by all immigrant children (see above; my Italian friends were also generally threatened by their mothers with an Italian malady similar to pneumonia when they played semi-naked ball hockey), is an infection of the lung tissue. The alveoli fill with inflammatory fluid caused by some infection or produced by an irritant. The patient usually has a high fever, a cough with thick, greenish sputum that is sometimes tinged with blood, and some chest pain.

Pneumonia is a severe infection that must be carefully monitored. Like all infections, pneumonia needs antibiotic treatment only when it is due to an organism that can be treated with these drugs. Even though we have antibiotics to treat most bacterial pneumonias, they can be such severe infections that they are still major killers of the elderly and the debilitated.

"Walking pneumonia" is a mild pneumonia in which the patient is often not too sick. This variant is due to either a virus, which does not require antibiotic treatment, or an organism called mycoplasma, which does require antibiotics.

More severe pneumonias may require hospitalization.

Chronic Cough

Chronic bronchitis is defined as any mucus-producing cough that lasts three months at a time for two years in a row. It is much more common in smokers than nonsmokers and is not very common in those under the age of fifty. You treat chronic bronchitis by preventing it in the first place, which means that you give up smoking.

If you have chronic bronchitis, there is some disagreement among medical people as to what you should do when you get sick with a cold or flu. There is some (debatable) evidence that you should be put on antibiotics as soon as you get sick, although you will frequently get better without any medical intervention. But presumably the early use of antibiotics will decrease the incidence of bacterial bronchitis and pneumonia, which is more common in people with this condition. And be prepared to receive a lecture on smoking along with the prescription. Often the lecture is more useful than the medication.

Chronic cough can also be a symptom of emphysema, although the main symptom of this disease is shortness of breath. The production of mucus and occasional chest pain are other symptoms of emphysema.

Emphysema is a disease in which the alveoli lose their elasticity and many are destroyed, so the lungs can't exchange oxygen and carbon dioxide as efficiently. It is very rare in those under fifty, but the groundwork for the disease is laid by smoking in the twenties, thirties, and forties. Emphysema is much more common in smokers, although some nonsmokers have a genetic predisposition to the disease as well.

Want to do something to prevent emphysema? Stop smoking. Are you getting the point yet about how best to prevent chronic damage to your lungs?

In many people chronic cough is due to mild asthma (see below). Chronic cough can also occasionally be due to a nervous habit. If there is no other obvious problem and the person does not seem to be ill or to be getting more ill with time, then the diagnosis of neurotic cough must be entertained.

The only treatment for this condition is to wait it out.

Tuberculosis (TB) usually appears as a chronic cough (often with a bloody sputum), accompanied by other signs of chronic disease, such as fatigue, weight loss, night sweats, and debilitation. Active TB is a serious infection, which is transmittable to close contacts.

The only time most of us ever have to think of TB is when we are asked to take a test to prove that we are not carrying this disease. This test is usually given when people switch jobs, especially in the health, daycare, and food industries.

There are two ways to test for previous exposure to TB. The first is to have a skin test (see chapter 3). The second is to have a chest X ray. If you are under thirty-five and have a positive skin test and you don't know when the test turned positive or why, you are generally advised to take a prophylactic antituberculosis medication (isoniazid). Isoniazid is not generally used for those oldies over the age of thirty-five because it has a greater tendency to produce liver damage in these aged people.

TB requires antibiotic therapy, but in contrast to the old days when TB patients were isolated in sanitoriums, the patient is usually able to return to normal life after a short period of treatment.

WHEEZING — A SYMPTOM OF ASTHMA

By far the most common cause of wheezing in young-to-middle-aged adults is asthma (and not swallowed whistles, as some may think). Asthma is caused by factors that irritate the lining of those airways below the level of the trachea. The most common factors include respiratory infections, allergies, cold air, exercise, smoke, reflux of stomach acid, and some drugs. Emotional stress can produce asthma, but only in some asthmatics some of the time. The irritation produces airway spasm and consequent narrowing of the airways, as well as inflammation and overproduction of mucus. The end results of all this spasm and mucus are the symptoms of wheezing, shortness of breath, and coughing.

Asthmatic attacks can be delayed for several hours after exposure to the precipitating agent. So some people who have occupationally induced asthma, for example, do not wheeze until several hours after work. As a result, the asthma is often erroneously attributed to other, more immediate factors.

Everybody recognizes wheezing as one of the main symptoms of asthma. Wheezing is often worse at night, especially between 3:00 and 7:00 A.M. The reasons for this are that the asthmatic response is delayed in some people, as mentioned above; there is less tone in the thin muscles of the bronchi during the early hours of the morning; and asthma is also often caused by the reflux of stomach acid into the esophagus when people lie down. Presumably, this acid irritates the bronchial tree and causes asthmatic symptoms.

Many people, especially young children, don't wheeze when they get an asthmatic attack; instead they cough. If the coughing is inter-mittent — that is, it comes and goes for a week or two at a time — the child is often erroneously diagnosed as suffering from repeated bronchial infections. Instead of getting the anti-asthmatic medication that he requires, this little cougher is instead given scads of antibiotics to take. The patient often improves while taking the antibiotic, mainly because the asthmatic attack has run its course, not because the antibiotic had anything to do with the patient's improvement. But because he got better while on this medication, he automatically gets more antibiotic the next time he is sick.

Remember, any person who coughs regularly and produces sputum should be suspected of having asthma, as long as other diagnoses have been excluded. The same is also true for the person who coughs persistently for several weeks after an upper respiratory infection. These people should be tested for asthma with lung function tests, in which the patient breathes into an apparatus that measures various lung capacities.

Every asthmatic attack must be carefully monitored. The rate of deaths from asthma has been rising all over North America. Part of the reason for this phenomenon is that we have become blasé about asthmatic attacks, mainly because we have excellent medications to treat them. As a result, both doctors and patients tend to delay treatment until the attack is relatively well advanced. The more severe the attack, the harder it is to turn around, sometimes resulting in irreversible airway blockage and death.

Although a small percentage of people can prevent asthmatic attacks by using a drug called sodium cromoglycate (Fivent), for most asthmatics, the main medications for asthma control are still bronchodilators, which are medications that can reverse airway spasm, or to put it in more technical terms, dilate the bronchi. For most asthmatics, a bronchodilator in a spray form is all that's required to keep the asthma in check. The most prescribed bronchodilator sprays include salbutamol (Ventolin) and fenoterol (Berotec).

When starting on them for the first time, most people complain of feeling a little more speedy, particularly at night. This symptom wears off after several doses. If you are not happy with the side effects of your medication, however, do try a different one before you give up on the sprays altogether.

It is important to remember several other details about bronchodilator therapy. Most important, you must learn how to use the medication properly — how long it takes to work in different situations, how many puffs you need when you exercise, and so on. The quality of the treatment is only as good as the "treater." I once read a study that analyzed the reasons for failure of asthmatic therapy in several dozen patients. I am not kidding when I tell you that several people who complained that the medication wasn't working had neglected to take the cap off the medication dispenser. (These are not the people who should apply for the head job at NASA.) The medication indeed doesn't work very well if you don't take the lid off the container, much as the banana generally doesn't taste very good if you eat it with its skin.

The aerosol sprays don't work well if there is already a good deal of mucus in the system, because the sprays cannot penetrate mucus well. So if you are already sick with a cold, for example, and you are an asthmatic, it is quite likely that you will require more spray than usual. You may also require an anti-inflammatory spray (see below) or perhaps some anti-asthma medication in pill form. One of these may also be required for a well-established asthmatic attack.

The maximum dose of most sprays is usually two puffs four times a day. If you need more than eight puffs a day, don't just increase the amount of spray you use — which is unfortunately what most people do. Check with your doctor instead. You may benefit from a change in medication.

If you get asthma with exertion, you should take your medication at least ten minutes before starting the exercise. Don't try to run through the wheeze.

Most anti-asthma sprays are only effective for about six hours, so people who rely only on these sprays for asthma relief at night still wake up wheezing in the early morning hours if they take their spray at bedtime. This type of asthma is best treated with oral medications that last at least twelve hours.

The most commonly used oral medications for asthma are the theophylline preparations. Everybody absorbs theophylline at different rates. Some people may need four pills of a certain preparation for a mild attack, whereas others may need only one pill for a similar attack.

Theophylline also has many side effects, not the least of which is that it speeds you up. You may notice a faster pulse, a racy feeling, agitation, and difficulty sleeping. If you use theophylline regularly, you generally can adjust to these side effects.

Because asthma is now thought to be due as much to inflammation as it is to airway spasm, the trend over the last three years is to use steroid sprays, which are anti-inflammatories, along with the standard bronchodilating sprays. Steroids are also being prescribed in significantly higher doses than they used to be. Among other potential side effects, these higher doses of cortisone may promote the growth of fungus, or yeast, in the mouth, so it is wise to rinse the mouth after using a steroid spray.

Want Dr. Hister's home remedy for asthma? (No, for a change it's not garlic.) But it is my other equally favorite substance, coffee. (My editor rebelled when I wanted to call coffee a food.) Caffeine, like theophylline, is a member of the bromine family. And it too can reverse mild airway spasm, although you probably have to make the coffee exceedingly strong (which is just the way I, but not my esophagus, like it).

Severe recurrent asthmatic attacks frequently require oral cortisone (prednisone) for treatment. Use of this drug should be carefully monitored by a physician.

HYPERVENTILATION

Hyperventilation is often mistaken for asthma, since the patient complains of shortness of breath.

Hyperventilation is a problem in which the patient, when anxious, takes many short, shallow breaths, resulting in light-headedness and dizziness, which lead to more anxiety and shallower breathing, and so on.

The treatment of this condition is (you must believe me) to breathe into a brown paper bag. (This is not the same as those people who wear brown bags to cover their faces at ball games because they don't want to admit that they're fans of the home team.) When you're hyperventilating, the brown bag around your mouth and nostrils collects the carbon dioxide that you are exhaling. You then breathe in this carbon dioxide, which has the effect of slowing down your breathing through an action on the breathing center of your brain. Now I realize that if you start to hyperventilate when you are riding home on a crowded bus, it is not too easy to get out a brown paper bag and breathe into it. The bus driver may just radio ahead for an ambulance with a couple of men in white coats, while the other passengers may all crowd to the other end of the bus. But if the symptoms are severe, it is the only thing that will work quickly. You'll just have to risk it. Let me know how it goes.

COUGHING UP BLOOD

Bloody sputum should always be discussed with a physician because there are serious possibilities like TB or a blood clot in the lungs (called a pulmonary embolus, a real medical emergency) or a tumor.

But surprisingly, most young-to-middle-aged adults who suddenly cough up a bit of blood are not very sick. The usual reason that blood is present in the sputum is that the patient coughed quite vigorously during a cold or some other upper respiratory infection and broke a few small blood vessels in the back of the throat. This usually shows up as a reddish tinge in the sputum, occurs once or twice, and disappears quickly.

CHEST PAIN

The lungs are not a common source of pain in young adults. The exceptions are infections such as pneumonia (see above) or infections that irritate the lung lining (pleurisy), as well as a problem called pneumothorax. All of these conditions should be monitored by a doctor.

The pleura are the linings of the lung. Pleurisy occurs as a complication of an infection, most commonly a pneumonia, in which the infected fluid collects between the lung and its lining. Pleurisy usually appears as a sharp pain of sudden onset that gets worse with each breath.

The pleurisy usually clears when the infection goes, but occasionally pleurisy can leave a permanently scarred area in the lining.

A pneumothorax is a hole in the lining of the lung. Because the hole allows air to rush into that closed space around the lung, the lung partially collapses in that area. If the hole is large enough, the entire lung can collapse.

Although it can happen to anyone, especially with trauma to the chest, pneumothorax tends to occur mostly in previously healthy, young, tall, thin males. (In other words, it's unlikely to happen to me.) It tends to occur suddenly, without warning, as a severe, sharp chest pain that worsens with each deep breath and that is accompanied by shortness of breath. In addition, a pneumothorax is often associated with pain in the shoulder area. There is no fever.

Anyone who has had one pneumothorax is much more likely to suffer a second. A pneumothorax is best diagnosed by a chest X ray.

Although a small pneumothorax can be managed with rest at home, many pneumothoraxes must be managed in hospital because the patient is so short of breath. The air is then actively drawn out of the space between the lung and its lining.

Tumors of the lung and its lining can cause chest pain, but luckily these tumors are rare in people under fifty years old. Lung tumors are of course much more common in smokers than nonsmokers. Any adult smoker with unexplained chest pain, a new cough, a cough that produces blood, or any weight loss that cannot be explained should be worked up for a possible chest malignancy. If a malignancy is strongly suspected, a chest X ray is not sufficient to rule out a tumor. A CT scan and often a bronchoscopy are also required.

CHAPTER 7

The Cardiovascular System

*In which the good doctor endeavors to show you
how not to lose heart*

A statistic you will hear quoted again and again is that cardiovascular disease is the number-one killer of adults in North America. This means that heart attacks and strokes kill more of us than any other disease, including all the forms of cancer.

So it is not surprising that this system has become a focus of great interest not just to doctors but to all North Americans who are concerned about their health. And because excess cholesterol in the bloodstream has been implicated as a major contributing factor to the development of disease in the cardiovascular system, how to lower cholesterol levels has become trend-item number one in medicine. These days we are all supposed to be monitoring our cholesterol level and changing our lifestyle to keep that level as low as possible.

I come from a more skeptical background than many, I suppose. After all, I am a Jewish male, brought up to question everything (except my parents, who were always right). I am still not convinced that we can predict many of the consequences of all the latest recommendations about cholesterol. In some Woody Allen film it was finally discovered in the twenty-first century that meat and potatoes are the healthiest diet for mankind. (Very few people know if a similar diet would be best for women as well.) Although I love meat and potatoes (my mother is the quintessential Polish cook — she serves potatoes and garlic with everything; occasionally they are the only thing), I doubt that this diet is the very healthiest one for us, but the point, I think, is well made. How sure are we of everything we believe? As someone famous once said, "Today's false gods were once true."

We do know that cardiovascular disease is not inevitable. There are a number of risk factors that can be altered to decrease our chances of developing these problems. One of the main risk factors is a very high level of cholesterol in the bloodstream. But what should we be telling people whose cholesterol levels are normal or only slightly or even moderately raised? Should these people also be put on diet patrol?

If you want to know my opinion, read on.

One word of explanation. Symptoms of cardiovascular disease are rare in fifteen-to-fifty-year-olds. For this reason, coronary heart disease, the major form of cardiovascular disease, is discussed at the beginning of the chapter, and symptoms of other problems that this age group may experience are discussed at the end of the chapter.

HOW THE SYSTEM WORKS

The heart is made up of four chambers, two atria (not atriums), and two ventricles. These chambers are separated by valves, which are composed of little leaflets that open and close with each beat. The sounds of the heart are produced by the closing of the heart valves.

Blood vessels include arteries, veins, and capillaries. The arteries carry oxygen from the left ventricle of the heart through the body. Starting with the emergence of the aorta, the largest artery in the body, from the left ventricle, the arteries branch into smaller and smaller arteries, eventually ending in tiny capillaries, which allow oxygen and other nutrients to pass through their walls into the cells of the body. The waste products from the cells, including carbon dioxide, then pass into other capillaries, which empty into veins, and are then transported back to the right side of the heart through a series of progressively larger veins. This venous blood, which is darker, enters the right atrium, from where it is dumped into the right ventricle. From the right ventricle, the blood enters the lungs, where it dumps its load of carbon dioxide and picks up its new shipment of oxygen to go back to the body.

And on and on, until you die.

Simple, wot?

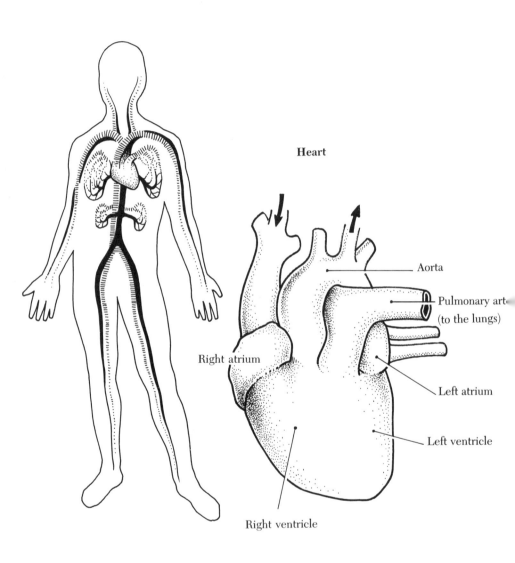

Heart

Aorta

Pulmonary art●
(to the lungs)

Right atrium

Left atrium

Left ventricle

Right ventricle

THE CARDIOVASCULAR SYSTEM

CORONARY HEART DISEASE

There are many different types of heart disease (after all, any injury to the heart can result in a type of disease of the heart tissue), but there is only one type that I will discuss in this chapter. Coronary artery disease (CAD) refers to that process that injures and clogs up the blood vessels that supply oxygen to the heart tissue. This type of heart disease is also referred to as coronary heart disease (CHD), which is the term I will use throughout this chapter. You will, by the way, see a lot of initials in this chapter.

Coronary heart disease *is* the number-one killer in North America. But most people think of CHD the way they think of Antarctica. It's a big thing, it's out there, but it's not too relevant for me.

Wrong.

It's a relevant problem for every North American adult because even if you yourself do not develop angina or a heart attack, there is a likelihood that someone close to you, a relative or close friend, will.

The arteries to the heart start life as smooth, wide-open channels. As we age and as our risk factors increase, the arteries become injured by deposits of plaque on the walls of the arteries. Plaque in your arteries is not like plaque on your teeth (you can't floss your arteries). Plaque in your arteries can kill you, whereas plaque on your teeth will only make you suffer from exorbitant dental bills. (Or leave you with that caricatured smile that Martha Raye has. Enough dental plaque, and you too can end your life peddling Polident on television.)

The plaque that injures arteries is made up of various substances but primarily of that substance that makes grown men tremble, cholesterol. The plaques lead to hardening, or sclerosis, of these arteries. Because the plaques are called atheromas, another term given to this type of heart damage is atherosclerotic heart disease. These atheromas in turn lead to a more turbulent blood flow through those vessels, sort of like speed bumps lead to a bumpier ride for a car. This turbulent flow, along with the narrowed arteries, increases the risk that blood will clot in these arteries.

When the arteries that supply the heart become clogged but not completely closed, the blood flow diminishes to the parts of the heart fed by those arteries. If the blood flow is too little, the heart does not get the oxygen it needs and signals its need for more oxygen by the symptom of angina. Angina pectoris is the name given to pain or discomfort in the chest that is associated with effort. With effort, the heart needs more oxygen, which the clogged arteries cannot supply. When the heart tissue does not get as much oxygen as it needs, it is said to be ischemic. (If the arteries are very severely blocked, you can get angina at rest.)

If the blood flow to a part of the heart is completely interrupted, that part of the heart dies. This is known as a heart attack, or in official parlance, a myocardial infarction, an infarct for short. When blood flow is interrupted to part of the brain, and that part of the brain is injured or dies, the resulting injury is known as a stroke. A heart attack or stroke occurs when an artery blocks up completely as a result of a blood clot on top of a cholesterol plug (remember those speed bumps and the turbulent blood flow mentioned above?) or when the plugged and narrowed artery goes into a spasm from some excess demand on it. Not all people with significant heart disease get symptoms from this problem. Unfortunately, many people with advanced CHD suffer from silent ischemia. Silent ischemia means that you may have significant blockage in your arteries without ever developing angina. According to some estimates, up to 10 percent of "healthy" adult males suffer from silent ischemia, which translates to about 200,000 to 300,000 middle-aged males in Canada, quite a boatload, you will admit (and a boatload that would have trouble getting insurance for its voyage).

Because silent ischemia by definition does not cause symptoms, people with this form of CHD are likely to die suddenly from heart attacks. Because of this risk, some doctors recommend that people with two or more risk factors for heart disease (see below) but no symptoms of CHD ought to check with their doctor about whether or not they should be tested for silent ischemia.

The rate of CHD varies significantly in different parts of the world. The highest rates occur in Britain, particularly in Northern Ireland, and in certain parts of Finland (which is practically the only fact I know about Finland, except that Finns ski-jump on their way to work), whereas the lowest rates for industrialized countries occur in Japan. As befits its political stance, Canada is in between (or as my dad used to say about everything, *comme ci comme ça*) although we're closer to Finnish rates than to Japanese rates. These rates are so vastly different that a Northern Ireland male, for example, has ten times more chance of dying of a heart attack than his Japanese counterpart.

Because these rates differ so much, and because many people who leave their homelands eventually develop risk profiles that are similar to those of the inhabitants of the country they have moved to, it also becomes obvious that the populations with the higher rates are doing something wrong that spurs the development of CHD. It is also probable that the people with the lower rates are doing the right things to diminish their risks.

The most important risk factors we know of for the development of coronary heart disease include high cholesterol, smoking, high blood pressure, lack of exercise, your sex (not the rate of intercourse but whether you are male or female), genetic susceptibility, stress, alcoholism, obesity localized in the abdomen rather than in the hips or thighs, and certain metabolic problems.

But there must be a whole lot more at work in CHD because even when we control all their risk factors, some people still die of heart attacks. The converse is that some people survive to ripe old age even when they pay absolutely no attention to sage medical advice and do all the wrong things. (Doctors usually dislike these people intensely, not only because they seem to rebut all we say just by staying healthy, but also because they never come into the office.)

The effect of cholesterol on the development of CHD seems to be particularly confusing. For example, despite the undisputed role of cholesterol in some cases of CHD, it is nevertheless true that half of all coronary events occur in patients with what are considered to be normal total cholesterol counts. (Coronary events sounds like something you would attend at Maple Leaf Gardens; the term really refers to "events" like infarctions.) This means that many people with completely safe and normal cholesterol counts have major atheromatous deposits on their coronary arteries. Dr. Michael DeBakey, the world-renowned cardiovascular surgeon, offers the sobering thought that throughout thirty years of observation in his clinic, there is no significant difference in the survival of coronary bypass patients between those who had high cholesterol levels (and no other risk factors) and those who did not have high levels. In other words, either our so-called safe levels are not really safe, or there are some other hidden factors at work promoting CHD that we are probably not yet familiar with. So when it comes to counseling people about significant lifestyle changes, especially the use of medication for high cholesterol levels, we should tread carefully, except with those people at particularly high risk.

FACTORS THAT AFFECT CORONARY HEART DISEASE

Cholesterol

In most people's minds, a heart attack occurs only because you have a high cholesterol level. This is wrong. A high cholesterol level is just one of several risk factors for CHD, although for many people it is probably the most important one. What is interesting about cholesterol is that many of the other factors that increase the risk of CHD (such as smoking and lack of exercise) also affect cholesterol levels. In fact, how these factors affect cholesterol is probably the most important manner in which they promote the development of CHD.

WHAT CHOLESTEROL IS AND WHAT IT DOES

Every doctor has his or her own way of approaching this contentious topic. Sit yourself down in a comfortable chair, favorite beverage at hand, and pay attention to my version. (It's long.) Remember that what you are reading is a mixture of fact and (my) opinion, and it's often difficult to separate the two.

Cholesterol is a naturally occurring body chemical that your body must have for a number of functions, which include the proper maintenance of the walls of your body's cells, the production of the acids present in bile to help with digestion, and the production of certain hormones. So even if you never took in any cholesterol, your body would manufacture its own supply in the liver and then transport that cholesterol to where it's needed.

Cholesterol travels in the bloodstream attached to a transport system called the lipoproteins. There are several types of lipoprotein. Those that are harmful to your arteries are known as low-density lipoproteins, or LDL. This form of cholesterol is deposited on the walls of your arteries and eventually leads to plugged blood vessels. The beneficial lipoproteins are known as high-density lipoproteins, or HDL. (I could confuse you even more by mentioning VLDL now, but I am not that cruel. For the moment, just think of LDL and HDL.) Cholesterol carried in your bloodstream in the form of HDL may actually protect you from heart disease. Many scientists now believe that HDL is a good guy, an arterial Zamboni, because it acts as a type of purifier by ridding the blood vessels of their LDL deposits.

If you've stayed awake till now, you should ask, "What does all this have to do with diet?" An excellent question. Enter now the infamous saturated fats. When saturated fats, such as palm oil or pork fat, or cholesterol from your diet are taken into your body, they are absorbed into the bloodstream through the intestinal lining. In the bloodstream, the saturated fat molecules are cleared out of the blood by attaching themselves onto those cholesterol totebags, the lipoproteins. Both saturated fats and cholesterol in the diet generally lead to increased levels of LDL in the bloodstream.

Saturated fats are now going through a reappraisal. It seems that not all saturated fats are created equal. Most saturated fats are bad for you, but some are not. There are saturated fats (such as those in some fish) that may actually be good for you because they promote the production of HDL.

CAN YOU TELL IF YOU HAVE A CHOLESTEROL PROBLEM?

Unless you have a strong family history of cholesterol-related problems such as heart attacks or strokes, or unless you have your cholesterol level measured, it is unlikely that you will ever know that it is high. There are few external signs of high cholesterol, except for xanthomas, white to yellow deposits of cholesterol on the skin near the eyes, on some tendons, or in some creases, such as the palms. In some people an extra crease in the ear lobe may also be related to higher levels of cholesterol.

CHOLESTEROL BLOOD TESTS AND LEVELS

Much of what follows is a matter of debate.

I think that every adult should know his or her cholesterol level. A lot of doctors and health experts disagree with this advice, arguing that the cost of this approach is excessive and that most adults under fifty have nothing to worry about.

I realize that my modest proposal would cost a lot of money, but I really can't see an alternative that makes sense. The debate about cholesterol is currently so contentious that the only way a person can make any sense at all of this issue is to at least know what his or her cholesterol level is. Besides which, I am willing to bet (and like Pete Rose, I really don't have a gambling problem) that every one of those doctors who doesn't think that it's necessary for you to know your cholesterol count has, however, had his or her tests done.

If you haven't had a cholesterol test, go get one done (before reading on). But what kind of cholesterol test you require is another matter. Unless you have specific risk factors, which I shall mention below, the screening test you should have is a random, *nonfasting* blood cholesterol level. That means that you leave the doctor's office, requisition form in hand, and go get tested. This test measures what is called your total cholesterol level.

If this random screening test comes back with a high reading, as it will in about 50 percent of the population, then you should have a more specific test, which is done after a twelve-to-fourteen-hour fast and after you have not had any alcohol for three days. This next test, called a lipid profile, should measure total cholesterol, HDL, LDL, and triglycerides.

What are triglycerides, the sharper of you will ask. Triglycerides are carried in the blood in the form of VLDLs, very low density lipoproteins. (As yet, we do not have very, very tiny low-density lipoproteins, but I am sure someone is working on finding them.) Very high triglyceride levels are probably independent risk factors for CHD, especially in women.

Now I am about to get really picky.

Your cholesterol level may depend more on where the test is done and less on your risk factors. The lab at which your cholesterol is measured matters a lot, because as has been shown in many studies, cholesterol results often vary greatly from lab to lab. I suggest that if your test result is abnormal, repeat the test at another lab unless the doctor can reassure you that the first lab's results were accurate. If the results vary a lot, you might consider having yet a third test.

What are desirable cholesterol levels? (It is important when talking about cholesterol levels to distinguish between *normal* levels in North Americans, which are generally too high, and *desirable* levels. The easiest way to understand the difference, according to one expert, is to say that it may be normal to get mugged in New York City, but it is certainly not desirable.)

To make this really simple, between the ages of fifteen and thirty, always aim to have your cholesterol level below 4.6 mmol/l (don't worry about what the units mean — most doctors don't understand them either), or 180 mg/dl under the old system. (I promise I'll leave the units out of the text from now on.) Between the ages of thirty and fifty, aim for a level below 5.2, or 200 using the old measures.

Levels of cholesterol between 5.2 and 6.2 are considered border-line, meaning that you should pay some attention to your diet, weight, and amount of exercise, but you don't really need to go beyond that. Any level above 6.2 should probably be treated with active intervention but not necessarily drugs.

How often should you measure your cholesterol level? I have patients who aren't happy unless their cholesterol level is measured daily, if not more often. Every change in diet means a request for "my cholesterol count." C'mon, guys, this is silly. If your cholesterol level is normal, then a measurement every five years is enough. If you have a high cholesterol count, then you should remeasure your cholesterol in about three months *but only if you change your lifestyle*. If you don't change your behavior, your cholesterol levels will not change. My taxes should be spent in a more efficient manner than that.

FACTORS THAT AFFECT CHOLESTEROL LEVELS

There are many factors in your life that can affect your cholesterol levels.

The first factor to mention is your genetic profile. It is too late to sue your parents. (No matter how unfair you think they were, and boy, were they ever unfair! Just look at how screwed up you are, and it's obvious that it's not your fault, so it must be the work of those dastardly parents of yours.) But in certain families, there are definite genetic defects in how cholesterol is eliminated from the bloodstream, defects that you may have inherited along with the family jewels. These defects lead to a much higher propensity to accumulate cholesterol deposits in arteries, and consequently there is a much higher risk of CHD in these families.

Your family history of cardiovascular problems is very important. If Uncle Sol died of a heart attack at forty-five, and your father had a heart attack at fifty-three, and another uncle on your father's side had a stroke, your family may very well carry a gene that results in high blood cholesterol. You should definitely have your complete cholesterol profile measured, and do it soon, because if you are at risk, the sooner you start to modify your lifestyle, the better the long-term results. You cannot change your genetic makeup. But you can try to change the effect that it has on your life expectancy.

At younger ages, men have more problems with cholesterol than women. The protective effect of female hormones disappears after menopause, however, when women tend to develop higher cholesterol counts. But at all younger ages, all other factors being the same, men develop more CHD than women, and this phenomenon is directly related to the higher cholesterol levels in men. Sex-change operations are not the way to handle this problem, by the way.

Smoking is probably the most easily manipulated risk factor for CHD. Smoking does the exact opposite of what you would like to happen to your blood lipids. If you smoke, your HDL level goes down and your LDL level goes up. Whatever risk of CHD you have from a high cholesterol level, you multiply that risk by two to four times if you smoke. Want a light?

We know that exercise increases HDL, but the amount of increase is not much. It certainly is not enough of an increase to explain the lower number of heart attacks in fit people. Exercise clearly confers other cardiac benefits.

A regular intake of small amounts of alcohol raises HDL (see chapter 1), but heavy drinkers have higher rates of other cardiac and vascular problems than nondrinkers.

There is no doubt that diet contributes somewhat to a high cholesterol level. But the significance of this contribution has gone through a reevaluation in the last few years. Much of our current thinking about the effects of cholesterol from the diet comes from studying various populations and charting mortality trends (what kills people and when) in those people. These trends periodically force us to reassess our beliefs. That is why we have changed our opinion about how harmful some types of shellfish are, for example. There was a time when shellfish, which are rich in cholesterol, were not permitted on low-cholesterol diets. But now shellfish that are bivalves, like oysters, clams, and scallops, are allowed in unlimited amounts on cholesterol-restricted diets because we have learned by studying people who eat a lot of this type of shellfish that they don't have high rates of CHD.

Olive oil has also gone through a reassessment. Olive oil is a mono-unsaturated fat, which means that it is a partially saturated fat. Research shows that populations that cook with lots of olive oil do not have a higher rate of heart disease. So, Greek and Italian food fans, olive oil is now allowed, even encouraged, on low-cholesterol diets, which is good news for anyone traveling to those countries because olive oil is simply unavoidable. (The only thing I ever learned to say in Greek was, pardon my Greek, *horeese lathee*, which is supposed to mean "without oil," although it may mean something entirely different, for all I know, because even when I ordered our food with this phrase, our dish invariably came to us swimming in olive oil.)

I wish that I could tell you that all the latest diet recommendations are God-given and not subject to change. But much like the disclaimers in those television commercials (only available in this book for a limited time, so act now), this advice could be withdrawn at any time.

In a book of this type, it is impossible to list all the foods that you should avoid and those foods that you should replace them with, so I won't even try. For a list of the general rules concerning saturated fats and cholesterol that you should follow, go back to the first chapter.

A word of warning to the converts. Do not become a cholesterol missionary. If your fiancée's family invites you over for a pre-nuptial dinner and serves you everything, including gefilte fish with a hollandaise sauce, eat it with relish. Forgive them, though. They are not trying to kill you prematurely (that comes after the wedding, when the wills are signed). That's just the way they eat.

But rather than rising at the dinner table and giving an impassioned Trotsky-like speech on the evils of such fat-laden meals, you should eat silently (you should always eat silently) and *enjoy it*. You should never worry about a single meal, or a day of meals larded with saturated fats, for that matter. The diet restrictions you should follow are general restrictions that apply over a lifetime, and there is surely room to cheat from time to time.

What are we to make of the latest fashion of consuming fish oils and oat bran (besides a fishy-smelling cereal)? Well, the easiest thing to say is the same thing you would say to a horse who wanted more oats than you thought necessary. Whoa! Fish is good for you. Eating fish does not lower cholesterol counts, but it does seem to protect against CHD. We know this from studies showing that some groups, like some Inuit, that eat lots of oily cold-water fish such as salmon, herring, and mackerel and also seal meat (not exactly a staple in the Hister household) have far less heart disease than people who eat no fish. This protective effect comes from the fish oils, the oily part of the fish. In addition, fish contains lots of good protein, doesn't have very many calories, and is easy to cook (overcook, actually).

Fish oils in capsules are another matter altogether. Remember that much of what we know about the benefits of fish comes from studies in which people ate the actual beast, Wanda the fishie, not little slimy globules of fish extracts. I write this as another warning to the some-is-good-more-is-better crowd. Do not go overboard on slippery fish oils until we know a whole lot more about them.

In the last few years, we have heard a good deal about oat bran (and recently, barley bran and rice bran). Oat bran can lower cholesterol levels, if you eat enough of it. But the latest studies seem to show that many nonfatty foods, not just oat bran, can have the same effect, so long as that food replaces fats in your diet.

It hurts me to say this, but if your cholesterol is high, you should probably watch your coffee intake because in some people caffeine may raise cholesterol. Surprisingly, however, even decaffeinated coffee, which is an aberration that all the purists seem to prefer, may also increase cholesterol counts in some people. So there.

Some drugs raise cholesterol levels. For people between fifteen and fifty, drugs that are commonly used and that will alter cholesterol levels include some birth control pills, Accutane for acne, and beta blockers and diuretics for high blood pressure. It is doubtful that by themselves the usual doses of these medications could do you much harm. But if you have a high cholesterol level to begin with, or if you have a family history of significant cardiac disease, you should consider the effect of these medications on your cholesterol level, and if there are alternative approaches to your problem, you may be wiser to select one of those.

TREATMENT

How should you treat a high cholesterol level? This is a Solomonic question. Scratch a doctor, and you win an opinion. If you get two doctors to match, then follow that opinion.

First you have to decide if your cholesterol level is legitimately high. Some people panic about a reading of 4.8; others are unworried by readings of 6.2 and higher. A lot depends on your other risk factors and your beliefs.

Once you've decided (either by yourself or in consultation with a physician) that your cholesterol level must be changed, the most important thing to do is change the factors in your life that you can control. So if you smoke, STOP. Today. Start an exercise program that gives you a good aerobic workout. Lose weight if you're overweight. Be conscious of your diet in a nonneurotic way. Eat more fish. Hey, life can still be fun. You're still allowed to chase members of the opposite sex as much as you want (as long as you don't catch them too often and as long as your wheezing and angina permit such exercise). And you're allowed to play the piano, if you have the energy.

If after doing all the above your cholesterol count is still in the high range, then you may require medical therapy. Medical therapy is just a euphemism for drugs, but we use the term because doctors like to talk in euphemisms.

The two most commonly used drugs are cholestyramine resin (Questran) and niacin. Both of these drugs have been around for many years, and all their side effects and potential complications are well known. For this reason, most doctors prefer them to the newer, less well known medications.

Niacin lowers LDL, raises HDL, lowers triglycerides, and makes platelets less "sticky," which means that they are less likely to produce a clot in a narrowed artery. Niacin must be taken in a dose of at least one and one half grams a day for this effect, and at that dose it tends to cause uncomfortable flushing for many people. This effect can be minimized by slowly increasing the intake over several days. Niacin can also cause liver damage, aggravate ulcers, and worsen both gout and diabetes.

Questran, which sounds like a video game, lowers LDL and increases HDL. But it causes gastrointestinal disturbances, most commonly some constipation, nausea, and farting. Nevertheless, many doctors are still surprised that patients don't like to take Questran. Think about it. You tell someone who has no symptoms that the new drug they're about to get may produce stomach cramps, constipation, nausea, and farting. A doctor who can successfully sell that to a patient is definitely in the wrong business. She should be flogging brushes door to door.

The newer drugs include gemfibrozil (Lopid) and lovastatin (Mevacor), both of which have a number of potential problems associated with their use. So anyone prescribed these medications should be carefully monitored.

Apparently, psyllium-containing laxatives like Metamucil can lower total cholesterol by up to 15 percent. Daily use of a laxative when you might not need one seems a rather dubious price to pay just to lower cholesterol. But because the side effects of psyllium are usually mild and pretty much restricted to the gastrointestinal tract, this may be a preferred treatment for some.

High Blood Pressure

The most frequently checked-off box on our routine health questionnaire is the one with the question asking if there is hypertension in the family. The usual answer is something like "Of course there's hypertension in my family! My mother is always screaming, my dad is always nervous, and you should see Uncle Max. He's the most hypertense of all!" Hypertension in medicine, however, does not refer to being "hyper" or tense. Hypertension in medicine means high blood pressure.

Hypertension is associated with a higher rate of strokes and heart attacks because the higher your blood pressure, the greater the wear and tear on both your heart and your arteries, particularly those arteries to the heart, brain, and kidneys. This wear and tear on the arterial walls allows the cholesterol plaques to build up much more easily, in turn allowing more clotting to occur in these injured vessels and leading to more heart attacks and strokes.

There are many possible causes of hypertension, but by far the most common is that old standby for most chronic problems: "Frankly, we just don't know." This "frankly, we just don't know" type of high blood pressure is called essential hypertension because as the old medical school joke goes, essentially, we know nothing about it. (The renaming police have now renamed this problem primary hypertension.) We know much more about hypertension now than when I went to school, but we are still very far from understanding why so many people without any obvious risk factors develop high blood pressure.

Blood pressure is measured with an instrument called a sphygmomanometer, which you are free to call a blood pressure machine. To measure blood pressure, a cuff is put around a limb, usually the arm, and the pressure in that cuff is pushed to a point that closes a large artery in the limb. The pressure in the cuff is released, and the person measuring your blood pressure then listens over the artery with a stethoscope for the sound of your heart emptying to fill your arteries with blood. This first sound is known as the systolic pressure. The sound eventually becomes muffled and disappears, corresponding to the relaxation of the heart between beats, and this is known as the diastolic pressure. Blood pressure is recorded as a fraction of systolic over diastolic — for example, 120/80 (and as usual, you don't have to worry about the units).

After all these years, we are still not certain about what is a normal blood pressure and what is not. We do know from following large groups of individuals that if as a young adult, your pressure (every older patient calls blood pressure "my pressure") is consistently above 160/105, you are more likely to die from a heart attack or stroke than if it were consistently below 140/90. It is the gray area in between that drives doctors nuts. The usually accepted healthy level that separates hypertensives from non is given as 140/90 for young and middle-aged adults (although some health authorities now argue that so long as all other cardiovascular risk factors are controlled, a blood pressure of 150/100 should be the upper level of normal).

I was taught, and have dutifully repeated lo these many years, that the diastolic pressure is much more important than the systolic pressure in determining your risk of developing complications from hypertension. This is not correct. It is now generally agreed that consistently elevated systolic blood pressure also increases your risk of cardiovascular complications.

So repeat after me. I want my blood pressure (I want my blood pressure) to be (to be) lower than (lower than) 140 systolic (140 systolic) and 90 diastolic (and 90 diastolic). Till death do us part. But I will not worry if it goes up from time to time.

Blood pressure is affected by many of the same factors that cause CHD and that raise cholesterol, and changing these factors can lower blood pressure. (There are also other ways, known only to wise old country doctors, to keep blood pressure down. One of my friends once did a summer relief for her dad, a small-town g.p. On her first day there, two elderly women came to see her to have their regular blood pressure checkup. My friend told them to go into the examination room, take off their coats, and roll up their sleeves. "But your father never makes us take off our coats," they both exclaimed. Which, I believe, is a very effective technique to maintain normal blood pressure levels.)

Being overweight increases blood pressure, and often in a person with mild hypertension, a simple weight loss (I know losing weight is never simple) of ten or fifteen pounds will bring the blood pressure down to a more normal level.

Stopping smoking will help blood pressure come down.

Heavy alcohol intake can increase blood pressure.

Exercise probably exerts some of its beneficial effect by keeping your weight within its normal parameters, but there is also evidence that even when your weight is normal, regular aerobic exercise improves blood pressure.

Stress contributes to high blood pressure. Stressful situations, such as visiting a physician's office, are enough to push the systolic pressure (and often the diastolic, as well) in many people into the abnormal range. This is supposed to be a temporary aberration and should be relieved when the stress is over. It is probable, however, that continuous stress can permanently elevate both systolic pressure and diastolic pressure in some individuals.

Excess salt intake is known to elevate blood pressure. Although there is some doubt that extra salt can increase normal blood pressure to high blood pressure, once you are hypertensive excess salt can worsen the condition.

There is emerging proof that in the occasional person (is an occasional person one who is only a person sometimes? a man for some seasons?) calcium intake can decrease minimally elevated blood pressure. Conversely, caffeine, a known stimulant, can increase blood pressure temporarily in those not used to taking their daily brew. It is doubtful that caffeine increases blood pressure in those who are used to taking it. (I have to believe this, or I would have to give up my cappuccino machine.)

You can't really tell if you have high blood pressure without having it checked. It's common for people to come to the office and say, "My pressure must be up, because I get flushed easily, and I'm getting headaches." In truth, these symptoms are unlikely to be due to hypertension, unless the hypertension is very severe (the exception is early-morning headaches, which are occasionally a sign of high blood pressure). The sad truth is that high blood pressure is a disease that is virtually asymptomatic in the great majority of people.

It has been customary for years to say that 20 percent of North Americans have high blood pressure. But in recent years, a great deal of doubt has been cast on this statistic. Various researchers have found that simply having your blood pressure measured by a doctor is enough to produce a high reading in a lot of people. It's not because doctors don't know how to measure blood pressure. Heaven (and the College of Physicians) forbid! It has more to do with how threatening doctors appear to be to many patients. When these people are remeasured in a more sympathetic setting — at home, for example, or even by a nurse, who is presumably less threatening to the patient than a doctor — the blood pressure reading tends to be significantly lower. This phenomenon has been tabbed "white coat hypertension." Some doctors estimate that up to 25 percent of people who have been labeled hypertensive only have the white coat version and that these people need to be treated by nothing more drastic than staying away from doctors (avoidance of Hister, so to speak).

What should you do if you have been labeled hypertensive? The first thing to do is question the reading. Ask to have it repeated. If it is still high, go home and try to determine how many risk factors you can easily change. If, for instance, you are the kind of person who inverts the saltshaker until it empties each time you eat, start by decreasing your salt intake. If you smoke, what can I say? ARRÊTEZ! STOP! MAINTENANT!

When you return in several weeks to get your blood pressure rechecked, do it under several preconditions. One of my eminent teachers always prefers to remeasure blood pressure late in the day, after a meal, with no caffeine intake, and on a day when there are no other pressing commitments. (I never have the time to go see him.) If your blood pressure is abnormal once more, ask to have it repeated yet again. You should still not accept treatment at this time. You should reassess your risk factors and change those that need changing. This time, think of losing those extra few pounds. Make a commitment to be more active. For treatment, do nothing more than book another appointment.

At this third visit, a lot should be decided. If your blood pressure is still high, it is time for both you and your doctor to make some adjustments. Your doctor should do the simple tests that are necessary to rule out correctable causes of high blood pressure, such as kidney diseases and thyroid problems. It is rarely necessary to go beyond simple blood and urine tests for adequate investigation of most hypertensives.

You can call this a "must" visit. You must get your weight into the desirable range, you must begin a regular aerobic exercise program, you must throw away the saltshaker for cooking and especially at the dinner table, you must stop smoking, you must moderate your alcohol intake, and you must learn to adjust your stress level (downwards, I hope).

The benefit of decreasing your stress level has become much more clear in the last few years. Dozens of studies show that for cases of minimally elevated blood pressure, relaxation techniques (yoga, meditation, biofeedback) are the best *cure*. If learned properly and adhered to, these relaxation mechanisms obviate the need for medical therapy, by which I mean drugs (euphemism, euphemism, all is euphemism).

Medical therapy is a hazardous road to start on, and you should never depart that way unless you have checked all the byways first. If you have had all the appropriate tests and have made all the necessary changes in your life and your blood pressure continues to hover in the high range, you must decide on one of several different medical therapies.

Until the late 1970s, the mainstay of medical therapy for hypertension was the use of diuretic medications. With diuretics, which are drugs that make you urinate more, you eliminate the excess volume in your blood vessels, and this reduced blood volume lowers the blood pressure. Wonderful, you say, except for the increased visits to the can. But not so fast. Diuretics also make you lose electrolytes, particularly potassium, so you may have to ingest extra potassium while on these drugs. Even if you eat potassium-rich foods such as bananas and strawberries, you can usually only get enough potassium by taking pills. Reducing your blood volume also means that the other chemicals in your blood get more concentrated. So for example, gout, a disease caused by a buildup of uric acid in the body, is more common in patients on diuretics because the uric acid concentrates more when you use these medications. Diuretics also raise your cholesterol and triglyceride levels. Most devastating, however, is that heart attacks don't seem to be decreased by the use of these products (although strokes are). Because of these limitations, diuretics have fallen somewhat from favor recently.

To replace diuretics there has been a broad shift to the use of a class of drugs known as beta blockers, particularly for the younger and middle-aged hypertensive. Beta blockers, the best known of which is propranalol (Inderal), lower the workload of the heart and consequently lower the blood pressure and the heart rate. But they also cause fatigue and sexual dysfunction (will no one rid me of these euphemisms?). Most of the beta blockers also lower your HDL, so if you have high cholesterol, these drugs should be used with caution. They may also (rarely) precipitate an asthmatic attack.

In the last few years, two entirely new classes of drugs, called ACE (angiotensin-converting enzyme) inhibitors and calcium-channel blockers, have emerged for the treatment of hypertension, and they are definitely poised to be major players in this huge market. ACE inhibitors interfere with a hormone mechanism based in the kidney that acts to control blood pressure. They have only been on the market for two years, but they are being promoted as virtually free of side effects (except for producing a dry cough in some users). As a result, many physicians are beginning to use them as first-line therapy, which seems a bit premature to me because we really do not know how safe they are in the long run. Calcium-channel blockers interfere with calcium channels in blood vessels, and this interference lowers blood pressure. They are also relatively new drugs, and each is somewhat different from the other — so use with care.

There are a host of other antihypertensives, but they are generally used only when one of the first-line drugs hasn't worked.

Stress

Although we really are not sure how or why, it is nevertheless clear that stress plays some role in the development of heart disease in some people.

Since the late sixties, it has been fashionable to divide the population into two large groups corresponding to different mental attitudes towards stress.

In the first group, there is me, and everybody like me. This is the type of person known as a Type A. Type A's love to talk about "me" and "I." After all, "I" is the most interesting topic in the world, *n'est-ce pas*? A Type A is the hard-driven, obsessive person who always seems in a rush because he or she frequently has taken on too much. We are described as hostile, impatient, tense, restless (and those are just the most complimentary phrases). We frequently interrupt people to finish their sentences for them. We sit tensely at the edge of the chair and drum our fingers on the desk. We drive too fast and curse at other drivers for being too slow (which they all are, of course). We constantly jump lines at supermarkets to get into the fastest line (which of course immediately becomes the slowest line as soon as we enter it). We eat quickly. We don't chew because it takes too long.

I am such a perfect Type A that some days in my office I seem to do away with any verbal input from the patients because it takes up too much time. One of my patients says that I generally diagnose her problem in the hall, before she is seated in my office, and frequently before she has finished her first sentence. Some Type A's keep their watch five minutes ahead of the actual time so that they will never be late for a meeting. God help the person who starts a meeting late at a Type A convention.

The mellow tones of the oboe will introduce our Type B's. They will stroll in, frequently late, figuring the meeting will start without them anyway, and it would be just as well. And besides, who needs this meeting in the first place? And we can always meet next week if it's so important. After all, we have to smell the flowers, both before and after the meeting.

Several years ago, Dr. Meyer Friedman from San Francisco proposed in a famous study that Type A's are much more likely to get heart attacks than Type B's. He further proposed that the best chance that Type A's had of surviving a "cardiac event" was to lose many of their driven personality traits and to slow down. In other words, Type A's should learn to smell the flowers rather than occupy themselves by timing floral growth rates.

For many years, this observation about the contribution of personality to CHD was taken as gospel and was repeated in all discussions of risk factors. But it has become increasingly obvious that most of us are not clearly in the one group or the other. We all have some traits of both types, although I can't for the life of me think of my own Type B traits. I hate anything to do with flowers, except receiving them.

Most authorities now agree that simply being a Type A is not that big a risk for early death from a heart attack. First, some people actually seem to thrive on stress. Second, many of the original differences noted in the earlier studies were due to the fact that Type A's tend to smoke more, exercise less, eat less healthfully, and be more overweight. Take away those controllable factors and Type A's do not have that much more coronary heart disease than Type B's.

In fact, some research shows that Type A's are likely to do better after a heart attack than Type B's, probably because a Type A will grit his teeth, swear, perhaps change his risk factor profile, and go out to prove that God was premature in His or Her expectations. A

Type B will more likely shrug her shoulders, mutter a "what the hell" because she can do much the same there as here (wherever she's going, there are likely to be flowers), and will go about business much as before.

It is also important to note that most cardiologists believe that stress can cause silent ischemia in some people with preexisting heart disease (and maybe even in a few people with no disease at all). What all this means is that it is not so important to figure out whether you are a Type A or a Type B. What matters more for most of us is to minimize the negative effects of stress in our lives.

Sex

No, sex doesn't cause premature heart disease (at least, every researcher hopes not), although sexual activity can be vigorous work that may occasionally result in a heart attack. What this heading really means is that men are more prone to coronary heart disease than women, at least until menopause, because estrogen plays a protective role in preventing this problem. But Father Nature evens the odds, so that postmenopause, in women who don't take estrogen replacement therapy, the risk of CHD soon becomes the same as for men of the same age. Women who do take hormonal replacement, however, continue to have a lower risk of CHD than men.

Diabetes

Uncontrolled diabetes leads to damage to the arteries of a number of organs, including the heart. This damage is accentuated by other risk factors, such as high blood pressure and high cholesterol. To prevent strokes and heart attacks, it is very important that diabetics keep their blood glucose levels under tight control and that they minimize other cardiovascular risk factors.

Smoking

What else is there left to say about smoking? Just remember that smoking increases the amount of CHD you will suffer through several different mechanisms. It is also important to remember that if you stop smoking, within a year and a half you begin to decrease your risks of cardiovascular disease so much that after several years of not smoking, you have only a slightly higher risk of a heart attack than a nonsmoker.

Alcohol

Although a regular intake of small amounts of alcohol is associated with a lower rate of heart attacks, larger amounts of alcohol increase the rates of several other cardiovascular problems, including strokes, high blood pressure, and damage to the heart muscle (see chapter 1).

Obesity

Being overweight is a distinct risk factor for the development of CHD. Part of the risk stems from the generally poorer diet of people who are overweight, part from the fact that overweight people have more diabetes and hypertension, and part from their more sedentary lifestyle.

What is interesting is that it seems to matter *where* you carry your weight (not in suitcases, but on your body). Someone who has a beer belly, or what doctors call abdominal obesity, has a higher risk for CHD than a person whose excess weight is on the hips or thighs. As Ricky Ricardo used to say, " 'Splain that if you can, Lucy."

Exercise

Exercise must be good for your heart because it tones you up, lowers your blood pressure, keeps your weight down, and raises your HDL (see above), right?

Probably.

Many studies show that people who exercise have lower rates of heart attacks and consequent death from heart attacks than people who are more sedentary. There are also studies comparing people who work in the same industry or profession, and the ones who do more active work have lower rates of CHD than the people who sit more.

But what confounds the experts who want to get absolutely objective proof of the benefits of exercise is that perhaps it is merely true that healthier people exercise more in the first place (or that they pick more active jobs). In other words, maybe the exercise doesn't protect these people all that much, because they really wouldn't be that prone to heart attacks in the first place. I doubt that this is true, but it has not been settled completely.

How much exercise is necessary? For cardiovascular fitness, the consensus among cardiac experts is that thirty minutes of aerobic exercise four to five times a week is sufficient (see chapter 1).

Medications

Recently a large American study showed that a group of doctors who took regular doses of ASA had significantly fewer heart attacks than a group that took no ASA, because the ASA prevented blood clotting and consequent blocking of the coronary arteries. So why not put every man, woman, and child on daily doses of ASA? In those words of my old professor that are so appropriate at so many junctures, "Not so fast, Dr. Hister."

There are a number of reasons to be cautious of that study. The study involved only male doctors; the study protocol eliminated many individuals from its research before the study began, such as those who had significant gastric (stomach) complaints because ASA can worsen ulcers; and the study also showed that precisely because ASA is an anticlotting drug, more of the ASA users died from a form of stroke known as a cerebral hemorrhage, caused by bleeding into the brain, than would normally be expected. With our current information, I believe that it's best to reserve the regular use of ASA for prevention of heart attacks to men over fifty, or those at very high risk of premature CHD.

So there you have it. If you want to protect yourself against coronary heart disease, eat properly, keep your weight down, don't smoke, exercise regularly, don't get diabetes (and if you do, make sure you treat it properly), keep your blood pressure down, be moderate in your use of alcohol, live a stress-free existence, and be a female. Some of these are obviously easier to do than others.

SYMPTOMS OF CARDIOVASCULAR PROBLEMS

Chest Pain

Aside from occasional cases of angina and heart attacks, chest pain in the fifteen-to-fifty-year-old patient is not often of cardiac origin. However, nearly all patients, especially those of the male persuasion, are convinced that every ache and pain in the chest area comes from the heart.

Chest pain in the adult under fifty usually occurs as a sharp pain localized in the front of the chest. This pain rarely worsens with effort, rarely wakes the patient at night (although it is not unusual to wake with it), rarely radiates to the arm or jaw or neck, and often worsens with anxiety or stress. We really don't know the source of this sharp discomfort, although it is commonly believed to be due to esophageal spasm or esophageal reflux (see chapter 8). No matter what the source, it is most important to stress that this type of chest pain is not due to cardiac disease.

Why are we so sure of this? Because the follow-up on this type of pain rarely ends with a cardiac catastrophe. This type of pain usually fades away if it is ignored, only to reappear when stress or anxiety builds up again.

What then are the types of chest pain that are associated with significant cardiac disease?

Angina is chest pain associated with effort and produced by disease in the coronary arteries. This type of pain is usually described as a heaviness or pressure or a tight kind of feeling in the center of the chest or on the left side. It can radiate to the jaw, back, neck, or left arm. But the cardinal symptom of cardiac angina is that the pain worsens with effort. The more you work, the more oxygen your heart needs. Angina is never a good sign. This pain indicates a severe problem that must be very carefully assessed and followed.

Now that I've described how angina should sound, it is likely that some people will develop this new symptom. Tonight. *C'est la vie médicale*.

The pain of a heart attack is usually described as a crushing or twisting pain or heaviness of sudden onset that generally starts in the center or left side of the chest and can radiate to all the same areas as angina. This pain is often associated with nausea, weakness, sweating, and a high level of apprehension. This is the classic picture. But as mentioned above, many cases of cardiac ischemia can be silent, and many heart attacks present with atypical pictures. For example, occasionally a heart attack can mimic a bad case of indigestion or just a sudden feeling of shortness of breath. In the high-risk individual, any pain in the chest should be carefully and quickly assessed.

As a last reminder, if you ever develop any chest pain that unduly concerns you, you should proceed to an emergency department as soon as possible.

Palpitations

Extra heartbeats are common in young and middle-aged adults. These beats are thought to occur more in stressful circumstances, and especially in people who drink a great deal of coffee (although evidence for this, as with most negative "facts" about coffee drinking, is weak). Most palpitations occur for no apparent reason.

Most people with extra beats develop a "funny" feeling in the chest or throat. The heart is something we generally ignore, but as soon as it beats abnormally, we become quite apprehensive about it, often expecting some morbid event to follow.

Most of these abnormal patterns and beats are benign. They should be checked by a physician who will make sure that there is no pathology to account for them, and then, unless they are very frequent or causing you any real problems, they can be safely ignored. (This is hard to do.)

Rapid Heart Rate

The sensation that the heart is beating too rapidly is a common symptom. But rarely in people under fifty does the heart beat fast enough (in the range of 150 beats per minute) to require medication to slow it.

If you suffer from a rapid heart rate, or tachycardia, time your heart rate. If it is below 140 beats a minute and if the rhythm is regular, which means that you are not skipping beats, relax, if you can. Relaxation really is the best therapy. Analyze what you could be doing to promote this symptom, such as drinking too much coffee or taking medications that might speed up your heart rate. If you can, reduce these factors and see what happens.

If the heart rate is above 150 per minute, it is likely to be due to a problem called paroxysmal atrial tachycardia (PAT), which means (surprise) rapid heart rate. This problem can occasionally be due to a metabolic problem such as hyperthyroidism, but it is often written off to stress. It is a benign condition that needs to be treated mainly because it makes the patient unduly anxious. Like most chronic conditions, PAT tends to recur, often suddenly and for no apparent reason.

Murmurs

A murmur is an extra heart sound that we hear when we listen to the heart. Believe it or not, heart sounds really do sound like *lup/dup*. A murmur can sound like *lup/shh/dup*. Is that clear?

Most murmurs are completely benign and just indicate incomplete closure of the valves in the heart. There are no known long-term harmful effects from having an innocent murmur.

Some murmurs, however, are due to heart pathology (guilty murmurs, so to speak). They result either from congenital defects, like holes between the chambers of the heart, or from a disease that developed on the leaflets of the valves, such as damaged valves from rheumatic fever. These pathological murmurs generally sound different from the innocent ones, but when we are not sure, an excellent noninvasive technique that can separate the two classes of murmurs is an echocardiogram, or an ultrasound examination of the heart valves.

Pathological murmurs must be followed carefully because they can worsen, sometimes suddenly, and heart surgery may then be required. If you have a pathological murmur, you should discuss with your physician whether or not you have to take prophylactic antibiotics at the time of certain procedures, especially dental work. The reason for this is that during dental work, bacteria spread through your body from your mouth. If there is a damaged heart valve, particularly one due to previous rheumatic fever, there is a tendency for these bacteria to attack that previously damaged valve, causing even more valvular disease. This type of bacterial spread can be eliminated by taking antibiotics just before the procedure and for several hours afterwards.

Mitral Valve Prolapse

This condition must be mentioned only because some people become alarmed when it is diagnosed in them. As with Lyme disease, the fear surrounding the problem is often worse than the problem itself.

Mitral valve prolapse (MVP) is a condition in which the mitral valve in the heart doesn't close properly. Do people with MVP actually have a disease? Very unlikely. MVP (which does not stand for Most Valuable Patient) should really be considered a variant of normal because as much as 15 percent of the population has it, and very few if any people have symptoms that can be proven to be due to this condition, although some people with this syndrome seem to suffer bouts of unexplained atypical chest pain, fainting, fatigue, palpitations, and shortness of breath — in short, all those symptoms that are also potentially related to stress.

CHAPTER 8

The Gastrointestinal System

In which the good doctor takes a look into the bowel, fore and aft, from a goodly distance, of course

No part of the body intrigues us more than the system known as the gastrointestinal (GI) tract — to wit, our stomachs and our bowels (although obviously a strong case can be made for the genitals). It is an inescapable fact of medical life that many people are both fascinated and troubled by their digestive systems to a far greater extent than any other body system.

As a Jewish male, I have a special interest in this part of the anatomy. I grew up in an environment pregnant with almost daily complaints directed at the "moogen." The "moogen" was a generic term in our house. Moogen complaints encompassed everything from eating to defecating and all parts and functions in between. Burping, gas, and bowel movements were all important indicators of health and behavior. In many immigrant Jewish families, a child merely had to hint at a stomachache and he was kept home from school and fussed over until his moogen magically self-corrected, a successful therapy that usually coincided with a missed exam. However, if self-healing wasn't quickly successful, the moogen was then treated with some barely palatable bitter mixture, which had never been, I am certain, approved by Health and Welfare Canada (although it may have been approved by H & W Poland). Moogen difficulties rarely needed more than one treatment. The need for a second treatment usually indicated a real medical problem.

This fascination with digestion and bowel movements is certainly not confined to one group or social class, or to a specific age. I interned in an area of Montreal that had a large North African population. At least once a night, a man (it was always a male) of about thirty or thirty-five would be dragged into the emergency department, hanging lifelessly on the shoulders of three or more family members. The women in the party would invariably wail, in various keys but in unison, that this man was suffering from a *crise de foie*, which literally translates as "a liver crisis." The literal translation, however, misses the flavor of the term. A *crise de foie* is a euphemism for any vague, ill-defined symptom, preferably associated with the GI tract — the French-African equivalent of a moogen disturbance. Two hours in emergency, three or four blood tests, sympathy from the family, a prescription for a placebo, and the patient had a remarkable recovery. He was, however, soon replaced by a compatriot with a similar problem.

In case any white Anglo-Saxons reading this think that these symptoms are confined to other ethnic groups, think back to the early years of television for a moment. Besides Lucy and Lassie and the Beaver, you may also recall all those ads for pills that were promoted to cure "irregularity." As a kid, I had no idea what irregularity was, but it was obvious to me from the people appearing in those ads (they were all solidly middle-class and overwhelmingly female) and their invariably sour expressions, that irregularity was the cause of much of the Western world's ills. I once asked my mother what irregularity was. She told me that I would eventually find out. My mother was always right. I did.

We have an incredible assortment of terms to refer to the bowel and how it works. Yet most of us don't seem to be able to use many of these words comfortably. Even doctors, who must ask about these problems dozens of times a day, are often left searching for euphemisms when questioning patients about defecation and other aspects of digestion.

This embarrassment with most terms intestinal starts early in our medical careers. I can never recall hearing the completely adequate word "fart" in medical school. It was always "gas" or "pass wind" or, worse still, "flatus." Can you think of any North American adult, apart from a doctor, who uses the word "flatus"? Can you picture any kid asking another, when that special scent fills the air between them, if his friend was flatulent? ("You flatulated!" "No I didn't. It was you." "Was not." And thus is perpetuated probably the world's oldest argument.) I remember asking one of the first patients I ever saw in the emergency department if he had flatus. He looked at me like I was the one who needed help. I looked away, swallowed hard, and asked if he was farting more than usual. "What's usual?" he asked. I suddenly became more interested in his chest than in his bowels.

Farts are not the only term we have trouble with. I have heard a perfectly sane physician ask a seventy-year-old woman if her tummy hurt. She hadn't had a tummy for sixty-odd years, we were told in no uncertain terms. Likewise, I once heard a medical resident ask an elderly gent if he had had a poo yet that day. That resident eventually became a radiologist.

In this book, a fart is what it has always been — a fart. A bowel movement is not a poo, at least not until I write a book on pediatrics.

HOW THE SYSTEM WORKS

To a large extent, the GI tract works on reflexes. In a perfect world, where we could eat when we wanted and defecate when we needed to, we would have a bowel movement after every meal. That is because eating stimulates a series of reflex contractions in the entire bowel system, and these contractions, left on their own, should end in a bowel movement. But as our living situations have evolved, we no longer are permitted to squat in the woods after berry picking. When is the last time you picked berries anyway? Or squatted any-where, for that matter? Can you imagine a school system functioning on the basis that each child would eat when he or she wanted and would go to the bathroom immediately afterwards? I can't recall any teacher of mine tolerating more than one visit a day to the boys' room, and then only after repeated requests, each more urgent than the preceding one.

So to function in modern society, we learn to suppress our urge to eat, just as we learn to suppress our defecation reflex. To this suppres-sion of normal reflexes we must add the other dietary adjustments we tend to make in our modern, "advanced" society. We eat too many rich and refined foods, too much saturated fat, too few vegetables, too little fiber. We eat on the run, wash the meal down with coffee or cola or alcohol, and jump right back into a harried existence of running a business or a household. We rarely exercise. We are always waiting impatiently in the McFast Lane. These adaptations to our advanced culture lead to many of the problems we experience with our GI tracts, problems that are rare in less advanced countries. Appendicitis, duodenal ulcers, reflux esophagitis, chronic constipation, and some types of bowel tumors (in short, practically the entire contents of this chapter) are much less common in other parts of the world. (In fact, so many of these problems are so uncommon in the third world that if a Canadian mother actually followed through on her threat and sent all her child's uneaten food to a child in Asia, the latter would be well advised to send the meal right back.)

The GI tract is a continuous tubular system that starts in the mouth and ends at the anus. This system is merely a long tunnel with light at the beginning and light at the end. In between, as every kid knows, the sun don't shine. The mouth connects to a long channel called the esophagus. The esophagus is a muscular, straight tube that is separated from the stomach by a tight band of muscle, called a sphincter.

The esophagus empties into the stomach, a J-shaped bag that collects what we eat and initiates the process of digestion through the action of stomach acid and digestive enzymes. The resultant mush enters a narrower channel called the small intestine.

The small intestine has three distinct parts, called the duodenum (pronounced duo-DEE-num), the jejunum (ji-JOO-num), and the ileum (ILL-ee-um). (I've always had nightmares that someday my sons would form a punk rock group called the Small Intestine and the members would be named after the various parts.) It is in this long, intricate system that most of the digestion and absorption of necessary nutrients occurs.

It is also into the small intestine that the gallbladder empties that awful-sounding stuff called bile, and the pancreas donates its enzymes. Both the gallbladder and the pancreas are necessary for proper digestion and absorption (although clearly the gallbladder is not essential, because it is often surgically removed).

The small intestine empties into the large intestine, or colon. The colon has four distinct parts, which (happily) are not given Greek names. They are the ascending colon, the transverse colon, the descending colon, and the sigmoid colon (likewise good names for punk rockers). These names merely describe how the colon ascends

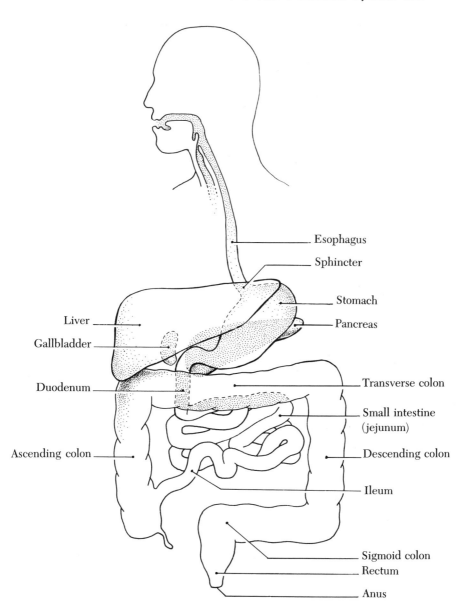

THE GASTROINTESTINAL SYSTEM

from the right side and then bends to traverse the body and descends on the left side to end in a sigmoid shape. Like the small intestine, the colon is also important in the absorption of nutrients.

The colon ends in the rectum, which is a type of chamber, or receiving room, that ends in the anus. The rectum is important for storing stool before it is excreted to the outside world.

THE ESOPHAGUS AND STOMACH

Take a second to consider your esophagus. I doubt if you have consciously ever done this in the past (so you may need more than one second). But you really ought to think of your esophagus every now and then because as you will discover when you read on, this long tube is probably the source of some chronic symptoms you may have had for years, most of which you have probably not attributed to this organ.

Hiccups

Anything (stress, some foods) that irritates the diaphragm will result in hiccups. There are dozens of home remedies for this problem. A particularly popular potion is a concentrated solution of glucose, which usually means pouring as much sugar into a cup of water as you can stand and then swallowing it. (If I forced my kids to drink this unpalatable concoction, they would just consider it an ideal desert.) Most hiccups pass without requiring any treatment, but occasionally heavy sedating medication is required for the intractable kind.

Burping

Most people just call occasional bouts of burping "gas" and assume that it was caused by something they ate and that the symptom will quickly pass. It invariably does (except if you happen to be a twelve-year-old who can burp on command at 70 decibels and even louder when guests are over for dinner).

Burping commonly accompanies many digestive conditions, including gallbladder problems, reflux, and ulcers. It can also be due to aerophagia, the swallowing of excessive air caused by anxiety, which is generally handled by some type of behavior therapy.

Difficulty Swallowing

The most common cause of a temporary pain with swallowing is a scratch to the esophagus from swallowing something sharp, such as a fish bone. This discomfort always passes within several days. When pain with swallowing continues, especially if it is accompanied by the sensation of food getting stuck in the throat, the symptom must be investigated for conditions such as diverticula, outpouchings from the esophagus, or cancer of the esophagus, which, as usual, is more common in smokers.

Heartburn (The Nonmusical Trio of Esophagitis, Gastritis, and Ulcers)

The most common type of "heartburn" is a burning kind of pain in the center of the chest behind the breastbone that occurs about fifteen to thirty minutes after swallowing any type of food and is definitely worsened by specific foods and beverages. These usually include raw onions, alcohol, caffeine, pickled foods, citrus fruits, fatty foods, and spicy foods (yes, amigos, you may be out of luck if you live for Mexican fare). The pain is often worsened by lying down after eating and is frequently exacerbated at night. It can radiate to the neck and left arm, and it can be accompanied by the regurgitation of an acidy mixture into the mouth.

This kind of heartburn is usually due to the return of acid from the stomach into the esophagus, where it irritates the esophageal cells, a phenomenon called reflux. (This sounds like the plot of a Canadian-made B thriller: *The Return of Stomach Acid, Part Two.*) If the end of the esophagus becomes inflamed from repeated reflux, the condition is known as reflux esophagitis.

Reflux esophagitis is extremely common. According to some estimates, up to 30 percent of adults suffer from reflux at least once a month and up to 7 percent suffer from this problem every day. Reflux esophagitis can also mimic other medical conditions. Thus, it can lead to a common form of chest pain that is often incorrectly treated as a cardiac problem. It may also produce asthma symptoms at night, when the patient is prone, probably because the acid irritates the airways or bronchi. This type of asthma often does not disappear until the reflux is treated.

Another type of abdominal discomfort, also often called heartburn, generally occurs one or two hours after a meal as a sharp or burning pain below the breastbone, at the top of the abdomen. This type of pain can radiate to either the right or the left side and to the back. It is generally not significantly worsened by lying down, but it too is often present at night and can be severe enough to wake the patient. This pain is also worsened by certain types of food and by stress. But curiously, filling the belly with the right kind of meal frequently relieves this pain. Regurgitation of acid is not a feature of this second form of burning, which is usually caused by an ulcer, in either the stomach or the duodenum.

Just to confuse the picture, many patients have a combination of the two types of pain, making it frequently difficult to distinguish between the two conditions purely according to the symptoms.

We have not yet indentified all the factors that cause these conditions, although smoking, stress, and diet can all be important factors for some people. Genes seem to play an important role in that some people seem programmed to develop ulcers, whereas others, no matter how badly they abuse themselves, rarely do. This latter situation is sometimes referred to as the Winston Churchill Syndrome. This is the kind of person all of us would (secretly) like to be — the one who smokes as much as she wants, drinks as much liquor as she wants, is grossly overweight, and dies in grand old age from a fall in the bathtub (and of course saves the Western world from a horde of transgressors). Old Winston did all the wrong things, yet history doesn't record that he had much abdominal discomfort.

Recently it has been found that some types of gastritis, an irritation of the lining of the stomach that may be a precursor to ulcers and that often has the same symptoms as esophagitis, are linked to the presence of a specific bacteria in the gastric tract. Most people with gastritis, as well as many with ulcers, have significantly more of this bacteria (*Campylobacter pylori*) in their stomachs than do normal people, which may mean that these types of gastritis and ulcers are transmittable from one person to another. (Think of that the next time you are sitting at a dinner with an obviously ulcer-prone business executive and he happens to want to taste your dish.)

Esophagitis, gastritis, and ulcers are notoriously recurrent. No matter how diligent you are in treatment, the symptoms are likely to return one day.

If you believe that your symptoms are due to reflux esophagitis, here's what you should do. Most important, avoid the substances that worsen the symptoms (see above). In addition, any food (such as chocolate) that decreases the tone of the muscles at the lower end of the esophagus worsens the symptoms of acid reflux because decreased muscle tone allows excess acid into the esophagus. Large meals, especially fatty ones, also increase stomach pressure and reflux. So don't be like me but try to eat moderate amounts at each sitting, preferably of nonfatty foods. (Something Hister men are genetically incapable of doing. There are parents who dread the thought of my younger son's staying at their home for supper. He must invariably be told when to leave the table after a meal, when presumably enough time should have elapsed for him to be full, even though he is rarely sated.)

Don't lie down for three to six hours after meals. Let gravity keep the gastric contents in the stomach where they should remain. (Isaac Newton would surely have discovered gravity earlier if he had had esophagitis.) If the symptoms are worse at night, raise the head of the bed three to six inches with blocks (or phone books) under the bedposts. Sleeping with more pillows generally doesn't work.

Be careful about what medications you are taking, especially ASA and the ASA-like medications known as nonsteroidal anti-inflamma-tories (NSAIDs), which produce gastric symptoms in practically everyone who uses them long enough. The higher the dose, the longer the NSAIDs are used, and the more alcohol you consume, the more severe the gastric problems will be. The range of complications associated with NSAIDs varies from mild gastric irritation to life-threatening ruptured ulcers. If you have to take NSAIDs, don't take more than the prescribed dose, check with your doctor periodically to discuss your use of these pills, and most important, always inform her or him of any new or persistent gastric symptoms you may have. Remember too that some OTC medications, like some cold remedies, also contain ASA.

If you continue to have symptoms despite these precautions, then you should try some type of medication. The most effective OTC medication is usually one that combines an antacid with a substance that prevents acid from coming in contact with esophageal cells. Thus, alginic acid compound (Gaviscon), which produces a foamy barrier between the stomach and the esophagus, is usually more effective for reflux than a simple antacid.

If you prefer to self-medicate with antacids, remember that they must be taken in larger amounts than most people think. Even though one tablet of Maalox, for example, may ease the symptoms, this dose is insufficient to help the irritation heal. You should really take antacids in a dose sufficient to produce diarrhea as a side effect. (Now isn't that something to look forward to?) Antacids should be taken after meals and at bedtime.

Complications of esophagitis, although rare, can be severe. One such complication is esophageal stricture, which is a hardened tightening of the lower end of the esophagus. A stricture can result in pain with swallowing or in a sensation that food keeps sticking in the throat. It is a very difficult problem to treat, often requiring surgical procedures that only work for a while and need to be repeated frequently. Another possible complication of long-term chronic esophagitis is cancer of the esophagus.

For gastritis and ulcers, the therapeutic approach is much the same. Always avoid the foods and medications that worsen the symptoms. If you are going to take an OTC medication for these conditions, you should start with an antacid rather than alginic acid. Again, take it in a dose sufficient to cure the problem.

If you cannot control the symptoms of any of these conditions, or if you have any questions about the diagnosis, you should consult a physician. When you visit the doctor, you are likely to be given a prescription for some type of medication to help the irritation heal.

The two most commonly prescribed drugs for these problems are cimetidine (Tagamet) and ranitidine (Zantac), both of which suppress the production of gastric acid. Cimetidine is known for its interactions with other medications, especially tranquilizers and drugs used for high blood pressure.

Although on rare occasions the symptoms of gastritis can be due to a gastric malignancy, most doctors still believe that because such a malignancy is so rare for people under the age of fifty, it is generally worth trying a trial of therapy before instituting any investigations. (A trial of therapy does not mean that it's a trial to take the therapy but is rather an initial attempt to alleviate the symptoms with some kind of therapy before doing tests.) Other doctors, however, believe that every patient with these complaints should be investigated immediately, either with a barium X ray or with a gastroscopy (sticking a tube down the gullet to have a look around). The problem with the latter approach is that these investigations are not innocuous procedures. The former involves radiation, and the latter requires sedation and is associated with possible complications.

To prevent the symptoms of esophagitis, gastritis, and ulcers from recurring, the most important thing is to be good little boys and girls (but not both at the same time). There is always a temptation to cheat when you're on a diet or a health regime, just to see if the symptoms come back. You don't need to cheat to find the answer. That's why you're reading this book. The symptoms will recur. And the more you cheat, the more often they recur.

The final word in this section will be given to the common entity known as a hiatus hernia. To understand what a hiatus hernia is, you must first review a bit of anatomy. The diaphragm is the muscle that separates the thoracic cavity, which contains the heart and lungs, from the abdomen, which contains the stomach and bowels. Because the esophagus travels through the diaphragm to enter the stomach, there is a hole in the diaphragm to permit the passage of the esophagus. When this hole widens, the top part of the stomach can, and frequently does, slide into the thoracic cavity. This condition is called a hiatus hernia. Symptoms, such as burning and abdominal discomfort, that accompany a hiatus hernia are due to the reflux that accompanies the hernia. Treatment therefore is much the same as for reflux esophagitis. Some people also tell you that tight belts make their symptoms worse. So buy a looser belt, of course.

Vomiting

Vomiting is a symptom that should always be carefully monitored (though from a distance). Many people, especially kids, vomit once or twice for no apparent reason. We usually write this off to "something you ate." The patient generally doesn't act too sick and bounces back relatively quickly (although if too quickly, he or she may vomit again).

Of much greater concern is recurrent vomiting, especially if it's accompanied by fever, and most especially if the patient looks ill. This type of vomiting should be evaluated by a physician. It can be due to something as simple as an intestinal viral infection, or it can be a sign of something as severe as meningitis. Don't put the burden on yourself for the proper diagnosis. Put the burden on that learned person with the degree who gets paid to figure these things out. See your doctor.

Of special importance is a type of vomiting called projectile vomiting. Projectile vomiting is just what you would expect. The vomit hurtles out of the patient across a distance. Projectile vomiting in an adult can be a sign of a serious problem, such as a brain tumor. (Of course American culture being what it is, if you aren't really sick, and yet you can vomit a great distance, you may earn a spot on "Geraldo," especially if you are a member of the Nazi party or have other weird habits.)

Food poisoning is a common cause of vomiting. Food poisoning is caused by the ingestion of one of several different organisms, most often either *Staphylococcus, Campylobacter* or *Salmonella* bacteria. The most likely source of these bacteria is food that was either improperly prepared or improperly stored. The most common food sources are turkey, eggs, chicken, salad dressings, and luncheon meats (your perfect picnic basket, in other words).

In the worst cases, food poisoning can result in horrible retching and vomiting every few minutes for several hours, and the patient must be hospitalized. But most often food poisoning acts like a relatively innocuous infection, with only some mild cramps and diarrhea.

There is no good drug therapy for most food poisoning, because most bacteria develop resistance to any antibiotics that we use. If you're vomiting, do not force yourself to eat or drink. Food or liquid intake often just provokes more vomiting. Except in children or debilitated persons, you generally do not need to be concerned about fluid loss. Make yourself a nice comfortable resting spot near the toilet and wait. (And close the door because you really don't want to explain to the visitors who always need to use the can as soon as it's occupied exactly why you are lying there. "An old family custom" will usually get rid of them nicely, and it's unlikely they will ask to stay for dinner.) If you're gradually getting more ill, if you develop a fever or significant abdominal pain, if the vomiting is not abating after twelve hours, or if you are just worried about sitting by the can for several hours, it is wise to consult a physician.

The best thing to do about food poisoning is not to get it in the first place. Nearly all commercially raised farm animals seem to be infected with *Salmonella* these days, so here are some simple rules to remember:

1. Don't eat eggs that have been cracked before you use them.
2. Don't prestuff a turkey (or any other bird) at feast time.
3. Don't thaw foods on the kitchen counter, especially in the summer.
4. Cook all foods, especially meat, thoroughly. A raw steak may taste better to you than a well-done one, but remember that it may also be home to a bunch of little critters who also prefer their steak raw. (Which is as good a time as any to ask how in the world anyone can eat a steak tartare.)
5. Don't allow anyone, but especially the kids, to eat those hamburgers that you cooked four hours ago and that have lain about near the barbecue since then.
6. Don't eat anything that looks "off."
7. On picnics, either refrigerate the food until serving or else eat only foods that do not easily spoil. If you're like my son, you'll rarely have trouble at a picnic. He usually eats his share as soon

as we get to where we're going and then asks every fifteen minutes, "When are we going to eat?"

8. With barbecues, be especially careful to cook the meats well. The Canadian male, that well-known burner of barbecued meats, often manages to torch the outside of a patty, leaving the inside slimy and undercooked — a perfect nest for bacteria.

9. Be watchful of your kids. They are more susceptible to certain infections (such as those caused by the bacteria E. coli, which can cause a severe complication known as hemolytic-uremic syndrome). Every parent has found out at some time or another that to a kid a cold hot dog is a gourmet item and often the hit of the afternoon (especially when served with soggy chips and some sickly, syrupy sweet beverage of vague parentage).

THE BOWELS (OR AS MY FATHER USED TO SAY, THE BOWLS)

The bowels are the source of many curiously interesting bodily functions that in North America at least often threaten the well-being of the owner. But much like a favorite car or an indispensable dishwasher, the bowels respond well to tender loving care. Be kind to your intestines and they will be kind to you, and much of the following information will then only be useful to you when you play doctor to your friends.

Abdominal Pain

Every human being has experienced a bout or two of crampy abdominal pain at one time or another. Usually we attribute this pain to gas cramps or constipation, and most of the time we are correct. We know that these guesses must be right because the pain is generally transient, mild, and rarely recurrent, so it is unlikely to be due to anything serious (the foregoing explanation is an excerpt from that school of medical theory known as the rationalization school, of which we are all, dean and intern alike, graduates).

But many people suffer from chronic abdominal pain. In fact, some researchers estimate that up to one third of North Americans are plagued by this condition. And although we can frequently guess at the probable cause of the pain, effective treatment is often elusive.

Before describing the more common conditions associated with chronic abdominal pain, a word about the pelvis (that should wake everyone up). In women, much more than men, it is quite important to differentiate pelvic pain caused by reproductive or urinary problems from other types of abdominal pain.

IRRITABLE BOWEL SYNDROME (IBS)

Irritable bowel syndrome, or spastic bowel, is the single most common cause of recurrent abdominal pain in North America. The name tells you most of the story — the bowel is easily irritated and subsequently goes into spasm, which in turn causes altered bowel movements and cramps, usually attributed to gas. The gas, however, is really a product of this condition rather than the cause.

The bowels are mainly a smooth muscle tunnel. Much like parts in a movable ramp (mixed metaphors, I know, but forgive me), the bowels must work in unison, pushing the load from the receiving end at the duodenum to the expelling end at the anus. This is done by a process called peristalsis. But if parts of the bowel decide not to cooperate, if parts of the bowel decide to start their own peristaltic waves, or if the system is overly sensitive to normal irritants, then the entire system can be thrown into spasm. As with the post office, when the unions work, you get your mail regularly, if late. When one of the unions strikes, there goes the mail.

The symptoms include a crampy, intermittent type of abdominal discomfort, not necessarily related to eating time, and farting (these people better have friends who are *good* friends). Because the bowel muscle movements can be so variable, sometimes quick and unified, sometimes slow and disorderly, another hallmark of this problem is intermittent diarrhea and constipation.

The causes of this condition include the usual suspects. Diet and stress are obvious culprits. IBS rarely occurs in cultures where bowel transit time (not the time it takes a #92 bus to move through your intestines, but the time it takes food to pass from your mouth to your anus) is not prolonged. Bowel transit time is affected by the amount of refined foods that we consume. Thus, a high-roughage diet (one that has lots of fiber in it, which decreases bowel transit time) is of some benefit to some people with IBS, although not all. An interesting finding in all studies of IBS patients is that they respond well to placebo. Anything, including daily prayer, should work so long as the patient believes in the treatment.

A recent report showed that peppermint oil could be effective for this condition. Since it has no common side effects, the oil is probably worth a try. (I believe you drink it, not wear it.)

But mostly, remember Mama, aproned, spatula in the right hand, severe look on her face, standing over you as you eat, cajoling. Take your time at meals. Don't eat so fast. What's the rush? Where's the fire? Chew well. Eat your veggies. Eat your whole grains. Don't worry so much. And write your mother more often. You know how she worries.

Do not start to rely on medications, most of which are available only by prescription, to help ease the symptoms of IBS. Some drugs will no doubt work somewhat, but if the problem does not go away, you will eventually become dependent on the medications and you will need stronger and stronger doses as time goes by.

BOWEL CANCER

One question comes up continuously in the office. "How can you be sure, Art, that my chronic abdominal pain is a benign condition and not the result of a bowel tumor, especially a malignant one?" The short answer is that you can never be 100 percent certain. But there are clues that can help in deciding which person with abdominal pain needs investigation for a tumor and which one doesn't.

First, bowel cancers increase in incidence directly with age. Malignancies are much more common at age sixty-five than at age forty, when they are still rare entities. For those between the ages of fifteen and fifty with prolonged abdominal discomfort, tumors are much less common than IBS.

Second, IBS has generally been present for a long time before the patient visits the office and is rarely described as worsening in severity. In contrast, if a bowel tumor produces pain, that pain should gradually increase as the tumor grows.

Changes in bowel movements can herald the development of a bowel malignancy. Pay special attention to bowel movements that have been gradually narrowing or bowel movements that are bloody or black (not dark brown, but black), what we call tarry. When these symptoms appear for the first time, they should always be discussed with a doctor.

However, the bottom line (a phrase that along with "networking" and "impacting" should be banned from the language, after this last punny use, of course) is that even if you have had spastic bowel complaints for a long time, if the pattern of your pain or your bowel movements has changed, you should see a doctor.

Certain people are at particularly high risk for bowel tumors and require close monitoring. These include people with a family history of bowel cancers, those with previous polyps (small benign growths) in the colon, people of Chinese ancestry, anyone with a long-standing history of ulcerative colitis, and those with other cancers, especially breast cancer.

But what about those people at average risk? Some doctors argue that everyone over the age of forty should have a yearly sigmoidoscopy (a peek into the bowel with a formidable-looking tube, a procedure that a gastroenterologist friend of mine describes as one arsehole looking at another) and occult blood testing (a test for hidden blood in the stool). Given the average North American's reluctance to acknowledge that she has a bowel and an anus, it is unlikely that this approach will ever catch on on this continent.

More sensible is the suggestion that those at average risk should have regular occult blood testing (perhaps every two years) beginning at age forty or forty-five (this will no doubt add even more trauma to the difficulty of turning forty). Sigmoidoscopy and colonoscopy should be reserved for those who develop other symptoms, such as rectal bleeding, or who have positive occult blood test results.

What can you do to prevent bowel cancer? Some studies have found that people who do physically demanding work have a lower incidence of bowel cancer than those who are more sedentary. Exercise is good fer ya, even for the parts that don't see the sun.

There is also good evidence that a diet excessively rich in both fats and calories increases the risk of bowel tumors. The richer the diet, the higher the risk. Nitrites, present in many smoked foods and luncheon meats, also promote the formation of bowel tumors. That's the bad diet news.

The good news is that foods that are rich in beta carotene may protect against malignancies of the GI tract. These foods include carrots, cauliflower, and other yellow vegetables.

Recent reports have also shown that the incidence of bowel cancer may be lower in people who get a lot of sun and in those who take calcium supplements (even in those who don't bare their butts to the elements). The sun is probably helpful because of its ability to help us make vitamin D. (See also "Protect Yourself from the Sun" in chapter 10.)

GALLBLADDER DISEASE

The gallbladder lies in the right upper part of the abdomen just under the liver. The gallbladder is a type of dishwasher in that it contributes a thickish solution (bile) to the digestive tract that is very important in helping break down fatty products of digestion. Bile is actually formed in the liver, but it is concentrated in the gallbladder before it is secreted into the small intestine.

The gallbladder gets into trouble when this sludgy solution collects on the inside of the gallbladder itself or in the ducts that connect it to the small intestine, where it can harden into mounds that are called gallstones.

Gallstones are more commonly found in middle-aged Caucasian women, especially those who are overweight. Gallstones are also more common in people who have a rich diet full of fat and in women who use the birth control pill.

Many people with gallstones complain that they have ill-defined trouble digesting meals that contain lots of fats. (So why do they eat them, I hear you asking. A good question, is the answer.) More serious complaints can include crampy pain, usually in the right upper part of the abdomen, especially associated with digestion, excess burping, feeling bloated, and farting. Your typical gallbladder patient, therefore, is female, fair, fat(tish), forty, full of air, and farty. (Please don't write me to protest. I didn't make this one up.)

What's interesting about many of these people, though, is that if their gallbladder is removed, many of them do not improve. Though they do have gallstones, the stones are not the source of their problems at all. In truth (which is a town just north of the borough of actuality) many if not most gallstones are silent. They produce no symptoms. That is why the gallbladder should not be removed for vague abdominal complaints or just because a few stones were found on ultrasound or X ray examination. You should always look for other explanations for vague abdominal complaints.

A specific group of patients, however, does experience great improvement when the gallbladder is removed. These are the people who have acute attacks of severe pain when a stone blocks the duct into the small intestine. This pain is often recurrent, occurring when the gallbladder tries to empty its load and cannot. The reason that we can remove the gallbladder without significantly penalizing digestion is that bile is produced in the liver, and the liver simply bypasses the missing gallbladder and empties its unconcentrated load directly into the small intestine.

An alternative to surgery is medication. There are some drugs that can dissolve stones. But most of them have significant side effects and cannot be tolerated by many people.

Another new type of treatment for gallstones is a machine, called a lithotripter, that can literally smash larger gallstones without damaging the organ. It works by emitting shock waves that presumably can pass through body organs without harming the tissue (I say presumably because these machines have only recently been loosed on the populace, and like all new medical toys, it is likely that we will one day discover something or other that these machines do that will surprise us. One hopes that only a minor price will be paid.) Back to the main story line. When these shock waves hit the stone, the stone explodes. The sludge that is left behind then passes out of the organ, although presumably that person continues at higher risk for developing a new stone.

THE ACUTE ABDOMEN

An abdomen that is acutely tender and may need to be operated on is called an acute abdomen. (We all have cute abdomens, but only sometimes do we have acute abdomens.) Every acute abdomen should be seen by a physician, but not every acute abdomen needs surgical therapy.

Even doctors sometimes have difficulty in distinguishing between an acute abdomen that requires surgery and its tender, nonsurgical counterpart. Thus, an inflamed intestinal diverticulum (an outpouching of the bowel) or a pelvic infection in a fallopian tube can present as an acute abdomen. Unfortunately, these nonsurgical conditions are sometimes operated on.

Never diagnose the cause of an acute abdomen yourself. You should always check the symptom of acute abdominal tenderness with someone who can tell you what to watch for.

Farting

Farting embarrasses and fascinates nearly everyone. I know one otherwise normal woman of about forty who giggles loudly every time she hears the word "fart." There must be a psychiatric name for this problem, but so far it has eluded me (she is definitely not fartophobic).

Farting can accompany practically any bowel problem. Farts are produced by intestinal bacteria breaking down foodstuffs and are a normal product of digestion. Depending on what you eat (and everybody can recall the Pulitzer Prize–winning verse that "beans, beans are good for the heart, the more you eat, the more you fart") and what kind of "mood" your digestive tract is in, you will produce varying amounts of gas.

But what about people who complain of excessive farting? This is a symptom that you often have to take the patient's word for. You wouldn't want to do otherwise. Luckily, few people can demonstrate their prowess on command in the office.

The first thing you must do is to minimize the amount of gas-producing substances you eat. These include beans, of course, but also many other foods, such as broccoli, onions, cabbage, and radishes. I make the most delicious roast chicken, for example. The secret is to put on a huge amount of onion salt. The price my family pays for this wonderful meal is that we must all occupy separate rooms for an hour or two later that night. I don't serve this dish for guests, unless they have to eat and run.

In some people, extra gas is a type of allergic response to some foods. Particularly implicated here are dairy products. If you — or even worse, your mate — are plagued by this problem, rent a home with a lot of space and good ventilation and then experiment by eliminating certain foods, starting with dairy products.

THE RECTUM AND ANUS — THE END OF THIS SECTION

Although the rectum and anus are really no more than a warehouse (with strong doors and gates) that stores the products it receives from elsewhere, it is amazing how many people have some type of complaint about the service they receive from this area. The complaints by and large are minor, but they are also usually recurrent.

Itching

I can think of very few people who do not complain of anal itching from time to time. Yet in underdeveloped countries, this is a rare symptom. They have anuses, same as us. Why are they lucky enough not to have to scratch continuously in a socially embarrassing place (not the dining room)?

The reason has to do with how we treat our rear ends, our waste-disposal systems. I can't believe that God ever intended man or woman to use toilet paper (which is as deep as I want to get). And if He or She did, it was surely not envisioned that we would rub as hard as we do for as long as we do as often as we do, that we would eat the kind of refined foods that we eat, leading to harder bowel movements, or that we would sit on a toilet seat for great lengths of time reading the latest issue of *Time* magazine, or on particularly tough occasions, *Gray's Anatomy*. All these factors produce a host of rectal and anal complaints, anal itching being only one.

The most likely cause of an anal itch is an irritated skin condition often called perianal dermatitis, followed closely behind by hemorrhoids. To a large extent, this condition is produced by either sensitivity to, or the overuse of, toilet paper.

You must be kind to your anus. Use the softest toilet paper you can afford. Wipe lightly. Better still, dab with a wet washcloth and gently dry the area. (In severe cases of rectal irritation I have told people to blow-dry the area, but this is not a treatment you would want to use in a communal shower, unless you are six-foot-seven and really don't care what people think.) Try not to scratch when it itches, although I personally know what a temptation it is to get that temporary relief, especially at night, when itching seems to be most prevalent. (In Yiddish this relief of discomfort is called a *mechayah*.) Take baths in warm water, allowing the area to be gently soothed. Remember to dry thoroughly afterwards. Avoid the foods that worsen the problem. If all else fails, this symptom may respond to medication, usually cortisone creams. But as always with cortisone, use it very sparingly and only for the most intractable cases.

PINWORMS

Very occasionally, especially in parents of young children, rectal itching is due to an infection with pinworms. The itching is very intense and is notoriously worse at night. A pinworm infection can also produce vaginal itching, especially in youngsters. The only good way to find these little critters is to swab your rectum first thing in the morning while the little guys are still struggling home from their nightly wanderings on your anal surface. Everyone in the house should be treated simultaneously because these infections are often asymptomatic.

Some people suffer from psychogenic itching. These folks just like to rub their backsides. Perhaps "like" is not the right word, but I am convinced that at least part of the reason for this nonpathologic itching is simply that it feels good to rub that area. What can one say about these feelings that a lounge singer couldn't express more movingly? Do not rub too hard or too often, or else you will set up a self-perpetuating irritation.

In my time I have also seen several cases of a different kind of psychological problem that centers on the rectum and usually involves itching. This is the problem in which the person is convinced that he or she has a parasite disease in the bowel, often described as little white worms, which are remarkably similar to pinworms. This usually occurs in someone who has actually had a pinworm infection that was successfully treated, but the infected party refuses to believe the medication has worked. Pinworm swabs are one of the few tests you should assume are nearly 100 percent accurate if done right. Do not convince yourself that you are still infected if the tests don't produce a positive result.

HEMORRHOIDS

Everyone thinks he or she has hemorrhoids. That is because so many adults have some type of rectal complaint and the only condition they have heard about in the rectum is hemorrhoids.

Hemorrhoids are varicose veins that occur in a network of veins called the hemorrhoidal plexus. A hemorrhoid occurs when some factor causes that part of the vein to stop functioning properly. The vein then fills with blood that just sits there, and the vein swells. Anything that puts pressure on the lower part of the abdomen, allowing blood to sit in the lower regions for a longer time, promotes the emergence of hemorrhoids. Thus, pregnancy, with its huge mass in the abdomen, is a common precipitating event for a lifelong bout with these troublesome veins. So too are strenuous physical activities such as weight lifting. (I'm so naive, by the way, that the first time I heard a weight lifter discuss "roids," I thought he was referring to hemorrhoids, although I couldn't understand how you could inject them into yourself.)

Hemorrhoids can itch, they can burn, they can hurt, and they can bleed (which almost sounds like a plea from some character in a grade B film asking you to feel sorry for these poor misunderstood blood vessels, who are only victims of their environment, after all). Mostly, they do none of the above but just sit there quietly. They often come and go, and they can be brought on by any activity that puts pressure on the rectum, such as straining with a bowel movement.

Mild hemorrhoids are easily treated. Sitz baths or baths in warm water with or without salt added are often very effective for mild cases. There are dozens of creams and suppositories that help the symptom disappear. Preparation H, the butt of so many jokes, works in the end.

More severe hemorrhoids (those that project out of the rectum in a large swelling and do not go back) need to be treated surgically.

Rectal Pain — The Real Meaning of a Pain in the Arse

Pain in the area of the anus and rectum is not uncommon.

Hemorrhoids can hurt, especially when they are newly inflamed or engorged. More commonly, acute pain in the rectum is due to a cut in the surface of the lining tissue, which is called an anal fissure. Fissures are common in every age group and are notoriously recurrent, especially when there is straining at bowel movements. Generally, the pain is a sharp pain on the outside of the anal area and is significantly worsened by bowel movements. Anusitis is a painful inflammation of the skin of the anus and is often worsened by certain foods and beverages, such as alcohol, citrus fruits, and coffee.

The same treatments apply to these conditions that you apply to all anal conditions — be kind to your anus and rectum. You only have one of each (usually).

There are several spaces around the rectum that can be invaded by bacteria and become infected, resulting in an abscess which causes sudden, severe pain in the rectum. Treat this condition as an emergency and see a doctor as soon as possible, since surgery may be required.

Rectal Bleeding

Rectal bleeding is a very common symptom in adults and is consequently easy to dismiss. This you should never do. Usually rectal bleeding is minimal and the blood can only be seen on the toilet paper. (And only if you look. Rectal bleeding does not send up a flare to tell you it's there.) This symptom is invariably due to a rectal irritation, such as anusitis, or to a hemorrhoid.

But if blood appears in the toilet bowl or covers the stool, then you should have a good rectal exam (there is actually no such creature as a good rectal exam). In the overwhelming proportion of cases, the bleeding will be due to a local cause, such as a hemorrhoid. But depending on other factors, you may need to be investigated for colon or rectal cancer. This investigation involves either a sigmoidoscopy or, less often, a colonoscopy (a look through the entire colon) or a barium-enema X ray.

More of a problem is recurrent rectal bleeding. How can you tell, if you have always had intermittent bleeding from a hemorrhoid, that any new bleeding is not actually due to a newly developed rectal tumor instead? The short answer is you cannot. That is why most gastroenterologists argue that you should have investigation with at least a sigmoidoscopy every year or two so long as the symptoms recur. The problem with this recommendation is that patients hate this procedure and avoid it as much as possible. In addition, rectal bleeding is so common that we probably don't have enough doctors around to do all those sigmoidoscopies, even if they did nothing else (perish the thought).

If you have recurrent rectal bleeding, and if there is any change in your bowel movements, such as the development of persistent constipation or narrowing of your stools, you should definitely investigate the cause. But if nothing else changes, then you must decide for yourself how often you want to let someone invade your nether regions, even if it's only your friendly family physician.

Changes in Bowel Movements

Satchel Paige once said something like, "Never look behind you. Someone may be catching up." Presumably, Satchel wasn't talking about bowel movements. You should always look behind you. You should also look at the toilet paper. I realize that this is not an appealing prospect for many, but it is necessary for maintaining good health.

Generally, the cause of altered bowel movements is obvious and can be simply corrected, or you can just wait for the problem to self-correct. If the altered pattern continues, and you have tried manipulating your environment to correct the situation and your treatment hasn't worked, then you should see your doctor. But you want to be sure that the results of any tests that are ordered will materially change your treatment or prognosis.

CONSTIPATION

Constipation is extremely common among adult North Americans. (One of my friends says it's because we have such a tough time letting go. But of what, I want to know, of what?)

There are people who have never known the psychic and physical pleasure of a soft, easily passed stool (another *mechayah*; see "Itching"). Often, their abnormal bowel patterns started in childhood and were perpetuated by our hurry-up lifestyle (like typical teenagers, the bowels rebelled, and rather than hurry up, they slowed down).

Constipation can be divided into two types — acute and chronic. We always ignore acute constipation for a while, hoping it will go away if we don't pay it any mind. Although this approach is proper, the unfortunate price that you frequently pay is that the longer the constipation goes on, the harder (literally) it is to treat.

Most recent-onset constipation is due to an acute change in lifestyle. Thus, being sick, changing your diet, dealing with greater stress than usual, and traveling to a different area can all cause temporary constipation. To correct the problem, all you usually have to do is sit and wait. And sit and wait. And . . .

If you continue to be constipated, always try a little diet manipulation to see if you can't unload your burden. Drink lots of water (at least six glasses a day), eat bran, other fiber-rich grains and breads, and dried fruits, drink prune juice, and stick to regular meals. You can also add in fiber products that you can purchase in the pharmacy, such as Fibryax and Fibermed. (Coffee is a questionable remedy, but it works for me.) Exercise frequently helps.

If these alterations don't work, then you should use a mild laxative such as Senokot, which acts by either bulking up the stool as it passes through the intestines or by softening the stool. Other useful laxatives for acute constipation include mineral oil or products that irritate and stimulate the colon like bisacodyl (Dulcolax). If all else fails, boys and girls, it's enema time.

Acute constipation that is not improving should be investigated, since you want to be certain that there is no other correctable cause for this change in the bowel pattern. The problems that can cause constipation range from metabolic abnormalities such as hypothyroidism to mechanical abnormalities such as a bowel tumor.

Chronic constipation is another problem altogether. Frequently people with this problem have seen a host of doctors and alternate healers with little help. Some people have intestines that just don't work properly, and medical science is unable to offer them much help. Do all the right things (water, foods, exercise), and if all else fails, you just may have to regularly take a bulk-forming laxative (like Metamucil).

DIARRHEA

Just like the weather, everybody seems to have a different opinion about what constitutes diarrhea. Some people assume that any increase, no matter how minor, in the frequency of their daily bowel movement is diarrhea, whereas others, perhaps more used to loose stools as a regular event, consider diarrhea to be only extremely wet, frequent bowel movements. I am a Wet, a member of the second camp.

The causes of diarrhea are legion. Any irritant can send the GI tract into overdrive and lead to more frequent, wetter stools. The most common are viral infections, bacterial infections when you are traveling, and food poisoning (which is usually a bacterial infection as well).

With mild diarrhea, all you ever have to do is to replace the lost fluids. Yes, Virginia, chicken soup is a good source of fluids and electrolytes (sodium and potassium that you require along with the liquid). So are most juices (although apple juice can actually make diarrhea worse in some people; if nothing else, this tidbit is worth the price of this book) and commercially available preparations like Gatorade and Pedialyte.

The previously healthy adult has a huge capacity to tolerate diarrhea before you have to start worrying about the implications. I am my own good example. I was diagnosed as a celiac (allergic to or intolerant of wheat) when I was twenty-eight years old. I was suffering with frequent, loose stools for several weeks, and in my wisdom I had been self-medicating with tea and toast, which of course made my diarrhea much worse. But I was able to tolerate up to thirty bouts of wet stools a day for a period of six weeks, involving a weight loss in excess of thirty pounds, before I needed to be admitted to hospital. (For those of you who like psychological contributions to diseases, my dad was a bread jobber, and I am allergic to wheat. Chew on that for a while.)

If the diarrhea is mild and the patient is not feeling too ill, you can be patient about investigations. Everyone has different standards, but my rule is that if the diarrhea is going on for two weeks, or if the diarrhea wakes the person at night, I do stool cultures. (The exception here is the patient who has recently returned from an area where parasite disease is common, like Asia. In those cases, I investigate more quickly.)

When diarrhea has been severe or prolonged, and especially if the patient is feeling ill, the possibility of a parasite infection or some type of inflammation of the bowel should be entertained. These inflammatory conditions include Crohn's disease, ulcerative colitis, and malabsorption diseases like wheat allergies. The tests usually start with cultures for bacteria and a search for parasites, followed by X rays of the small intestine and large bowel, and sigmoidoscopy. Even after these investigations, sometimes even including a biopsy of the small intestine to look for absorption problems, the cause of the diarrhea is not apparent for some patients. We then usually write this symptom off to irritable bowel syndrome, or to "nerves."

Remember that the speed with which you want to be investigated (I know nobody wants to be investigated) for diarrhea depends on how sick you are and what you expect to find. A sick patient needs tests quickly, especially when you are looking for treatable infections. The patient who looks well can safely wait a long time.

You treat diarrhea by being kind to your gut and replacing fluids. This kind of diet manipulation is usually sufficient. With significant diarrhea, always cut your diet down to what is easy to digest and remember to do that for a few extra meals after the symptom passes. It always amazes me what people will stuff into their gut as soon as they show any improvement. In your diet, avoid anything that may worsen the symptoms, like raw fruit and vegetables, spices, alcohol, pickled foods, caffeine, and milk products. Reintroduce well-cooked foods gradually and in small amounts, and the diarrhea is not likely to recur.

If the diarrhea is more chronic but not severe and you are satisfied that you are not dealing with a parasite infection, you can treat the diarrhea with a product to harden the stool, like loperamide (Imodium).

Several parasites that cause diarrhea are common in Canada. The best known is *Giardia lamblia*, which causes the well-named beaver fever. The name stems from the fact that this parasite is present in certain wild animals (five bucks if you can guess which ones), and these animals deposit the parasites in water supplies, which humans then drink. (Isn't that a lovely thought? Next time you bend over to take a nice cool sip from a running brook, picture a bear squatting just upstream from you.) This infection is particularly common in people who have camped in the wild. Giardiasis is also commonly passed as a sexually transmitted infection, especially in gay men, through anal intercourse. This parasite is very difficult to find in stool specimens, since it seems to appear in the stool only intermittently. If stool tests do not reveal any organisms and there is a high suspicion of giardiasis, then the best way of finding it is to take a sample from the small intestine. The most successful treatment for this infection is metronidazole (Flagyl).

Other parasites occasionally found in travelers include whipworm, roundworm, tapeworm, and amoebas, which cause amebic dysentery. Each infection is treated differently, so it is important to have proper stool tests to nab the guilty party.

BLACK BOWEL MOVEMENTS

Unless you have eaten something like blueberries or taken vitamins with iron, both of which can make the stool appear dark, black bowel movements are always a source of concern. Black bowel movements indicate some source of bleeding high in the GI tract. In people under fifty, the source is usually a silent ulcer, rarely a tumor. But this is one symptom for which the cause *must* be found.

NARROW BOWEL MOVEMENTS

Bowel movements that change either from wide to narrow and back are usually due to irritable bowel syndrome. But bowel movements that are generally narrowing more and more can indicate a bowel tumor. (You and your bowel movements *can* be too thin.) This symptom also requires investigation.

CHAPTER 9

The Musculoskeletal System

*In which the author takes a trip through that enchanting forest
of ligaments, tendons, muscles, bones,
and most enchanting of all, joints*

The musculoskeletal system, or as some would have it, the locomotor system (LMS), is the seat of many complaints in adults between fifteen and fifty. As a matter of fact, it is often the more healthy among us (a group that does not, of course, include your author) who tend to have more musculoskeletal problems than the less healthy of us. That is because the healthier specimens in our culture tend to do more exercise, and exercise, as any couch potato is only too happy to tell you, is the source of many injuries, nearly all of which occur in the musculoskeletal system. (It is considerably more difficult to develop an injury if the only part of your anatomy that moves is your thumb as you flip channels and take the tab off another can of brew. The exception is when the can falls to the floor and you strain your back or your shoulder when you bend over to retrieve it.)

But aside from sports injuries and other causes of acute musculo-skeletal complaints, the LMS is also the source of many chronic problems in the young to middle-aged adult. In this age group, this system is the cause of many visits to doctors, many of which can politely be called a waste of time (the visits are a waste, not the doctors) because the treatment of the underlying condition is gener-ally routine and one that the patient can usually initiate himself or herself without a physician's care.

HOW THE SYSTEM WORKS

The Vertebral Column

The spinal column is composed of bones (vertebrae) that are separated by cartilaginous pads (discs) that act as shock absorbers for the column. Nerves run out from the spinal cord to the periphery through openings in the vertebral bones. These nerves run very close to the discs, which is why protruding discs (see pages 181–82) can cause pain along those nerves.

As a result of an injury, an infection, or a genetic predisposition, the disc material can change consistency and produce pressure on the nerves that run out of the spinal cord. This pressure produces pain along those nerves.

The largest nerve that emerges from the spinal cord is the sciatic nerve, one to innervate each leg. So when people complain of pain in the back that extends along a sciatic nerve, we say that they are

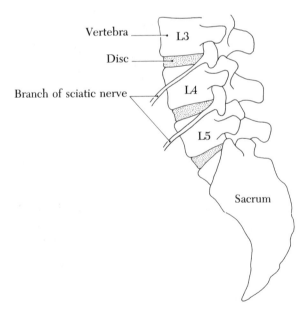

A PORTION OF THE VERTEBRAL COLUMN

suffering from sciatica. The pain of sciatica can be felt anywhere along the tract of the sciatic nerve, which ends in the toes.

Muscles and Tendons and Ligaments and Bursas

A muscle is a group of elastic fibers that can contract and relax and that are united together for a common purpose. Muscles move bones and protect parts of the body, acting as a sort of shock absorber.

A tendon is the tough, fibrous structure at the end of a muscle that attaches the muscle to a bone.

A strand of fibrous tissue that connects bones is known as a ligament.

The best way to think of a bursa (which you need to do only when you have bursitis, because otherwise why should you care?) is to consider it as a collapsed balloon. A bursa is actually a *potential* space enclosed by a lining, which surrounds certain bony prominences, tendons, and joints. The linings around bursas are slippery and smooth, permitting less friction when that particular body part moves.

PROBLEMS OF THE LMS

Low Back Pain

It has been estimated that 90 percent of North American adults will suffer from low back pain at least once in their lifetime. This statistic applies to acute low back pain, a sudden onset of moderate to severe pain, usually in the middle of the lower back, which is generally caused by excessive lifting or straining (although a large number of people will tell you that their backs started hurting after a relatively innocuous event, sometimes even during sleep). Acute low back pain is usually the result of a "soft tissue injury," meaning that one or more of the soft tissues — a muscle, a tendon, or a ligament — has been stretched or pulled. There are no reliable laboratory tests to confirm this diagnosis. X rays are invariably a waste of time and should rarely be ordered for this kind of injury, although for various reasons, legal ones being prominent, X rays are often taken.

Most people who have strained their back require nothing more than a few days of rest. Recently there has been much emphasis on combining rest with early mobilization. This means that you can pamper your back by not lifting anything very heavy and by avoiding activities that strain the back, such as those requiring twisting or repetitive bending, but you should otherwise try to live as normal a life as possible. Prolonged bed rest is counterproductive in most of these situations. You must not lie around feeling sorry for yourself for too long, or else the condition will take much longer to improve. Early mobilization is the clarion call of all back specialists.

Chronic low back pain affects as many as 500,000 Canadians and is the second leading cause of time lost from work for adults in full-time employment. (There's no truth to the rumor that boredom is the number-one cause.) It's often difficult to narrow down the exact cause of chronic low back pain. And it's even harder to treat.

Like acute low back pain, most chronic low back pain originates from problems in the soft tissues of the lower back. The factors that contribute to recurrent pain in this area are leading a sedentary lifestyle, being overweight, having poor posture, sleeping on a soft mattress, and using incorrect lifting techniques.

There are also several other, less common causes of low back pain, including a type of arthritis known as ankylosing spondylitis, which is more prevalent in young men, and facet impingement syndrome, in which the bones in the vertebral column do not seem to ride properly on each other.

Frequently people who have recurrent pain in the low back diagnose themselves as having a "disc problem." They are usually wrong. Although disc damage in the lower back may cause recurrent bouts of pain, this condition is a lot less frequent than most people think.

X rays are often useless in establishing the cause of chronic low back pain because plain X rays do not pick up soft tissues (which are the most frequently injured tissues) and they are also not very accurate at picking up disc damage. Much more useful for the diagnosis of a disc injury, but much more expensive and much less available, are CT scans.

There are three complications of low back pain that must be treated as acute emergencies because they indicate a sudden deterioration of the disc pressing on the sciatic nerve. These include interference with bladder or rectal function or a weakening in the muscles of the foot (foot drop). No matter how long you've had your back pain, if you develop these symptoms you must see a doctor right away. If treatment is delayed, these complications can result in permanent damage to the sciatic nerve.

As long as there are no complications, both acute and chronic low back pain of any cause should be treated conservatively for as long as the person can stand it (if standing is hard, try sitting). Conservative treatment does not mean listening to the speeches of Brian Mulroney to see if any two are consistent. Rather it means physiotherapy, rest, medications such as nonsteroidal anti-inflammatories (NSAIDs) for the inflammation, manipulation therapy, ice for swelling, heat for increased blood flow, occasional use of muscle relaxant medication or analgesics, even praying to your particular deity. In short, anything that you believe in, so long as it does not make you worse.

Therapy for chronic low back pain must be individualized. There are no magic bullets. If you believe in a particular therapy, it is much more likely to work. It doesn't really matter what you use so long as the therapy does not take too long and so long as it returns you to some semblance of normal. Quickly.

To prevent back problems in the first place, or to prevent frequent recurrences of preexisting back pain, take precautions. Keep your weight down. Most therapists advise you to sleep on your back or side (something that I simply cannot do), since this seems to minimize strain on the back muscles. Lift properly by bending your knees every time (just picture your spouse standing over you to monitor your technique every time you have to lift something heavy). Do back exercises regularly. And stay in shape — walk, bike, swim. Doing any exercise that builds muscles is helpful.

If the pain is due to a protruding disc and has not improved after an adequate trial of conservative therapy, then you should consider an operation on the disc. In certain centers, doctors treat this problem by injecting an enzyme called chymopapain into the disc to dissolve the protruding part of the disc. This therapy has several hazards, including the risk of improper injection and allergy to the chemical.

But the benefit of this therapy is that it involves very minimal surgery and so recovery time is very quick.

The operation that is done much more commonly now is to shave off the protruding part of the disc, using a microdissection technique. If this doesn't work, a more complex procedure on the entire disc must be done.

Neck Pain

Two types of neck pain are common in youngish adults. These include an acute syndrome of pain that accompanies an accident — the condition that we commonly call whiplash — and the more chronic, recurrent ache in the neck that accompanies stress and is a frequent companion to a headache.

Whiplash is as much a pain in the butt as it is a pain in the neck. We really don't know what happens in whiplash except that there is some kind of injury to some of the soft tissues of the neck. The overwhelming proportion of people improve in one or two weeks. But there is a small group of whiplash patients whose pain lingers and lingers, sometimes for many years. Although many books have been written on this subject, the truth is that we don't know why this occurs and who is most likely to suffer lingering pain.

Like all types of pain, whiplash should be treated with any therapy that is effective. This includes physiotherapeutic treatments (manipulation, lasers, ultrasound, transcutaneous nerve stimulation, and traction), neck collars, exercises, appropriate rest (but as with back pain, there should be an emphasis on early mobilization), massage therapy, yoga, acupuncture, various medications used for a short period to help with pain and inflammation, and anything else that will work.

Chronic neck pain that accompanies stress is treated in much the same way as whiplash, but there should also be an attempt to minimize stress. You should be very reluctant to use medication to control these symptoms, since this chronic condition is likely to lead to addiction to the drugs that will have to be continuously used.

Pain in the Joints — Arthritis (Not, As Some of My Patients Have It, Arthuritis)

Arthritis refers to any process in which the tissues in a joint become inflamed. There are many different types of arthritis, including septic arthritis, in which a bacterial infection in the joint can rapidly destroy the tissues and lead to permanent damage in a few days. Luckily, septic arthritis is rather rare.

Only three types of arthritis occur with any regularity in fifteen-to-fifty-year-olds. These include rheumatoid arthritis, osteoarthritis, and gout.

RHEUMATOID ARTHRITIS

When most people think of arthritis, they think of the variant known as rheumatoid arthritis. This type of arthritis results in the deformed, turned joints, especially in the hands, that we have all noticed on some older people. But as the television ads stress, arthritis is a disease that can and does strike at any age, and it is frequently more devastating in the younger person. We don't really know what causes rheumatoid arthritis, although there are all sorts of theories. The most prevalent is that it is caused by a viral infection. The inflammation starts in the joint and later spreads to the cartilage and the other tissues surrounding the joint lining. When these other tissues become inflamed, the joint can become permanently deformed.

Rheumatoid arthritis can affect any joint, but it has a predilection for the joints in the hands, wrists, and feet. A cardinal symptom of rheumatoid arthritis is morning stiffness. The affected joints feel worse after a period of rest, such as sleep overnight, and frequently improve as they are used more throughout the day.

It is important to keep the inflammation in the joint to a minimum because the longer the inflammation lasts, and the more severe it is, the greater the likelihood of permanent deformity. Part of the essential treatment of arthritis is regular exercise that keeps the joints and limbs supple. Keep the parts moving, and they won't freeze up on you as quickly.

Recently there has been a flurry of interest in the use of fish oils to prevent and treat rheumatoid arthritis. Fish oils contain substances that inhibit inflammation, and it certainly never hurts anyone to eat more fish. We still can't say that taking fish oils in any other fashion, such as high-dose capsules, is beneficial, but eating cold-water fish like salmon can only do you good (and you help foster a Canadian industry at the same time).

The mainstay of arthritis therapy is still medication and variants of physical therapy, such as hydrotherapy and manipulation therapy.

A drug that has often been used for the treatment of rheumatoid arthritis is the old standby, ASA. ASA is very effective when used properly, but it has drawbacks. To treat arthritis, ASA has to be used in doses high enough to control the inflammation. And when it is used in those high doses, it eventually causes gastric problems, including bleeding, and in the worst-case scenario, rupture of a gastric ulcer. High-dose ASA can also cause ringing in the ears.

Because so many people complain about stomach irritation with ASA, other NSAIDs have largely replaced ASA for treatment of arthritis. These include such well-known drugs as ibuprofen (Motrin), sulindac (Clinoril), piroxicam (Feldene), diclofenac (Voltaren), keto-profen (Orudis), and tiaprofenic acid (Surgam).

Although we promote NSAIDs as having fewer side effects than ASA, the truth is that the NSAIDs, when used long enough, will all cause the same stomach problems as ASA. In fact, these problems are so common with these medications that many doctors believe that all long-term users of NSAIDs should take anti-ulcer preventive medication at the same time.

Anybody who is prescribed a NSAID drug should avoid the use of alcohol (which worsens the gastric effects of the NSAIDs), should maintain regular contact with his or her physician, and should certainly report any new symptom right away. Don't just ignore those stomach complaints. Report them and see what can be done about them. When NSAIDs are not sufficient, many other medications can be used, but a discussion of these medications is beyond the scope of this book.

As with all inflammatory conditions, physiotherapy can often decrease inflammation in an affected joint. Good physiotherapy also often makes the difference between managing at home and needing hospital care.

OSTEOARTHRITIS

Osteoarthritis is a degenerative disease of the cartilage in a joint. It occurs in joints that are overused, abused, or malaligned in some way, or in joints that have had some trauma to them — for example, a knee joint in which there has been previous ligament damage. Osteoarthritis also tends to occur in the joints of the back or in people who are overweight because of the strain on these joints from the excess poundage (kilogrammage?). Other common areas of osteoarthritis are the joints in the hands and feet.

Osteoarthritis tends to show up with pain that worsens when the affected joint is used. In contrast to rheumatoid arthritis, the pain in osteoarthritis is worse later in the day and often better in the morning. Osteoarthritis tends to worsen with age, and the only good preventive measures are to maintain proper weight and not to tax the joint unduly.

As with rheumatoid arthritis, medical therapy of this condition includes anti-inflammatory medications and physical therapy.

GOUT

Hands up all those who remember that Jiggs suffered from gout. (Leave the room if you never heard of Jiggs.) Maggie's treatment was to wrap his foot in a bandage resembling swaddling clothes and to hit him with a rolling pin. We have slightly better treatments now.

Gout is an acute arthritic inflammation, caused by the deposit of uric acid in a joint. As with Jiggs, gout often occurs first in the large toe of one foot. Gout attacks tend to come on suddenly and quite severely and need to be treated with high doses of anti-inflammatories. Many people also need to take medication that lowers the level of uric acid in the bloodstream. These medications include allopurinol (Zyloprim) and probenecid (Benemid). There is some correlation of gout with the ingestion of purine-rich foods, such as organ meats and sardines and especially port wine, which was presumably Jiggs's problem. (Picture, if you will, a diet consisting of sardines, liver and kidneys, and port wine. Gout would simply be God's way of laughing at you.)

The other concern about gout is that the uric acid can also be deposited in the kidneys, leading to eventual kidney damage.

Just to confuse the picture, of course, there are many people who have high amounts of uric acid in the bloodstream yet never have gout attacks. These people do not need to take medication for lowering uric acid.

Softening of the Bones — Osteoporosis

Osteoporosis does not affect many women under the age of sixty, but it has its roots in the younger female, so it should be mentioned here.

In osteoporosis, the bones soften, in part due to the reabsorption of calcium from the bony tissue. Although it can happen to men as well, osteoporosis is much more common in women, especially Caucasian women, who lead a sedentary life and in women who are thin, who smoke, and who have a poor diet. It is also more prevalent in those women who did not take in enough calcium while younger.

A woman who has osteoporosis is much more likely to fracture certain bones as she ages, particularly the bones in the vertebral column, in the wrist, and in the hip, which is a common cause of death in the elderly.

The best treatment for osteoporosis is to prevent it in the first place. Prevention includes adequate calcium intake in the premenopausal years (about 1000 milligrams a day, and not much more, as higher doses are associated with higher rates of kidney stones), regular exercise, (probably) estrogen replacement therapy after menopause, and perhaps fluoride.

SPORTS INJURIES (NOT INCLUDING THOSE ASSOCIATED WITH CHESS)

Several times in this book, I refer to how old I am. Just exactly how old are you, Art? Well, I'm so old, boys and girls, I remember back to a time when there was no specialty called sports medicine (and the Dodgers were still in Brooklyn, and the Russians were evil, etc.). There was a time — you youngsters won't believe this — when if you were injured as an athlete (which was not a word that my generation used a whole lot when we were growing up), the team coach (who was also probably the guy who taught you math or socials), told you one of two things: to tough your way through it and resume training, or the converse of that admonition, if it hurts, don't do it. That was the sum total of sports medicine advice then, in those days before we had fire.

In the last ten or fifteen years we have seen a major expansion of knowledge in all aspects of sports, including equipment, training methods, physiology and kinesiology, and particularly prevention and treatment of injuries. Today it is a rare athlete, competitive or recreational, who doesn't make use of this new knowledge.

Even couch potatoes seem fascinated by information about sports medicine, although they're usually only interested in the type of information that justifies their sedentary existence. Ever notice how people who are bloated from excessive time on their backsides always pin the latest counterfitness article, the one that shows that even one minute of exercise can ruin your sex life or your career or your stamp collection, to the staff bulletin board? Or what about the difference in response between the lean and the fat to the death of Jim Fixx? I think I can guess someone's weight just by asking that person why Jim Fixx died. (It is a proven *Reader's Digest* fact that it is more relevant to yuppies to ask where they were and what they thought when Jim Fixx died than to ask the same about John F. Kennedy's death.)

Types of Injury

Get set for some more definitions.

When a muscle is acutely strained by a force that is greater than the strength of the muscle itself, some of the fibers become stretched too tautly. This stretching is known as a muscle pull or muscle strain and results in pain and tenderness along the path of those particular fibers.

Tendonitis (which is also spelled tendinitis, although I have no idea what a tendin is) is an inflammation of the tendon, usually from overuse. A pulled tendon is called a tendon strain.

Bursitis is the condition in which the lining of the bursa becomes inflamed either through direct trauma or with overuse.

A partial tear in a ligament is known as a sprain. (The sprain in Spain happens mostly in the rain on wet terrain.)

An overuse injury is caused by increasing the rate or intensity of your exercise so rapidly that your body cannot accommodate itself to this change. The medical way of putting this is to say that overuse injuries are caused by accumulated minor injuries from repeated exposure to excessive loads, or overloads. (I like the first explanation better.)

An overuse injury stands in contrast to a traumatic injury, which results from an acute episode that is (surprise!) traumatic to some body part, such as an ankle sprain when landing inappropriately in volleyball.

A stress fracture is an overuse fracture, or break, to a bone that occurs through repeated overload. (This is not the same fracture that a spouse may threaten her mate with if he continues to cause her so much stress.)

Bones can be violently ejected from their joints. This injury is known as a dislocation.

"Shin splints" is an inexact term that is applied to any pain in the leg between the knee and the ankle. This nondiagnosis can encompass any of the following: stress fracture, tendonitis, muscle strain, compartment syndrome (in which muscles cannot move smoothly inside their sheaths), infection, and several milder difficult-to-diagnose conditions. Usually pain in the shins develops from sports in which it is easy to land too hard, especially on shoes that are not right for your feet. Thus, pain in the shins is common in people who participate in volleyball, basketball, running, and hard aerobic classes that involve a lot of jumping.

Preventing Injuries — Stretching and Strengthening

Stretching muscles, especially in the older athlete (sorry, but that's anyone over forty), is said to reduce most sports injuries. Every activity and every participant requires their own unique set of stretches, which are readily available from any good book written for that sport.

For muscle strengthening, you can use all sorts of new (and expensive) equipment, but often you can do just as well at home with a few homemade gadgets. For example, lifting a purse with some type of weight in it, such as small rocks, is a good way to build up some of the leg muscles.

Treatments

RICE

Rest. Ice. Compression. Elevation. RICE is all ye need, and all ye need to know.

1. *Rest the area.*
   There is no better treatment for an injury than rest. By rest we mean that you modify the activity (or stop it altogether) and you cut down on the load that you put on the injured area. This means that even though you can run for an hour, though with pain, you should still *not* run for that hour. Whatever is producing the pain will merely become chronic if you take a stoic attitude and try to outrun the pain. In addition, you run the risk (even if running is not your sport) of developing new areas of pain as your body compensates to relieve the pressure on the injured body part.
   Rest allows the injured area to recover. There is no substitute.
2. *Ice the injury.*
   Although heat makes you feel better by increasing the blood flow to an injury, it doesn't reduce the swelling. Ice, however, decreases inflammation, swelling, and pain. So the main form of thermal therapy for an injury should be ice, except in the neck and back, where many therapists prefer to apply heat.
   Ice should be applied in the form of a pack (cheap and easy-to-use packs include a bag of frozen peas, but you must remember not to eat the peas after they have been thawed and refrozen several times, or a paper cup containing water that has been frozen) for about fifteen minutes at a time, several times a day, if

possible. Don't apply the ice for much longer than that, however, because too much cold causes inflammation as well.

People with a preexisting problem with blood flow to an area (such as those with Raynaud's disease) shouldn't use ice, because it will only aggravate the problem.

3. *Compress the injury.*

It often helps to tape or bandage an inflamed area, such as a sprained ankle or a bad thigh bruise. You must always insure that the taping is not too tight, however, so as to allow adequate blood flow to the injured area.

4. *Elevate the area.*

Blood collects in the lowest parts of the body. If an injured limb is elevated, preferably above the level of the heart (although you will look awfully silly walking around with your leg above your heart if you have suffered an ankle sprain) there will be less swelling and pain because it is then easier for the blood to return to the heart.

MASSAGE

Which one of us doesn't feel better after a massage? The fact that it probably doesn't help with healing too much is secondary. Never refuse a gentle massage to an inflamed area. But a vigorous massage can occasionally make a swelling worse.

MEDICATIONS

When an injury is acute, anti-inflammatory medications, particularly the NSAIDs, help the swelling to settle. They also act as mild analgesics. In more chronic pain, except for specific conditions such as Achilles tendonitis, shoulder tendonitis, and plantar fasciitis (see below), these drugs are not nearly as useful. (Doesn't the word "fasciitis" make you think that surely there must also be a problem known as communiitis?)

For proper pain relief with acute injuries, there is often a need for strong analgesics, usually those containing codeine. These medications should be given to help you sleep or if you absolutely require them to function at work or at home. They should never be given for prolonged periods for acute injuries.

Muscle relaxants are rarely useful except for back and neck conditions, for which they should be carefully prescribed because they can cause drowsiness in the short term, and some can produce addiction in the long term.

ORTHOSES

Orthoses are mechanical devices that are meant to shift weight away from an inflamed area. They alter the way you bear weight on that area. The most common orthoses are inserts that you put into your shoes while you participate in your chosen sport.

Specific Sports

RUNNING

Lots of people run, and lots of runners develop injuries.

First the good news. Running is a very effective form of aerobic exercise. Running is also a very effective way to lose weight and to keep your weight down. Running gets you out of doors. Running can be a social activity but often isn't, mainly because too many people who run seem to be miserable nontalkers.

Running provoked many of the improvements in sports medicine that we've developed over the last few years. Think about those high-topped black runners we all grew up with as children and then compare them with the latest runners offered by Nike or Brooks, and you realize just how far we've come. (Of course, high-tops are back in, but for an entirely different reason. Why are my childhood runners, which I could wear now and be cool, and my complete collection of all those baseball cards, which I could sell now and retire on the profits, the only things from my childhood that my mother didn't keep? She has, however, kept my first pair of skates. Any offers?)

But despite the advances in equipment and techniques, many if not most runners still develop injuries. And many of these injuries are not minor little aches that pass with one night's rest. Many are chronic injuries that interrupt that person's running schedule for a significant period of time.

The most frequently injured joint in runners is the knee. The patella, or the kneecap, rides in a groove on the front of the knee. It is held in place by tendons and ligaments. If the patella does not ride properly in its groove and you stress the knee with overuse, you will develop pain in the knee when you run. The pain can occur on either side of the knee, in the front of the kneecap, or behind the knee. Usually there is not much swelling or tenderness, and the knee generally doesn't hurt at rest. This kind of "runner's knee" is due to patello-femoral syndrome, and it is the most common form of knee pain. An important sign of an overuse injury to the knee is what is called the theater sign, in which you get pain not from thinking of going to a play but from prolonged sitting with the knees crossed.

Treatment is geared towards reducing the pain and preventing it from recurring. For immediate treatment, the usual RICE modalities are used. But the most important part of treatment is to reduce the running to a point where the pain is not happening. This may mean as little as intermittent thirty-second runs interspersed with periods of walking.

You should build up your quadriceps muscle, which is that huge muscle that runs along the front and sides of your thigh and which is underdeveloped in most runners. Partial knee squats are a good exercise for strengthening the quadriceps muscle. You should, at the same time, also build up your hamstrings, the big muscle mass on the back of the thigh, so that you don't develop an imbalance between these two large muscle masses. The best way to build up the hamstrings is with an exercise in which you lie on your stomach and have a weight at each ankle, which you lift by bending your knees. Most important, after you recover, increase your running intensity *slowly*, preferably by alternating short periods of running with longer periods of walking. If the pain recurs, you may require orthoses to correct the problem.

The most common ankle injury in runners is a sprained ankle, from turning the ankle during a run. To treat a sprained ankle, use RICE and keep your weight off that foot. That often means crutches for a few days if you are limping, whether you like it or not. Sprained ankles are easily turned again. Don't be surprised if the ankle doesn't feel quite right for as long as a year after a severe sprain. To prevent sprained ankles, always wear good runners and always run on as smooth a surface as you can. (Paved surfaces are preferable to paths through the woods.)

Several foot injuries are common in runners, including several types of tendonitis and ligament sprains.

One common foot injury is plantar fasciitis. The fascia is the layer of connective tissue under the skin, which tends to become inflamed with overuse. This condition causes a sharp pain on the heel or sole, which is tender with pressure. The fascia attaches to a small projection off the heel bone, the calcaneus. An inflammation of this attachment is known as a heel spur, or a calcaneal spur. The treatment is RICE, along with the use of anti-inflammatory medications. You may also require orthoses to prevent the problem from recurring. Occasionally, cortisone injection is helpful for this condition. And as usual, your return to running must be modified.

Another foot problem that can occur with overuse is a stress fracture in one of the long, thin bones of the foot, which are known as metatarsal bones. The symptoms of this condition are pain and tenderness in the area of the fracture. It is important to return to running slowly after one of these injuries.

The huge Achilles' tendon that runs down the calf to the back of the foot is a common source of problems in any sport that involves taking off and landing hard on the feet, such as running (especially downhill) and basketball. Many of these problems are due to inflammation not of the actual tendon but of structures around or near the tendon. The treatment, however, is always the usual.

Hip pain is usually due to a bursitis or a tendonitis in the hip. Hip pain due to bursitis often hurts if you lie on that side. Both inflammations are worse with running and better at rest. Hip pain can also occasionally be a manifestation of a back disorder. The inflammations are treated in the standard manner.

AEROBICS

Aerobics is not my idea of a sport, but then what do I know? It certainly is a popular pastime, although I suspect that participation is dropping off as members of the fitness generation become slightly less concerned with how they look and somewhat more concerned with how they age.

Aerobics facilities have greatly improved over the last few years, so many of the injuries that we used to see from landing too hard on surfaces that were not built properly and from workouts that were too vigorous for the level of fitness of the participants are now not nearly as prevalent. These injuries still do occur, however, in people who do not buy proper shoes or who participate too rigorously in high-impact aerobics, which involve a great deal of jumping and landing. Common aerobics injuries include knee problems like patello-femoral syndrome, ankle injuries from repeated ankle sprains, shin injuries, and foot problems like plantar fasciitis.

The easiest way to correct these problems is to buy proper footwear, to gradually build up the intensity of your workouts, and to not participate in high-impact aerobics, unless there is a compelling reason to do all that jumping.

BASEBALL

Curiously, baseball, one of America's favorite pastimes, that laid-back sport reserved for lazy summer nights in cities with ghettos, like Toronto, results in many injuries.

The most common source of injury in recreational baseball is sliding into a stationary base. This practice can result in severe ankle, foot, and knee injuries (as well as severe scrapes to the skin, as my competitive son discovered the day he slid into *first* base with short pants on). If you don't know how to slide, don't. Better still, get your park to order detachable bases.

Other common injuries in baseball include sunburns, eye injuries, muscle pulls, and tendonitis and bursitis in joints such as the shoulder after they have been in hibernation all winter.

If you want to play baseball, oil those joints. Do your own spring training, and don't throw hard until you've thrown for a few days. Warm up and stretch each time you play.

One last word about baseball. It is one of those sports that seems to bring out the hero in many a man. In mixed softball, there are many men who can finally be that star they were not able to be in their youth. So they throw harder than they need to, they swing harder than is required, they slide more, they knock the catcher over when running into home plate on a close play (one of the worst brain injuries I ever saw occurred in a pickup softball game, where a runner ran into the catcher's head with his knee). Using such poor judgement, these players cause many injuries to themselves and to others.

Now the real final last word (which has nothing to do with the musculoskeletal system but must be included somewhere). Too many adults drink alcohol and play ball, often participating in both activities at the same time. Baseball is a dangerous sport, both for the drinker and for his or her potential victims. If you have to drink, do it after the game. And don't drive home.

CYCLING

Cyclists seem to suffer from a genetic defect that attracts them to a horribly ugly array of funny uniforms and weird little hats, which may look good when worn while cycling on the back roads of France (although I doubt it) but certainly look bizarre when worn on the streets of Canadian towns and cities.

Cycling is an excellent aerobic sport, although it is frequently expensive. It also provides you with beautiful scenery, unless you are in the habit of cycling through downtown anywhere. The most common injury from overuse in cyclists occurs in the knee. This problem can invariably by corrected by proper muscle strengthening and changes in technique that involve gradually increasing the load and easing spinning of the wheel.

Although the head is not, by my criteria, part of the musculoskeletal system, it must also be mentioned that cycling can be a dangerous sport for the head. Yet it is truly amazing how few cyclists wear helmets. Too many cyclists suffer head injuries, and some suffer permanent brain damage. I realize that helmets don't offer perfect protection, but what else do you have? If you have spent several hundred dollars on a bike, what's the reluctance in spending another hundred or so on a good helmet? It may not be as macho, but it could save your life.

RACQUET SPORTS

Although eye injuries tend to be the most serious injuries in racquet sports, injuries to the musculoskeletal system are also common, especially those to the shoulder, ankle, and elbow. Invariably these are due to improper technique.

In the shoulder, there is the usual cast of problems, including tendonitis and bursitis.

In the elbow, the most common injury with racquet sports is tennis elbow. The pain in tennis elbow occurs from frequent inappropriate trauma to the tendons that insert in the bone that protrudes on the outside of the elbow. Contributing factors, are, as usual, not training properly before beginning rigorous play, improper technique, especially that most poorly played stroke, the backhand (if you ever want an evening of cheap, light entertainment, go to the nearest public tennis courts and watch people serve and hit the backhand), and in some people, an overstrung racquet. Treatment is the usual RICE, as well as investment in a few lessons to improve your technique.

The ulnar nerve runs down a groove near the inside of the elbow. You know you have hit your ulnar nerve when you get that electrical-type shock we call hitting your funny bone. In sports that involve using a racquet or throwing, it is not uncommon to injure a ligament in the area of the ulnar nerve, causing pain along the nerve. Again, there is no substitute for RICE, followed by a gradual return to the sport with a new and proper technique.

SKIING

What fascinates me most about skiing is that so many novice skiers seem to be injured the first time they ever participate in the sport and that even many experienced skiers get injured the first or second time they resume skiing that season.

Skiing is no different from any other sport. You must prepare yourself for this sport just as you would for any other. Do all the appropriate preseason muscle preparation and stretching that you know you should. Just as important, use the best equipment you can afford. A binding that doesn't give when it should is a guarantee of a severe injury.

And unfortunately, skiing injuries far too often involve severe tears to tissues in the knee that can only be repaired with surgery.

Surprisingly, the most frequently injured joint in skiing is the thumb. Always hold your poles properly, and try not to fall on an outstretched hand (try not to fall, period).

SWIMMING

Swimming is an excellent aerobic exercise with the advantage over running that it does not jar the joints. The main disadvantage is that you have to get wet, which is something that I am genetically programmed to hate. If a dry form of swimming is ever developed, I will be the first person to sign up.

Some research shows that swimming is not an effective way to lose weight, probably because swimming in cold water stimulates people to eat more to keep extra fat on their bodies for insulation. Have you ever seen a thin seal, I ask you?

The most common problem that interferes with freestyle swimming is a shoulder injury, either a bursitis or a tendonitis, or an impingement syndrome, in which some tissue in the shoulder is caught between the moving structures in the joint. These problems are invariably due to poor technique or overuse. They produce pain in the shoulder when the arm is swung through a specific arc. There is usually no pain at rest (except for some types of bursitis, which may hurt more when you lie on that side), and usually no pain through the first few degrees of arm swinging. But when the shoulder, which is a ball-and-socket joint, swings through the part of the arc (as the arm begins to swing overhead) that uses the inflamed tendon, or impinges on the inflamed bursa or other structures, the pain can be quite sharp and severe.

Treatment consists primarily of correcting the stroke that is causing the problem, and RICE (rice goes with everything). It's the same as for tennis elbow. Admit that you are not Mark Spitz. Pay for a lesson, or several. It will save you a lot of trauma in the end.

WALKING

We live down by the beach in Vancouver. What has been most noticeable about the shoreline over the last three or four years is the remarkable increase in the number of vigorous walkers there.

You can't take five steps without being passed by some gray-haired couple swinging their arms wildly and smiling a "Have a good day" at you. They actually look happy, compared with the often miserable-looking runners who frequent the same routes.

Walking is the fastest-growing participation sport in North America. According to all the experts, it is an excellent, nontraumatic way to get aerobic exercise.

Walking vigorously, as opposed to strolling, does burn a lot of calories. It taxes your heart in a positive way. And it seems to be virtually injury-free. For one thing, walkers do not land as hard as runners, and for another, they tend to be more sensible people than runners. Walking is a sociable sport. You *can* walk and talk at the same time. Walking is cheap. Walking can be done anywhere, on any surface. Walking takes no coaching, requires no clinics. The only problem with walkers as far as I can see is that they smile too damn much.

You can of course develop stress fractures and overuse injuries from walking, but these injuries are rare.

CHAPTER 10

The Skin

In which the dear reader will finally find out how deep beauty really goes, and if that doesn't satisfy you, then how you can change it, for a slight fee, of course

My son likes to ask his friends, "What's the largest organ in the body?" He's clearly not your average boyo, I must add. A very sick kid, I keep telling him in private. The answer, which always stumps his friends, who have very erotic (and misguided) ten-year-old imaginations, is the skin.

The skin is an organ that has the important job of protecting the other organs so that they can do their work. The skin is also important in the distribution of blood, the metabolism of vitamin D, the regulation of body heat, and the evaporation of some waste products. In short, our skin is not there just to make us look good.

In the last few years, as those of us born in the late forties and early fifties have slunk, not boomed, into middle age, the skin has become the focus of much more attention. That beautiful, glowing epidermis that all of us Greek gods and goddesses once possessed has begun to sag and droop and hang in places where it ought not to sag, droop, and hang (which just happens to be the name of my cut-rate clothing firm). Because we thirtysomethings and fortysomethings (will we be eightysomethings, I wonder?) tend to monopolize health expenditures and issues, a great deal of time and effort and dollars is being expended to discover cures, remedies, and stopgaps for these cosmetic concerns.

More important, those of us who once believed that it couldn't happen to us ("it" being skin cancer) are now carefully checking our outer layers periodically because it is happening to some of us. Or as Queen Victoria once put it, we are not immune.

HOW THE SYSTEM WORKS

Beauty is only skin deep, it's true, but that means that beauty goes much deeper than you think. What you see on top is only the outer layer of the skin, called the epidermis, which varies in depth in different areas of the body. Below the epidermis is the thicker dermal layer, and below that is the subcutaneous fat, the shock absorber of the skin. It may comfort you to know that even if your epidermis isn't perfect, below it lies a perfect dermis, which is, after all, the real you.

The skin contains glands that produce an oily secretion called sebum. These glands are very imaginatively called sebaceous glands. The skin also contains hair follicles, which are sort of sleeves for the hairs, as well as sweat glands.

The skin also contains cells that produce a darkish pigment called melanin, which colors the hair and the skin and helps block the damaging effects of ultraviolet light. Melanin concentrates in patches such as freckles, which are completely benign and which tend to darken in the summer and fade in the winter.

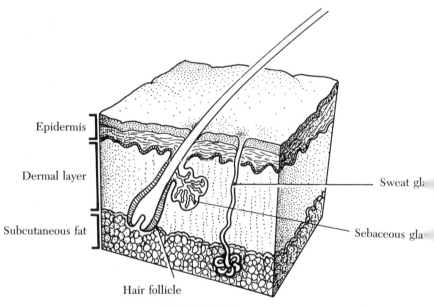

THE SKIN

HOW TO TAKE CARE OF YOUR SKIN

There are several things you can do to keep your skin smoother (or as Henri Richard used to say in Gillette commercials, "smooooder"), younger looking, and healthier.

Keep Your Skin Moist

One of the worst things we do to our skin is dry it excessively by washing too much, overusing soaps and cleansers, and overexposing ourselves to the sun. The best way to keep skin moist, as it should be, is to avoid the factors that dry it out. (See how hard it is to be a doctor?) If you don't need to wash your hands as often as you do, then don't. Protect your face from direct wind and sun. If you absolutely can't avoid such provocations to the epidermis, then always wear protective clothing, such as rubber gloves when you are washing dishes. (Always practice safe soap.) Greasy ointments may help, although most protective ointments for the hands are not very effective.

If you can't avoid excessive dryness, the next best thing is to moisturize the skin frequently. Most moisturizing creams are fairly effective at restoring some moisture to the skin, especially to the face. If you need medicated moisturizing agents, then creams containing lactic acid or urea are useful.

Bath oils work for mild dryness when the skin over the entire body is very dry.

Protect Yourself from the Sun

How can the sun harm thee? Let us count the ways. Sun exposure can burn the skin, cause wrinkles, promote pigmentary changes, decrease immunity to certain (perhaps all) viruses, especially herpes simplex, cause reactions if you are taking certain drugs concurrently (some antibiotics, Accutane, anticonvulsants, antidepressants, tranquilizers, and vitamin A cream, just to name a few of the more commonly used drugs), and of course promote both precancerous and cancerous changes in the skin.

To protect the skin from the sun, the best thing to do is not go out in the sun. Mad dogs and Englishmen . . . (Noel Coward was, among other closet personas, a closet dermatologist.) If you do have to expose yourself to the sun, wear a sunscreen with as high a protection factor as you need. The sun protection factor (SPF) is a measure of how well a sunscreen protects your skin from burning. The higher the SPF, the longer you can stay out in the sun without burning. The cream or lotion does not protect you forever; it merely delays the impact of the sun on your skin. If you stay in the sun long enough, your skin will still burn, even with ten layers of cream on. In Canada, the minimum SPF you need on a summer day is 15, although this may change if the hole in the ozone layer (a hot topic that is on everybody's lips) enlarges.

All creams and lotions rub off with sweat and dry with time, so they should be reapplied every few hours. Sunscreens also wash off in water, so if you swim, you will have to reapply some lotion after emerging from the water, no matter how much reassurance the manufacturer provides that its product is waterproof. Also bear in mind that PABA (para-aminobenzoic acid), the active ingredient in most sunscreens, stains cotton clothes. If you are allergic to PABA, there are several alternatives.

Protect Yourself from Chemicals

Chemical contact with skin can lead to problems that vary from mild irritation to severe burns. Even household chemicals can be toxic or cause dryness or induce contact irritations. Do not let any chemicals come into direct contact with your skin. When working with a chemical, you should always wear appropriate protection, such as gloves. This warning is particularly relevant for artists, who frequently take no precautions with the materials they work with, which can cause both respiratory and dermatological problems.

Don't Smoke, Watch Your Diet, and Exercise (Natter, Natter, Natter)

Don't smoke. Smoking ages skin prematurely, as you can see by examining any photo of the wrinkled Marlboro Man.

Although diet and exercise are not known to produce specific benefits to your skin, it just makes sense to eat properly and to exercise, if only because it keeps the rest of you in better shape. If you are in good shape, you won't worry as much about aging skin.

SKIN CHANGES WE ALL HATE

Wrinkles

Death and taxes are not the only things that are unavoidable. So are wrinkles (unless your name is Dick Clark). The skin naturally loses its elasticity as we age and bunches up in those nasty little wrinkles all of us baby boomers have begun to notice.

The surgical treatment of wrinkles is a medical growth industry. You can smooth 'em out; you can fill 'em in. You name it, some plastics specialist will do it for you (for a fee, naturally). The trouble is, I think, that no matter how much money you spend, you still end up looking like a sixty- or seventy-year-old, but one with shiny, smoother skin.

Until recently, we have had no effective cream or ointment that could delay this seemingly inevitable chain of events. Now, however, vitamin A acid cream is being promoted as a miracle wrinkle treatment. It seems to work mostly for those wrinkles produced by photodamage, or damage from the sun. Vitamin A acid cream can also remove "aging spots" (those darker patches of skin we all get as we age) and perhaps prevent certain types of skin cancers. If this proves true in larger, more extensive studies, and if there are no long-term negative effects, then run, don't walk, to buy shares in the companies that make the stuff.

When using vitamin A acid cream (which is only available by prescription), always start with a weak dosage (for most people, 0.01 percent is enough) and apply it once a day, preferably at night, until you adjust to it. You may then increase the strength of the prescription, as required, although you should not apply it more than twice a day. Remember to avoid excess exposure to the sun when taking this treatment.

Does it work? Well, you and I have seen miracle cures come and go before, Amanda, so let us not hold our collective breaths.

Spidery Veins (Telangiectasia)

These are those thin little blue-to-purple spidery veins that increase with age and with the overuse of cortisone creams. On the legs, they can be treated by injection with certain chemicals; on the face, by electric burning.

Varicose Veins

Strictly speaking, these have nothing to do with the skin, but where else could I include them?

If your mom or dad had varicose veins, then chances are you will. Varicose veins are superficial veins that have a diminished ability to return blood to the central circulation. Varicosities are worsened by anything that decreases blood return from the periphery, like prolonged standing at your job or pregnancy. They can cause pain but are usually asymptomatic. Clots can occur in a varicosity, causing a superficial inflammation of the vein called phlebitis, but this is not the serious life-threatening form that phlebitis takes in the deeper veins in the legs.

Some varicose veins can be injected with hardening solutions that close them off. Subsequently they shrink. Or they can be removed in that bloody procedure known as a vein stripping. It's actually a vein ripping, because that's what is done.

Sebaceous Cysts

When one of the sebaceous glands cannot empty its secretions, the gland swells. This swelling is known as a sebaceous cyst. The gland continues to swell until it stops producing sebum. Sebaceous cysts can reach the size of golf balls, but most of them are less than one centimeter in diameter. They are painless swellings unless they become infected, in which case they become suddenly tender and look inflamed.

Cysts are most prevalent in areas where there are many sebaceous glands (which is only logical, don't you think?), such as the scalp and face. They can shrink on their own, but most of the time if they are a cosmetic concern or if they repeatedly become infected, the only way to get rid of them is through surgery. They have a nasty habit of recurring, though.

Cellulite

Cellulite is one of those things, like a real Vancouver hockey team, that may or may not exist, depending on your point of view. The term is used to describe the bulging "orange peel" skin that some people seem to accumulate on the hips, thighs, and buttocks. We don't know what causes it and we don't know how to treat it, except with certain plastic surgery procedures. And no, Virginia, you can't exercise it off. It's the real you.

SKIN DISEASES

The Heartbreak of Zits (aka Acne)

Nearly every adult who seeks medical care for acne introduces the topic by saying "I don't understand it. I'm not fifteen anymore. Why am I still plagued by pimples on my face?"

Look around the next time you're at a beach, and without being too conspicuous (or you may get arrested), notice how many adults have acneiform eruptions on the face, chest, and upper back. You will likely notice that a lot of adults do, and the closer you look, the more acne pimples you'll see. Acne can go on well into middle age. It tends to die down in old middle age. (Is "old middle age" an oxymoron, like "the comedian Bob Hope"?)

Acne is a disease in which androgen hormones cause changes in the sebaceous glands of the skin. These changes include increased production of that oily secretion the sebum, and also excess shedding of cells inside the sebaceous gland. Both this increased "oily crap" (courtesy of a very articulate patient) and the increased cells in the gland itself make the sebaceous secretion thick, and it tends to block the gland. Bacteria in the skin then act on this thickened secretion, and depending on how much of the fluid is broken down to irritate the surrounding tissue, you can develop whiteheads, blackheads, or inflamed cysts and abscesses.

There are many factors that contribute to acne and some that just as certainly do not. The hormonal changes that accompany puberty lead to excessive circulation of androgen in both boys and girls. This we all know as the pimply phase of teenagehood. In some women acne can be aggravated by normal changes in the menstrual cycle. Drugs that can induce acne include birth control pills (although most pills actually improve acne), steroids, cortisone, and phenytoin (Dilantin). Hormonal diseases like polycystic ovary disease can also cause acne. Stress is a definite acne promoter in some individuals, as are many cosmetics.

Much to the chagrin of most mothers, acne is *not* promoted by eating greasy or sugary foods, or chocolate. If diet does aggravate acne, this effect varies from individual to individual. So if you notice, for example, that artichoke and bologna sandwiches make you break out, then avoid them (which is good advice even if they don't give you acne). Likewise, acne is not caused by dirty skin.

The way to treat acne is to somehow unblock those plugged glands. Exposure to the sun is generally helpful. But remember that excess exposure to the sun can produce certain reactions if you are taking some acne therapies, such as Accutane, concurrently. In mild cases, just washing the skin can unplug those glands that are lightly plugged. Many OTC lotions, gels, and creams are quite effective for mild cases of acne. The best known of these is benzoyl peroxide, which comes in varying strengths.

No matter which self-therapy you choose, always start with low doses to see how you will react and then slowly increase both the frequency of use and the dose until you get the desired effect.

The most widely used prescription creams and lotions are either antibiotic preparations like clindamycin or erythromycin, or vitamin A acid cream, which has recently become the stuff of folklore (see above). If you are using both benzoyl peroxide and vitamin A acid cream, they should be applied at opposite ends of the day because of possible interactions.

Again, it is always wise to increase the dose of these medications slowly and to be patient because these creams, when overapplied, can all irritate the skin and cause it to dry and turn red. Better to camouflage the pimples with the judicious use of makeup than to increase the dose of anti-acne medication too quickly. (Of course a man using makeup should be somewhat cautious about where he is seen.)

More resistant cases, especially those that result in inflamed cysts or outbreaks in areas where it is hard to apply lotions, are usually treated with an oral antibiotic, the most common one being tetracycline. Some types of tetracycline are more effective in some patients than other types, so it's worth experimenting with the various forms of this drug.

Once tetracycline has worked — and this often takes four to eight weeks — you can decrease the dose to the lowest dose that still suppresses the acne cysts. Many people have to continue tetracycline therapy for years. Although it is considered safe even in these large quantities over a long period, you should always ask yourself whether or not using a drug over many years is worth the cosmetic improvement you may have achieved.

Tetracycline doesn't work in everyone. Thus, there is always a need for more effective medication, especially for the more severe forms of cystic acne. We have this now in the form of isoretinoin (Accutane). Accutane is very effective medication but comes with several very strong warnings. It can cause inflamed linings in various organs, most especially the liver, so it is prudent to have periodic liver function tests if you are on this medication. It can also minimally increase blood cholesterol levels. It can cause severe irritations with excessive exposure to the sun. Most important is that Accutane causes birth defects in over 25 percent of the women who take it while pregnant. Any woman of childbearing age who is on Accutane should insure that she doesn't get pregnant and should instantly report any abnormal period to a doctor.

Occasionally, for an isolated acne cyst or two, injecting the cyst with cortisone can decrease the inflammation. The injection must be done carefully to insure that the skin over the lesion doesn't thin, or atrophy.

For the more resistant cases, especially those in whom scarring has occurred, dermatological surgery can be of some benefit.

Dermatitis

Dermatitis is an irritative condition of the skin that can be due to many causes. Contributing factors include allergies, stress, fungi, certain irritants, medications, wetness, and foods. Depending on the irritating factors or the appearance of the lesions, each type of dermatitis has a separate name. Thus, we have neurodermatitis (caused by stress), atopic dermatitis (a genetic form), contact dermatitis (this is obvious), nummular dermatitis (appearing as round patches), and so on. The term "eczema" is often used interchangeably with the term "dermatitis," although strictly speaking "eczema" should be reserved for atopic dermatitis only.

There really is not a single picture to give of these lesions. The skin can flare up with an irritation that varies from a small, round patch that is slightly red and barely noticeable to irritated, weepy, crusting lesions that cover extensive parts of the body. Some forms of dermatitis, like that caused by contact with poison ivy, can produce fluid-filled blisters. Itching, which is often very intense, is a prominent symptom of most types of dermatitis. Itching can be present even without any obvious lesions on the skin. When dermatitis has been present for some time, and when the patient has scratched the lesions excessively, the skin in that area often thickens.

The reasons that all dermatitic lesions can be lumped together in one section in this book are that first, they all have the same pathological profile, and second, all forms of dermatitis are treated in much the same way.

It is important to try to identify the causes of a dermatitic eruption. This is relatively easy if you have walked through a field and developed a rash along the parts of the body that were exposed to the foliage. It is considerably more difficult if there is no obvious precipitating event, since the cause is often what we call multifactorial, which does not mean many factories but rather that many factors have to combine to cause the symptoms. Thus, the person may have a food sensitivity that by itself may not produce dermatitis. But in the presence of stress, on a Tuesday, with the moon in Capricorn, after sweating, the food sensitivity may make the dermatitis flare up. (One of my dermatologist friends told me that there are people who will actually take this seriously. I hope they don't come to see me.) Often the patient can identify an aggravating influence better than the doctor can, through the tested formula of trial and error. "Every time I wear that nickel bracelet, I get a rash, doc." "Hey, man, stop wearing the bracelet. Next."

Despite this multifactorial aspect, we do know some of the common agents that cause specific forms of dermatitis. Contact dermatitis is often caused by soaps, cosmetics, drugs such as neomycin and thimersol, which is present in eye drops, jewelry, especially that made of nickel, which includes all costume jewelry, preservatives containing formalin, coins with nickel in them, adhesives, and plants like poison oak and poison ivy. Textile contact dermatitis is caused by certain formaldehyde resins used to make crease-resistant finishes in clothes.

Allergic dermatitis usually occurs in a person who has other allergic symptoms, like asthma or rhinitis. In children, foods that most commonly cause dermatitis include dairy products, corn, wheat-based foods, shellfish, and citrus fruits. In adults with atopic dermatitis, it is usually futile to try to isolate a food-based cause, although everyone does try.

Neurodermatitis is often an easy diagnosis to make in the office, even before the patient undresses, because the obviously tense patient keeps rubbing body parts while sitting there. Often the doctor starts scratching too when confronted with a scratching patient. Neurodermatitic lesions generally occur as thick, itchy areas on the ankles or shins, the arms and wrists, and the neck. The sun can also produce a photosensitive dermatitis in persons who ingest certain products, especially medications.

Seborrheic dermatitis usually appears as a scaly, reddened, patchy eruption in the areas where there are a lot of sebaceous glands. These include the scalp (where seborrhea is partly responsible for that plague of all dark-suited persons — dandruff), the face, behind the ears, and parts of the torso. It now seems that seborrheic dermatitis is often caused by a skin fungus. As a result, appropriate antibiotics should insure that it doesn't recur too easily.

The hands are especially prone to recurrent bouts of dermatitis that vary from tiny blisterlike swellings between the fingers to very raw, fissured skin all over the hands. This is invariably worsened by frequent washing (dishpan hands) and is often aggravated by a concomitant fungal infection. It is imperative that people with this problem keep their hands as dry as possible (and if enough people cure their problem we'll stop seeing those awful ads with Madge promoting Palmolive soap).

All types of dermatitis should be treated, as usual, by avoiding the known precipitating causes to the extent that you can. This advice reads like a Little League tract on good behavior. Avoid stress. Do not let plant poisons contact your skin. Do not work with chemicals to which you are sensitive. Do not wear jewelry made of materials to which you react. Avoid eating foods that make the dermatitis flare up. Avoid excessive moisture to the skin, particularly to the hands. Don't bunt with two strikes, and never throw behind the runner. Don't worry. Be happy.

If none of this works, the next best thing is to take medication. The most effective medication is topical cortisone cream or ointment, which decreases the inflammation and stops the itching. But when the cortisone is stopped, the condition often recurs.

The use of topical cortisone should always come with precautions attached. When overused, cortisone can thin the skin and produce those tiny little purple blood vessels that everyone hates, as well as reddened skin and stretch marks. This thinning effect is particularly evident on the face, where cortisone should always be applied sparingly and only if absolutely necessary.

Cortisone applied to the skin is also absorbed into the bloodstream. Too much absorption of cortisone can (rarely) inhibit your body from producing its own necessary supply of cortisone.

Topical cortisone comes in many types and strengths. The most potent forms are known as fluorinated cortisones. You should always use the weakest cortisone, in the weakest dosage that will do the trick. And do not reapply the cream every time the condition flares up. In very recurrent conditions, it is important to tolerate a certain amount of ineradicable disease.

Psoriasis

Psoriasis is a disease in which the rate of new skin formation is greatly accelerated, resulting in "silver" patches of thickened, scaly skin that are found predominantly on the elbows, knees, scalp, and back. A quick test to see if you have psoriasis as opposed to other, similar-looking conditions is to scrape one of the scales. If it is a psoriatic scale, you should see some bleeding spots after you scrape it.

We are not at all sure about what produces flare-ups of psoriasis, but as usual, many psoriatics can point to some stressful or dietary provocation.

Psoriasis is on the whole a treatable disease. It is often improved by the ultraviolet rays from sunlight. Cortisone creams and anti-inflammatory creams with sulfur and other compounds can be very effective. For more widespread disease, anthralin in various forms, or a form of untraviolet-light therapy under special lamps, often improves the condition.

Up to 5 percent of psoriatic patients develop psoriatic arthritis, most commonly in the joints of the fingers. This is treated with the usual arthritic medications and therapies.

SKIN INFECTIONS

Fungal Infections

The best way to think of fungal skin infections is to divide them into those that are most common in warm, moist areas of the body and those that occur elsewhere.

In the groin, a fungal infection usually has a distinct border that is often slightly raised and darker than the middle of the lesion and usually itches a lot. Some fungal infections caused by candida also have satellite lesions, small, discrete islands that are separate from the main body of infection. These infections can be spread by sharing towels and clothing. They are also worsened by friction, so they are more common in overweight people who rub their thighs against each other and in athletes who do the same.

Between the toes, athlete's foot manifests itself by cracks in the skin, which has a scaly, irritated appearance. The infection often extends to the soles of the feet, where it tends to show up as little irritated blisters that run together, or as a dry, silvery irritation that is called a moccasin-foot infection. The latter often resembles a type of dermatitis, and it is not unusual to confuse the two. Athlete's foot is often very itchy. The same fungus that causes athlete's foot causes a similar infection of the fingers and hands, especially at the border of the nail to the finger.

For infections in areas like the groin and between the toes, the best prevention and therapy is to keep the areas as dry as possible. Wear clothing that permits the sweat to evaporate. (Often wearing no clothing is the best answer, although you must be careful about where you do this.) Powders can be useful to help keep some areas dry. A good drying method after a shower is to gently blow-dry the infected area, although if you are blow-drying your groin, you'd better have a good story ready should anyone wander over to ask you what it is you are doing.

OTC antifungal preparations are available as powders and creams (tolnaftate, or Tinactin; undercyclenic acid, or Desenex). These often have to be applied for a long time before they work.

Ringworm is a common fungal infection that can occur anywhere on the body. It is often caught from an infected animal, so always inspect old Fido carefully after you have been diagnosed with ringworm. If it ain't Fido, better check your mate. Ringworm on the torso occurs as a round to oval lesion with a distinct red raised border and a paler center. On the scalp, it looks like a round area of hair loss. On Rex, ringworm occurs as a patchy area of hair loss (which is not like the patchy area of hair loss that is occurring over the entire patch of my scalp).

Tinea versicolor is a unique infection of small oval to round lesions that fail to tan. They usually cover the upper torso and the arms and are most noticeable in the summer, when the rest of the skin tans. They often look like darker patches in the winter. For tinea versicolor, a good treatment is to use Selsun shampoo (with selenium) applied three times a day to the upper torso and arms, or left on overnight (ugh!). This should be done for at least a week, and then you should wait until the next tanning season to witness the effect.

The most common fungal infection of the nail is known as onychomycosis. That's that ugly thickened nail, usually on the big toe, that so many of us will get as we age.

Topical therapy for onychomycosis is still not available, although it's in the pipeline, as they say. Currently, despite the claims of the drug companies that promise quicker cures, you must take some sort of oral antifungal medication for at least six months and often much longer to get rid of that ugly nail.

When fungal lesions are persistent, as most invariably are, you will require prescription antifungal medications, usually in the form of topical creams.

Viral Infections

HERPES SIMPLEX

Herpes simplex infections around the mouth and gums produce cold sores (see chapter 13). The great majority of North Americans have antibodies to the herpes virus in their bloodstreams, indicating that they have been exposed to this virus at one time in their lives. Yet few of us can actually recall having had a cold sore. This means simply that many people have a transient herpetic infection when they are still very young. This mild infection may be barely noticeable and only last a few days, but it means that they harbor the virus for the rest of their lives. Although most people have one infection and never have another, once you've had any herpetic infection, it can come back at any time. Flare-ups are especially associated with stress, exposure to sun, and the presence of other illnesses.

For about 10 percent of patients, a herpetic sore announces its imminent return by producing a numbness or tingling sensation just before it erupts. In these cases, you may be able to apply a solution of idoxuridine (Herplex-D Liquafilm, Stoxil) as soon as you feel the tingling and thereby avert the infection. You have to apply it every two or three hours for best results. The only other effective therapy is oral acyclovir (see chapter 13).

Herpes infections are transmittable to any close contact, especially a sexual contact. When an oral herpes infection is transmitted to the genital area, it acts exactly like the venereal form of herpes in its new locale.

SHINGLES (HERPES ZOSTER)

Shingles (now often known by the single name of zoster) is a reactivation of an old chicken pox infection. Although the first name of this virus is herpes, it has nothing to do with its more notorious cousin herpes simplex.

Shingles usually comes on suddenly as a painful, wet eruption along a very specific distribution on one side of the body, rarely crossing the midline. The wet lesions usually dry and crust in a few days. Interestingly, significant pain often precedes the infection by as much as two days.

The new treatment developed for herpes simplex, acyclovir, seems to be effective in some cases of zoster as well, but it has to be given early and in very high doses. No currently available cream is effective at relieving the very intense pain that sometimes accompanies this infection or at shortening the course of the illness.

A zoster outbreak on the face should always be monitored by a doctor because it can lead to blindness if it invades the eye.

Most people recover in two to three weeks, but a significant percentage of people complain of persistent discomfort for many months afterwards.

PITYRIASIS ROSEA

Pityriasis rosea is a skin disease that every doctor has misdiagnosed at one time or another.

Pityriasis rosea occurs as a number of oval, small pale lesions over the torso and upper arms and legs, which may or may not be itchy. These lesions are often preceded by one very large, ringwormlike lesion, called a herald patch (herald, not Harold, who appears elsewhere in this book). This patch is often misdiagnosed as ringworm, and the patient is given a prescription for an antifungal cream, which doesn't work. Pityriasis rosea acts much like a viral infection in that it tends to occur in the spring and fall, when many viruses wake from winter hibernation or summer slumber, it tends to last for four to six weeks, and it departs without any treatment. But it is clearly not very catchy, because most people exposed to someone with this problem will not get it.

Treatment: relax. This too will pass, although it can last several months.

WARTS

Warts are caused by viruses. There are several different kinds, including the garden variety or common warts and the pearly molluscum contagiosum. Common warts include the slender skin tags commonly seen on the face and neck, plantar warts on the bottoms of the feet, palmar warts on the fingers and hands, and venereal warts. (For more on venereal warts, see chapter 13.) Molluscum contagiosum are small, pearly lesions that have a tendency to appear in bunches, especially in the pubic area.

The most frustrating aspect of warts is that they can incubate on your body without evident symptoms for years. So even when therapy seems successful for any individual wart, there may be others lurking, ready to erupt as soon as you become complacent. You should always use appropriate protection when exposed to warts because all warts are catchy, although many people seem to be quite resistant to them.

In theory, you don't need to treat your warts (except for venereal warts, which should always be treated). Because warts are viruses, your body should eventually develop antibodies to them, which will cause the warts to disappear. According to the experts, over 60 percent of warts disappear without treatment within two years. But try telling that to the person who thinks that the entire world is staring at her warts. This woman wants her warts gone, yesterday.

Warts can be treated in several ways. Solutions such as salicylic acid and lactic acid have to be applied frequently and carefully.

Because there are many layers of skin through which the wart is growing, in most areas the skin over the wart should be thinned by paring with a blunt knife. This is especially important in areas where the skin is thick, such as the bottoms of the feet.

Warts can also be treated with freezing therapy, known as cryotherapy. This is most often done with liquid nitrogen. Warts can be surgically removed, and they can also be treated with lasers. But no matter what therapy is chosen, all warts can recur. And always beware the incubating wart.

Plantar warts especially should *not* be treated unless they are spreading, or unless they hurt. The reason for caution with these warts is that frequently the treatment hurts more than the wart. Most cases of molluscum contagiosum also do not need treatment, since most of these lesions disappear within one year. If the molluscum occur on the inner thigh, however, it is advisable to treat them because these warts seem to be particularly contagious. Even if you don't care about them, your partner likely will (your bedmate, that is, not your business partner).

Bacterial Infections (The Plagues of Boils, Impetigo, and Cellulitis)

Bacterial infections of the skin are usually caused by a strain of either *Staphylococcus* or *Streptococcus* and often by both. This type of infection can take several forms.

A crusty, wet type of bacterial infection, most common around the mouth, especially in little kids, is called impetigo. In theory, you should scrape the crust off an impetiginous lesion so that a topical antibiotic cream or lotion will penetrate better. I dare you to try that on Rambo. It hurts. Instead of scraping the lesions, you may choose to just soak them with warm water and see if the crust will separate on its own. When it does, you can apply an antibiotic cream such as mupirocin (Bactroban), which is able to penetrate the crust somewhat. Or you can wash with chlorhexidine (Hibitane), but you often have to dilute the strength of the solution. If the lesions are not clearing, then oral antibiotics will work well.

A superficial but serious spreading infection of the skin is known as cellulitis. It usually follows some minor injury like a sting or bite and shows up as a hot, red, swollen area, just under the skin, that spreads rapidly. For cellulitis, you must use an appropriate antibiotic. You should also try to keep your weight off the infected area to keep the swelling down. Treat this infection seriously because it can spread rapidly.

A superficial infection centered in the hair follicles of the skin is called folliculitis. When the infection extends into the subcutaneous tissue, it is known as furunculosis. When several furuncules, or lesions, coalesce, a small abscess may result. The lesions are reddened inflamed areas, or boils, in the hairy parts of the skin, especially the scalp and back. Individual inflamed cysts or follicles occur most frequently on the nose and on the eyelids. In the latter location, they are called styes.

Do not squeeze pimples, boils, or styes, no matter how tempted you are.

I put that into its own paragraph because an amazing number of people know they shouldn't squeeze these lesions, but they do anyway. Perhaps if they read it in a separate paragraph, they will recall this advice more easily.

Soak all styes and boils to bring them to a head so that they will rupture through the surface of the skin rather than spread inward. Use warm water. Add salt to the water if you like (to taste). All abscesses that do not clear quickly should be lanced. Antibiotics are often required for these infections. Red swollen "lines" extending out from an infected area mean that the infection is spreading along the lymph channels that are present all over the body. These lymph channels can spread the infection to all the internal organs (a similar infection killed Norman Bethune). This is a lymphangitis, and it requires prompt medical attention, as it must be treated with antibiotics. Occasionally lymphangitis requires hospitalization.

Some people get recurrent boils because the staph bacteria that cause the boils like these people and love to inhabit enclaves on their bodies, in what you can think of as staph condos, and from where the bacteria tend to spread to other parts of the skin. To prevent recurrent boils, the best medication is a prescription antituberculosis drug, rifampicin (Rifampin). This drug must be taken with care because it tends to cause liver inflammation.

One other bacterial skin infection that is common and that responds particularly well to antibiotics is peri-oral dermatitis. This rash presents with small red spots around the mouth, which often extend into the folds near the nose. This rash is often treated with cortisone, but it responds better to tetracycline, given for about eight weeks.

Parasite Infections

LICE AND SCABIES (THE A TEAM)

These are the skin infections that people hate most, partly because the thought that your lovely epidermis is home to a colony of disgusting, homeless parasites is rather obnoxious, and partly because of the (erroneous) impression that only dirty people get them. But as a liberal thinker, don't you feel that everything needs a shelter, and aren't you comforted even partly by the fact that you are now that shelter? No matter. I can at least reassure you that a parasite infection does not mean that you are unhygienic. It just means that you were unlucky enough to be exposed to these little bugs, no matter how clean you are.

Parasite infections of the skin include pubic lice, head or body lice, and scabies. Pubic lice are also called crabs, and these are dealt with in the chapter on STDs (chapter 13.)

Head lice are usually transmitted through shared brushes and combs. Body lice are transmitted through shared clothes or bedding. These little creatures live off your body by biting your skin and ingesting the blood (a ghoulish, not goulash, thought). Lice cause itching in two ways. First, the bite on the skin itches. Second, they leave "louse droppings" behind in the puncture wound, what has been delicately referred to by several patients as crab shit. Both head and body lice lay eggs, or nits, that attach themselves near the base of hairs.

Scabies is a parasite that burrows under the surface of the skin. The infection is usually recognized as small, discrete, very itchy red lesions that gradually increase in number. The classical sign of a scabies infection is two very itchy red spots connected by a track, caused by the parasite's burrowing in one end and leaving by the other end — sort of a commuter tunnel for the bug. The lesions are often said to start on the wrists or arms but in truth, they can start on any body part. They are very common in the pubic area, particularly on the penis. No self-respecting scabies bug would be caught dead on the face, so scabies infections are rare above the neck.

The therapy of choice for both lice and scabies is lindane (Kwellada). Lindane must be used in the appropriate dosage because overuse can cause itching. The patient, thinking that the treatment hasn't worked, will apply more lindane, resulting in even more itching, which will result in even more application of lindane, and so on. Get the picture?

It is very common to itch for a few weeks after a treatment for scabies has been effective. Do not apply more lindane. There are creams such as crotamiton (Eurax) that can work on small areas where you are convinced that your strong-arm tactics haven't evicted every last scabetic tennant.

Your clothes and bedding must be treated as well. Regular washing at very high temperatures of all clothes, towels, and sheets used over the preceding week usually suffices.

If the lesions keep recurring, however, you must carefully examine the reasons for reexposure, which may include inadequate sterilization of clothing. Also check your partner. Even if he or she has only one or two not very itchy lesions, they may be the source of your infection.

With lice, you must nitpick. And remember that lice will inhabit any body hair. So you have to carefully examine chest hair, armpits (hold your nose), eyebrows, and even that thin hairline that extends up from the pubis to the belly button. A good way of getting rid of nits on the eyebrows is to suffocate the devils by applying a thick cover of petrolatum jelly.

Lyme Disease

You can't pick up a magazine without being scared to death by the prospect of getting (Horrors!) Lyme disease. Lyme disease (not to be confused with that illness that affects certain persons who order even a glass of water with a twist of some citrus fruit) is named after Lyme, Connecticut, the town in which many cases were first recognized. Lyme disease is an infection caused by a bacteria called *Borrelia burgdorferi*, which inhabits the body of a little parasite called a deer tick. Deer ticks do live on deer, but they also live on many other small mammals, including field mice. Anyone walking through the woods where the deer tick live can be the next meal ticket for the tick (a tick ticket in the thicket, so to speak).

Lyme disease has three stages. The first stage occurs within a few days of the bite, when a flulike illness appears, accompanied in 50 percent of people by a characteristic rash called a bull's eye or target rash. This rash consists of a series of alternating reddish and pale circles that radiate out from a center, where the bite occurred. Treatment is most successful in the first stage. Either penicillin or preferably tetracycline can kill the bacteria and prevent further complications.

If Lyme disease goes unrecognized, or if treatment is unsuccessful, from a few weeks to a few months later the disease enters the short second stage, which involves cardiac or neurologic complications, such as a temporary facial paralysis, heartbeat irregularities, double vision, profound fatigue, or difficulty with concentration and speech. Most people recover fully from these complications.

In the third stage, Lyme disease causes arthritis (and perhaps some neurologic complications). This condition can be permanent.

There is no really good blood test for Lyme disease as yet. Diagnosis depends mostly on a high index of suspicion and an ability to recognize the typical rash.

Prevention is the key to this problem. If you go out in the woods today, tralalala, cover as much of you as you comfortably can. When you get back from your excursion, lalala, check yourself for the presence of bites or ticks. The ticks, like picky diners choosing the perfect place to eat, will frequently walk over a good part of you before they bite. So you can occasionally discover a tick that has not yet supped upon thee.

The animal that should be most carefully checked is the family hound, that treader in all parts woody (although how you check a thick-coated husky like mine, even if she'll let you, is beyond me). Insect repellents containing DEET (such as Off!) are also useful (although I well remember my first and only trip to Algonquin Park, and how the mosquitoes and blackflies considered the insect repellent simply delicious).

SKIN CANCERS

Luckily, skin cancers in adults under fifty are still rare. That's the good news. The bad news is that their rate is increasing rapidly, and it is likely that we will see many more cancers, particularly malignant melanomas, in adults under fifty in the near future.

There are three main types of malignant skin tumor. These include basal cell carcinomas, squamous cell carcinomas, and malignant melanomas. But only the dreaded malignant melanoma occurs with any frequency in the fifteen-to-fifty-year-old.

A malignant melanoma is a melanin-producing cell that has become malignant. The malignancy spreads rapidly and has a very poor prognosis if treatment is delayed.

A malignant melanoma is most commonly thought of as a black spot that suddenly appears on the skin and begins to enlarge, or as a mole that suddenly turns much darker and likewise begins to expand. In truth, a melanoma can be any color, even colorless on rare occasions (which ought to keep everyone up for several nights figuring out how you can spot a colorless growth on your skin). They are most common in people who have fair skin, and especially those who had repeated severe sunburns in childhood. Indeed, there is a study that shows that every severe burn in childhood raises the risk of melanoma by 10 percent (so if your parents sent you out to play in the sunshine, which all kids instinctively know is bad for them, when all you wanted to do was prevent future melanomas by watching television indoors all summer long, you now have another reason to sue your parents.). Melanomas occur most frequently on sun-exposed areas of the skin. They are *not* related to freckles.

Any lesion on the skin that is enlarging or has changed color or texture (crusts, ulcerates, raises up) or has begun to itch (which all your spots will be doing while you read this chapter) or has begun to bleed should be quickly evaluated by someone proficient at this type of inspection.

There is much emphasis these days on removing certain moles

prophylactically because it has been noted that certain moles, those known as dysplastic nevi, have a greater tendency to become malignant. These generally include the larger moles, on sun-exposed areas, with irregular borders or with irregular consistency of color within the mole. We usually tell people to inspect their moles using an ABCD guide. A stands for asymmetry, B for irregular border, C for irregular color, and D for a diameter greater than six to eight millimeters (so tonight the ruler will no doubt be in full use in your household).

The current feeling is that these should all be removed prophylactically (which doesn't mean that the surgeon is wearing a condom), even if you have thirty or forty of them.

HAIR PROBLEMS

Male-Pattern Baldness (I Used to Look So Young)

Baldness, believe it or not, can be a matter of dispute. (Something I tell my wife every time she points out my rapidly retreating hairline. I'm not balding. I just like my hair short.) Baldness is in the eyes of the hair counter, so what can look like a good treatment result in the eyes of the executive of the company selling a baldness cure may not look like such a good result in the eyes of an aging, insecure male.

Yes, minoxidil (Rogaine) does work. But alas, it doesn't work as well as the early reports would have it. Minoxidil probably works well for 10 to 20 percent of the men taking it, and somewhat for about another 20 to 30 percent. The rest are doomed to look like me. (There are compensations. You shower more quickly, you don't have to spend as much money on new hairbrushes or blow-dryers or haircuts, and best of all, you don't have to worry about whether or not you will eventually be bald, because you already know.)

Minoxidil does have some drawbacks, not the least of which is that it is expensive. It also takes a few months to judge whether or not it will work. It must be applied continuously because if you stop, the new hairs will fall out. It works best on newly bald areas. Because minoxidil in its other life was developed as an antihypertensive, there have been worries about potential heart damage from this product. Currently, however, it's believed that this product is safe for everyone.

All other baldness treatments work slightly for some men, but none work universally, or even for a majority of males. Save your money and adapt. You're still beautiful, just bald.

Hair Loss

Occasionally some people, especially women, lose significant amounts of hair from all areas of the scalp: "Every time I shower, the tub is full of loose hairs." (Not showering is not the solution, by the way.) Although stress is commonly said to be a strong contributing factor, the evidence for this is slim. Other, proven contributing causes include pregnancy and the postpartum period, surgery, and high fever.

Occasionally, the loss of hair occurs in distinct patches, which can sometimes involve the entire skull. This condition is called alopecia areata. The hair generally regrows completely, which is why these people are often used as the miracle "before and after" patients in ads for hair restorers. Hey, send me a few dollars, and I'll pray for you, and I guarantee that if you are suffering from alopecia areata, your hair will regrow like new. Money refunded if you're not happy. Write me in Rio. Hair loss from alopecia areata unfortunately tends to recur.

Occasionally, hair loss can also be due to scalp infections or to other metabolic conditions, such as thyroid disorders.

Shampoos for Hair Problems

All shampoos are the same, except for those that aren't. So unless you are one of those rare people who really needs a medicated shampoo, when you are spending extra dollars for shampoos that theoretically protect your hair from God knows what horrible hair problems, you are basically wasting your money.

Medicated shampoos are different in that they contain sulfur or tar or some other product that lessens the inflammation of the scalp that can accompany conditions such as seborrheic dermatitis. But most people do not have an inflamed scalp and really don't need medication in their shampoo.

Hirsutism

Hirsutism is excessive hair growth in a male pattern (so obviously this should only be a noticeable problem in women). The hormones that cause hirsutism are known as androgens. Most cases of hirsutism are due to excess androgens from the ovaries, but the adrenal glands can also be the source of this problem.

The excess hair growth is usually most evident on the face, especially the upper lip and the sideburn and beard areas. Excessive growth may also occur around the nipples, on the abdomen, and in the pubic hair, which tends to extend upwards in a male pattern. Many women with hirsutism also suffer from anovulation, or absence of periods, as well as acne. A woman who develops new, excessive hair growth should always be checked for gynecological and other metabolic abnormalities.

Besides treating the underlying cause, there are other things you can do to camouflage excess hair. You can bleach it, shave it, wax it, pluck and pull it. You can also use chemical treatments and electrolysis. Plucking hair is only a temporary solution because it doesn't remove the root, so the hair regrows. Bleaching with 6 percent hydrogen peroxide works until the hair grows out. With electrolysis, you do destroy the root, but it can occasionally result in scarring.

MISCELLANEOUS SKIN PROBLEMS

Itching (aka Pruritis)

Itching can be caused by diseases that affect only the skin or by diseases in other systems that also cause itching. The first group includes dry skin, fungal infections, various kinds of dermatitis, hives, parasite infections, and bites, for example. In the second group, liver diseases, kidney diseases, thyroid disorders, anemias, and lymph-omas, or tumors of the lymph glands, are also well known to cause itching.

In addition, there may be absolutely no pathological reason for the itching. This has been called psychogenic itching (which is what happens to me every time I have to assist at an operation). Obviously treatment should be geared to eliminating the cause when possible. Keep your skin from drying out and avoid excess bathing, which tends to make the problem worse. Use only mild, preferably nonallergenic soaps.

When you have to treat the itching because it is driving you nuts, be cautious about what you apply because some ingredients in anti-itch lotions can make the problem worse. This is true even for home remedies and especially for topical anesthetics. Otherwise, strong antihistamines, of which hydroxyzine (Atarax) is most commonly used, are effective, probably mostly because they have a sedating effect.

Corns and Calluses

Corns and calluses are thickened pads of skin that are produced by repeated pressure on that area of skin. They are especially common on the bottoms of the feet. Corns have sharp borders; calluses don't — but since both are treated the same way, who cares? Treat them by redistributing the pressure away from them with appropriate inserts in your shoes or by changing shoes. Also, debride (take de bride off) the lesion either surgically (with a blunt knife) or with some kind of softening chemical.

Pigment Changes

There are three common types of pigment changes in the skin. Vitiligo is the loss of pigment-producing cells, resulting in white patches (you *can* be too white). This usually occurs for no apparent reason in younger patients (under twenty) and is often permanent. There are not many successful therapies (except for camouflage). Ultraviolet-light therapy is used for the more severe cases.

Postinflammatory discoloration is, not too surprisingly, the name given to brownish (occasionally other hues) patches that occur after some inflammation in the skin. These often fade with time.

Chloasma is excess patchy, pigmentary changes on the face, and it occurs principally in women who are on birth control pills, are pregnant, or are on steroids. Get rid of the cause, and the color reverts to normal.

Hives

Many cases of hives are due to allergies, but they can also be caused by stress, exposure to cold, infections, bites, drugs, and exercise. Then there is that old favorite, the idiopathic hive, which means we don't know why it occurs. When foods are to blame, the common sources include berries, nuts, shellfish, fish, eggs, chocolate, dairy products, and food additives. In those people who are easily prone to hives, ASA is notorious for producing them. Each hive lasts about twenty-four to forty-eight hours, but frequently new ones start forming while the old ones are fading. The most disturbing aspect of hives is that they itch.

Most hives are caused by the release of histamine, which means that antihistamines in appropriate doses should stop the reaction as well as relieve the itch.

Dermographism

This is a weird one. There are people who, if you put pressure on their skin with something like a scratch, will develop a hivelike reaction along the scratch line. You can literally make the hives appear as letters or numbers. In other words, it looks as if you can write on the skin. Because the hives are due to the release of histamine, suggested treatment is to use an antihistamine, but only if the condition bothers you. (You can also print messages on your skin, a practice that would be useful at final exam time, except that you would look rather strange lifting your shirt every few minutes to look for an answer.)

Bites and Stings, Stings and Bites

Bites are usually easy to recognize, although occasionally the patient resists the diagnosis if he or she can't remember having been bitten. There are insects, especially spiders and (ugh) bedbugs, that bite at night, when presumably you are less able to identify the little buggers. Bites often appear in several bunches in one area, in what is called the breakfast, lunch, dinner, and dessert pattern. Bites can become infected, so clean the area well if it looks as if the bite is becoming more inflamed.

Stings can lead to anaphylactic reactions (see chapter 4), but this is rare. To treat a sting, make sure the stinger is gone. Trample the insect to get rid of your anger. And then go and ice the area around the sting.

Nail Abnormalities

Brittle nails are extremely common. They occur more in people who keep their hands wet a lot and those who smoke. Guess what the recommended treatment is? Calcium and vitamins are a waste of money. Some people can keep the nail from breaking by applying nail polish, but avoid products that contain formalin.

Ingrown toenails are the stuff of legend. ("You think you had a bad ingrown nail? You shoulda seen the one . . . ") To prevent them, you will hear that you have to cut the nail straight across, but in people with very curved nails, this technique is rarely successful. Soaking the nail to soften it and pulling up on the edge, or inserting a small piece of cotton under the ingrowing edge, does lessen the chances of an infection.

People who bite their nails are particularly prone to developing a chronic inflammation at the edge of the nail. (Surprisingly, I have never seen anyone who developed this problem in a toenail.) It is much more common in people who also wet their hands frequently. The fungal infection usually responds to antifungal medication but recurs unless you stop doing what it is you do that keeps this area inflamed.

The side of the nail can also become acutely infected with a bacterial infection, which requires antibiotics and often minor surgical drainage.

The easiest pain relief to offer in this business is to that poor soul who has traumatized his or her finger and has a collection of blood under the fingernail. The blood produces intense, throbbing pain until it is either reabsorbed (which will take several days) or released, which will take one minute. You can do this procedure at home, with a little courage and a lot of cooperation from the chicken who is the injured party. Heat the end of a paper clip or other sharp, thin metal object until it is red hot. Then stick it through the nail. (Have a cloth handy to catch the spurting blood.) It won't hurt, honestly. Would I lie to you? And the pain relief will be instantaneous.

PLASTIC SURGERY

I am going to mention this topic briefly even though it has nothing to do with good or bad health, mainly because we get so many questions in the office about plastic surgery. I think you should look as good as you want to, so if you have the bucks and you can stand the risk (all surgery has risks, my dear), go right ahead and become that beautiful person you know you really are. I once referred a woman to have a microscopic lesion removed from her cheek because she had already seen three physicians who had refused her the referral. She was convinced that she couldn't get a better job unless this lesion, which to her looked as big as the moon, was removed. The surgeon, bless him, took it off (the lesion), and within weeks this lady had a new, better job. I cannot recall refusing any plastics referral since.

You can have practically any part tucked, plucked, or (lipo) sucked. Things can be made larger or smaller.

But I will reiterate that all tinkering has a potential cost.

CHAPTER 11

The Female

In which the good doctor thanks God for women because otherwise he'd be left taking care of only kids and men and would consequently look even older than he already does

Women are much better health consumers than men. (I was going to say that doctors prefer women, but that doesn't seem like a completely safe statement, so I'll stick with the other.)

Women are not afraid to approach a doctor to ask his or her opinion when something seems amiss. Unlike a man, who often pretends that he is not the least bit nervous about a symptom that is totally consuming his thoughts and who always insists that he is in the doctor's office only to satisfy his wife, a woman frequently arrives at the office with an apology, saying that she knows this symptom is not a major problem but that she wanted to check it out nonetheless.

In general, most women have learned their health lessons well. They do come in, no matter how reluctantly, for their routine Pap tests and pelvic and breast examinations. These visits also frequently serve as occasions to ask a question or two about a symptom that has been bothering them. On these routine visits, a good rapport is often set up between the patient and her physician, so she has less fear about coming to the office in the future, when perhaps the symptom is not routine and may even be a little embarrassing.

Women also have more health problems and concerns than men in those years between fifteen and fifty. The reason is that contraception problems (nearly exclusively) and complications from sexually transmitted diseases (STDs) tend to gather more on the doorstep of the female. And let us never forget that currently only women can get pregnant, with all the visits to doctors that that condition produces. Because the years between fifteen and fifty are times of generally good health for the population at large, birth control, STDs, pregnancies, and period changes account for a disproportionate number of visits to the doctor. Unless there are specific diseases or risk factors, men seldom have to see a doctor before the depths of middle age, and they seldom do.

Don't despair, ladies. God is pretty fair. The prostate is a great equalizer as the years slip by.

HOW THE SYSTEM WORKS

The female reproductive system can be divided into two regions, which are completely interrelated (the original free trade). One region is above the waist (in the brain, actually), and the other is below the waist. The breasts are like the forty-ninth parallel.

Female anatomy in the southern region is more complicated than it seems. Moving outwards, the anatomical parts of the female reproductive tract include the ovaries, fallopian tubes, uterus, cervix, vagina, and vulva (all of which may come as a surprise to those men who think that there are only two parts to the female reproductive tract).

The ovaries are often described as walnut sized. They contain thousands of eggs, most of which will never be released and which eventually disintegrate.

Those eggs that are released make their way into the fallopian tubes, which are two arms on either side of the top of the uterus. The ends of the fallopian tubes are composed of very thin tubular extensions, the fimbria, which pulsate and vibrate in a sort of samba-like dance to help them gather in an egg when it's released.

The uterus is often described as being pear shaped, with the thinner part pointing down. The uterus can be anteverted, which means that the bulky top end points forward and turns into the abdomen and can generally be felt through a normal pelvic examination. Or the uterus can be retroverted, which means that the top end turns backwards towards the rectum and cannot be felt in a normal pelvic exam, unless a rectal examination is done at the same time (something neither the doctor nor the patient volunteers for too often). The bladder sits directly on top of the uterus, which is why you need to urinate so

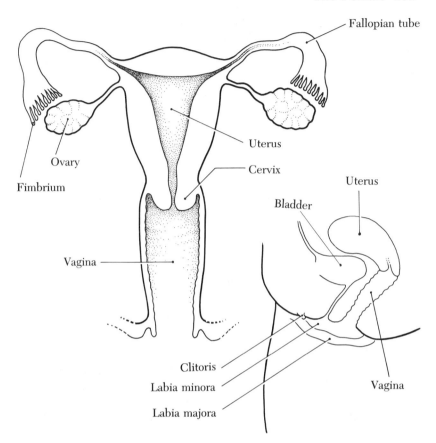

THE FEMALE REPRODUCTIVE SYSTEM

badly when the doctor is feeling for your uterus by pressing on your abdomen.

The cervix is the fibrous and muscular end of the uterus. The cervix has an opening to permit the passage of blood and sperm and, of course, the fetus during childbirth.

The vagina is a tube into which the cervix enters at the back. The vulva includes those exotically named parts, the labia majora and the labia minora. On either side of the vagina are the two Bartholin's glands, which supply secretions to the vagina. Above the vaginal opening, also known as the introitus, is the opening of the urethra, and above that is the hooded clitoris.

Now for the northern parts. The brain is the seat of the two glands that govern female hormone output, the hypothalamus gland and the pituitary gland. The hypothalamus is the real governor, while the pituitary is more like the lieutenant governor (sort of like the hypothalamus's gofer). The hypothalamus releases hormones that in turn stimulate the pituitary to release other hormones that start the ovaries into action.

THE FEMALE CYCLE

The easiest way to understand the female reproductive cycle is to start with the first day of a period and follow the changes through to the next period.

Right after a period begins, the pituitary increases the release of two hormones: FSH, or follicle-stimulating hormone, and LH or luteinizing hormone. FSH primes the ovary to prepare an egg for release from the ovarian penitentiary (or ovarian day care, or ovarian college, depending on what perspective one takes). At the same time, the ovary also starts to release the female hormone estrogen. Meanwhile, back at the ranch, the uterus starts to build up a thicker lining to make a home for its potential tenant, the fertilized egg. After about fourteen days (in a regular twenty-eight-day cycle), an egg is released from the surface of the ovary. At this point, much like *The French Lieutenant's Woman*, the story has two possible endings — the egg may be fertilized, or it may not.

Scenario number one: nothing happens.

If the egg is not fertilized, it will disintegrate within about twenty-four hours. Where does the egg go? It may pass through a fallopian tube and down the uterus, or it may just drop into the pelvic cavity. Meanwhile, the area on the ovary that released the egg forms a little structure called a corpus luteum, which starts to release the hormone progesterone. At the same time, the level of estrogen from the ovary begins to fall. The progesterone level gradually increases until two or three days before the next period, when it drops abruptly, while the corpus luteum degenerates. This sudden drop in the progesterone level prompts the uterus to shed its lining, producing the next period.

Scenario number two: a potential new person is formed.

If the egg is fertilized, it will travel for a week or so through a fallopian tube and then implant in the gradually thickening uterine lining. (Like any teenager, it wants to see the real world before beginning its new life.) Occasionally, like an accidental tourist, the fertilized egg may implant in the fallopian tubes (or other structures in the pelvis) to become an ectopic pregnancy.

When the egg implants, the tissue that connects the uterus to the egg becomes the placenta of the developing fetus. The placenta produces increasing amounts of progesterone, a process that continues well into the pregnancy.

Back to scenario one. (Like any good movie, this is a story that fades from present to future and back again.) A normal period varies from three to seven days. Often there is a day or two of spotting or light bleeding before the period starts. The amount of blood lost with a period varies from woman to woman, but it generally averages about 50 to 100 milliliters. (You can figure out how little that is the next time you have to measure out 100 milliliters of oil for a salad dressing.)

The length of a monthly cycle also varies a lot. Most women think that a "normal" cycle is twenty-eight days. This is true for those women who have a twenty-eight-day cycle. It is just as normal for some women to have a thirty-five-day cycle and for others to have a twenty-two-day cycle. In some women, the cycle normally varies a few days from month to month.

Ovulation occurs about fourteen days *before* the next period. In a twenty-eight-day cycle, this means that ovulation occurs in the middle of the cycle. But in a thirty-three-day cycle, ovulation usually occurs about nineteen days *after* the last menstrual period, which corresponds to fourteen days before the next bleed. Ovulation time is a lot like dinnertime in the Hister household in that it generally occurs at the same time, but it can also vary a lot (and it can be accompanied by discomfort). It doesn't have to happen exactly fourteen days before a period, which is one of the reasons that the rhythm method of birth control has such a high failure rate.

There are many other changes that occur regularly, but if you remember only the foregoing, that is sufficient information to help you understand the most common gynecological complaints. (And for all the male readers who have trouble distinguishing estrogen from progesterone and the cervix from an elbow, do not despair. I will repeat the important facts at the appropriate spots in the text, so you don't have to continually flip back and forth.)

VAGINAL DISCHARGE

It is normal to have some vaginal discharge. It is also normal for the discharge to be heavier at midcycle or just before a period. For some women, this change can be quite dramatic, but it still does not indicate any pelvic disease.

Anything that changes the pH (the acid-base balance) of the vaginal secretions can cause a change in discharge. Factors that commonly do this include normal bacteria from a new sexual partner, a change in birth control, illness, too much douching or bathing, stress, and the use of antibiotics.

Common organisms that cause vaginal infections with a change in discharge include *Gardnerella vaginalis, Candida albicans*, and *Trichomonas vaginalis* (see the section on these infections), although any pelvic pathogen can produce this symptom. If a discharge changes in smell, becomes significantly heavier, causes excess itching, irritation, or pain, or becomes more pus-sy, it should be cultured for the presence of an infection. Also, if you have a new sexual partner and your discharge is different, you should always get a culture taken, even though most of the time there will be no pathology to account for this change.

Besides a culture from the vagina, a Pap smear may also be warranted to determine whether the discharge stems from changes in the cells of the cervix (see the section on Pap smears later in this chapter). Even if the Pap smear is normal, the cervix may still be inflamed, a condition known as cervicitis. Cervicitis can be due to a specific infection (with an organism such as *Chlamydia*), in which case it can be treated with appropriate antibiotics. Cervicitis can also be due to a postpregnancy inflammation that persists. In that case, the cervicitis should be treated only if symptoms such as heavy discharge or bleeding with intercourse bother you. The treatment can include burning the cells with a laser or cryotherapy (freezing the cells).

Sometimes the doctor cannot discover the cause of a persistent, troublesome discharge despite the best attempts at testing. A patient with this problem would be well advised to try to find "natural" solutions, such as acidophilus douches or herbal remedies, and to concentrate on discovering the events that trigger a worsening of this symptom.

Although a discharge tinged with small amounts of blood is rarely due to a major problem, this type of discharge should always be carefully evaluated because it can be the first signal of a malignancy, especially in the aging patient. (Sorry, but aging is anyone over forty. You knew I would say that.) Usually there's an obvious explanation, such as very vigorous intercourse with trauma to the vaginal tissue (if you've never had this happen to you, you will of course be surprised to hear that a lot of women have) or a cervical polyp (a small, benign growth in the opening of the cervix) or an inflammation of the cervix. But never ignore that symptom without finding the cause.

One last hint. Be sure not to wash in the vagina or douche before visiting the doctor with a vaginal discharge. (It's not the doctor who has the discharge, but you know what I mean.) I appreciate that most women want to visit the doctor when "clean," but if you clean the vagina, you may eliminate enough of the organisms to make a culture virtually useless.

Gardnerella

There was a time when the growth of *Gardnerella* in the vagina was not considered an infection. In fact, it wasn't even called *Gardnerella* back then. Its old name was *Hemophilus vaginalis*, and it was considered by most people to be a normal constituent of the vaginal flora.

Something happened in the early eighties. Someone named this bug after a guy called Gardner (it's hard to believe his name may have been Gardnerell), and the organism turned into a vaginal pathogen. (A pathogen is sort of like the bad guy in a bad Hollywood movie —

nobody likes pathogens because they cause infections and they wear black hats.)

A gardnerella infection is generally thought to cause a foamy, milky discharge with a fishy odor. (One of my patients once asked me what kind of fish. Farm-raised salmon, I think.) The discharge may also cause a burning sensation in the vagina. However, the great majority of women who have *Gardnerella* cultured on a routine pelvic exam have no complaints of excessive or smelly discharge. In fact, they have no complaint at all. With our current knowledge, those women should not be treated.

Because health workers can't even agree whether *Gardnerella* really causes any problems in the first place, an overgrowth of this organism is called gardnerella vagin*osis*, which is an indefinite term that leaves you in doubt as to whether you have an infection or not, instead of gardnerella vagin*itis*, which indicates a definite infection. (This is an old diplomatic trick — if you can't cure it, rename it, and maybe someone else will figure out what to do with it.) In other words, if you want to consider it an infection, go right ahead, but you may not be right.

If you decide to treat your vaginosis, try to do this with some type of douche that you can make up yourself. One of the best is a vinegar douche, in which you add two tablespoons of vinegar to one quart of warm water. (Another patient once asked me, "What do you do then?" Well, you don't drink it.)

If you have to use medication, there is much controversy about the most appropriate treatment regime. Part of the reason for this confusion is that if *Gardnerella* is a normal constituent of the vaginal flora, any treatment you choose is likely to fail because the organism will regrow after the treatment is discontinued. So if you feel you must treat, be prepared to do this often.

The most effective treatment in my experience is metronidazole (Flagyl) for seven days. If the infection recurs in a short period of time, I treat the partner as well, assuming that some men carry this organism even though they have no symptoms.

If left untreated, vaginosis is not thought to cause any long-term complications, such as PID (pelvic inflammatory disease) or changes in the Pap smear.

Candida

What woman hasn't experienced at least one yeast infection, caused by the organism *Candida albicans?* (Do I hear the sound of one hand clapping?) Luckily, most women only get an infection every so often and are easily able to get rid of it with appropriate treatment.

There are an unfortunate few, however, who are plagued with yeast infections on a recurrent if not semiconstant basis. In fact, these infections are so common that the first diagnosis I learned to make in French was *champignons* (mushrooms, or yeast).

Traditionally, yeast infections are said to cause a thick, white, "cheesy" discharge, which we usually describe as a "cottage cheese discharge." This is accompanied by a vaginal itch, which is often very intense, swelling of the vulva, and often an irritation when urinating.

There are as many theories about why yeast infections occur as there are books about these theories (and there are lots of books, I assure you). Yeast grows normally in most human vaginas, and the simple presence of these fungi does not constitute an infection. An infection is diagnosed only when the owner of that yeasty vagina complains of symptoms that are compatible with a yeast infection.

Yeast infections can be caused by anything that changes the normal acidy pH of the vagina to allow the ever-present yeast to multiply and produce symptoms. So, for example, in some women, normal changes throughout the menstrual cycle can allow yeast to flourish at various times in the cycle, usually just before menstruation. Various types of birth control, stress, the use of antibiotics, excessive use of tampons, a new sexual partner, concurrent infections — all these and a host of other conditions can also precipitate a yeast infection. (Some women are so prone to these infections that jaywalking can probably bring on a new outbreak.) In very recurrent cases of yeast, diabetes should always be checked for.

We really don't know why most of these women get recurring vaginal yeast infections, whereas others, exposed to the same situations, don't. A certain segment of the population believes that recurrent yeast infections are mostly due to our lifestyles and diets (see chapter 15). If you want to experiment by changing your diet or by bowing three times a day to some exotic deity, who am I to argue with you? Whatever works is fine by me.

Most women treat mild yeast infections by waiting, the old tincture-of-time therapy, and this often works. Thus, many women who get a little itchy a few days before their period have learned that the onset of menstruation generally takes care of the problem. As with gardnerella vaginosis, if a yeast infection is lingering, try a homemade douche, such as one with vinegar and water. Some women recommend a douche with yogurt or acidophilus, which you can buy in a health food store. The lactobacillus present in the yogurt counteracts mild yeast growth. (There are other people who tell you to shove the yogurt in the other end — to wit, to eat it — but it is doubtful that these little lactobacilli are hardy enough to survive a trip through the GI tract and then to find their way into the vagina.)

None of these douches are very effective in well-established infections. In such cases, you must use one of the many anticandidal antibiotics that are available in both cream and suppository form. These medications come in varying doses that can be prescribed for as little as one day or as long as fourteen days. In very resistant cases, some doctors recommend using these medications for up to six weeks in a row.

It rarely pays to treat the male partner concurrently, although when the male has obvious symptoms (such as a fungal-type rash on his penis), it's always wise to at least try to eliminate this obvious source. It is clear that some women with recurrent yeast infections are "allergic" to their sexual partner. For some reason, these women develop yeast infections every time they have intercourse with that partner. This is a dilemma that is rarely easy to deal with. In those cases, you should invariably try any manipulation related to diet, sexual activity, lifestyle, or any other factor that you can think of to try to minimize the recurrences. But don't hold your breath (breath holding is not known to change vaginal pH).

Trichomonas

Unlike the two other types of vaginitis mentioned above, a trichomonas infection is a sexually transmitted disease (but it's included in this section at the whim of the author because I wanted to keep the common vaginal infections together).

Traditionally, the discharge associated with a trichomonas infection is described as thin, watery, and having a foul odor. However, many cases are asymptomatic and are detected purely by accident, when the person doing the pelvic exam decides to test for this little critter. Trichomonas is asymptomatic in most men. Thus, all male partners of a woman with a trichomonas infection are probable carriers and should be treated at the same time. Otherwise, you can get the Ping-Pong effect, in which the partners give this infection back and forth to each other. (This has nothing to do with Ping-Pong diplomacy, or does it?)

The most effective treatment is metronidazole (Flagyl). In fact, I have rarely seen any other medication work for this infection, although many antibiotics (including the commonly used ampicillin) are proposed as useful.

This is the only form of vaginitis in which homemade douches don't seem to work well. However, a commercially available douche containing povidone-iodine (Betadine) seems to work somewhat for some women.

Even if left untreated, trichomonas is not thought to do you any long-term harm. But who wants to walk around with a smelly discharge if you don't have to?

PAIN

Pain in the Vagina

Most of the time, pain in the vagina occurs only with intercourse, a symptom known as dyspareunia. If dyspareunia is new, the most likely cause is a local irritation, such as a cut; a vulvar or vaginal infection; or an allergic or a hypersensitive reaction to one of the lotions or potions that so many women seem to use to beautify their bodies.

If everything looks normal, then attention should be paid to techniques of intercourse with your partner. Experiment. Not only is it fun to discover positions that only *Penthouse* or *Kama Sutra* readers have known about before, but new positions might also relieve the pain (and even if they don't, look at what you've learned about what your body can do, which may be a great consolation to those heading into — or out of — their forties).

Pain from the Cervix

One of my first (male) medical teachers, Dr. K. (this is my Kafka imitation), informed me that the cervix "never hurts." This was in reference to the fact that a Pap smear never "really" causes pain. It's those neurotic women, Dr. Hister, who complain just because they don't like to have this done.

I wanted to pass that course. I believed him. The second woman that I did a Pap smear on (and you do, do a Pap smear *on* someone), informed me that the procedure was uncomfortable. "What do you mean?" I asked. "Dr. K. said it doesn't hurt." "Oh yes it does," she said. She did not finish the sentence by calling me a moron or worse, but she could have.

The cervix can indeed hurt if provoked. Thus, in intercourse, if the penis hits the cervix, the woman may complain of dyspareunia. The obvious answer is to find positions that are more comfortable. The cervix also hurts when it's inflamed and when pressure is applied to it.

Pain in the Pelvis and Abdomen

The causes of pelvic pain are many, so I will only deal with the common ones, except for pelvic inflammatory disease (PID), which is an STD and is discussed in chapter 13.

ENDOMETRIOSIS

Endometriosis is probably the most common undiagnosed gyneco-logic problem in young to middle-aged females.

Endometriosis is a disease in which the normal cells that line the inside of the uterus — the endometrial cells — are found in other areas of the pelvis. Thus, endometrial cells can be found on the ovaries, on the fallopian tubes, on the pelvic walls and ligaments, on the bowel, and on the bladder.

How do the cells get there? The most accepted theory is that some menstrual blood washes back up from the uterus into the fallopian tubes and spills into the pelvic cavity. This retrograde uterine blood flow then stimulates endometrial deposits in these other organs in the pelvis to become active.

It is estimated that up to 15 percent of adult women have endometriosis, but most never have it diagnosed. It has been called working women's disease because it is more common in women who delay their first pregnancy. (And I'll bet you thought that working women's disease was a syndrome in which a woman complains of excess fatigue because she has to run a household as well as do her own job. That's not a disease. That's called normal.)

The most common symptom of endometriosis is pelvic pain associated with periods or with intercourse. Depending on where the cells are found, endometriosis can also cause diarrhea, abdominal cramps, pelvic pain throughout the entire monthly cycle, infertility, and symptoms of bladder irritation such as excessive urination.

The reason that pain is such a common feature of endometriosis is that the endometrial deposits go through all the same hormonal changes that the cells would if they were still lining the uterus. Thus, they swell and shed blood, and in the unusual areas in which they now find themselves, these endometrial deposits inflame their new homes, causing pain.

The only accurate way to diagnose endometriosis is through a laparoscopy. Blood tests and X rays do not help.

A number of hormonal therapies have been proposed. The first recommendation is always to get pregnant (and no, not just male physicians advocate this particular therapy). Being pregnant rids the patient of pain because the cells do not go through their changes anymore. But pregnancy seems a high price to pay for pain relief, so other therapies are often more attractive.

Some women get relief by going on the birth control pill or by taking progesterone. Much more effective is a medication called danazol (Cyclomen), which in theory not only treats the symptoms but can also cure the disease. But because of potential side effects, danazol should be reserved for severe cases.

For simple pain relief (which is never simple, of course), the usual armamentarium of analgesics is available. With pelvic pain that originates in the reproductive organs, there is often good response to one of the NSAIDs like naproxen sodium (Anaprox).

OTHER CAUSES OF PELVIC PAIN

An ovarian cyst can occasionally produce pain when the cyst bleeds, when it ruptures (rarely), or when it twists on its stalk or pedicle. (A dog has a pedigree; you can rent a pedicab; a cyst has a pedicle.) The pain in all three situations is usually severe and of sudden onset. If a cyst has ruptured, the pain usually subsides within several hours and requires no other treatment. If a cyst has twisted on its pedicle — a condition known as torsion of an ovarian cyst — the cyst must be surgically removed, unless it untwists.

Never forget that other organs, such as the bowel, might be the source of pelvic discomfort. Always try to ascertain whether or not your recurrent pelvic pain is connected with other bowel symptoms, such as changes in bowel movements.

A fibroid, a benign growth on the uterus, can also produce pain occasionally, especially associated with a period, but this is rare. Even when a fibroid is present, one should always try to find more likely explanations for the pain.

And last, of course, there is pain of psychological origin. This is a diagnosis that should only be made after a vigorous attempt to find physical causes for the pain has failed. Sadly, this attempt has not always been made. For years (centuries?), women were told that many, if not all, pelvic pains were "in their heads." (A variation on a theme by Python, Monty. "I'm sorry, Mrs. Gumby, your uterus is what hurts, but the problem is that it seems to be in your brain. It will have to come out." "Out of my head?" "No out of your pelvis." Which is what was done.) The last thing in the world anyone needs to be told is that she is "neurotic," what my old psychiatry professor, a South American liberal, called crazy, only to discover later that the cause of her discomfort was really something wholly physical and correctable.

CERVICAL CANCER

Risk Factors

Cervical cancer is the second most common cancer in the world. There are many factors that put a woman at high risk. The younger a woman is when she first has intercourse with a male, the greater the number of male sexual partners she has over her lifetime, the younger she is when she has her first pregnancy, the more sexually transmitted diseases she has had (especially venereal warts), the more she smokes, and the more sexual encounters she has with men who are themselves at higher risk for STDs, the greater that woman's chance of developing cervical cancer.

Although a number of other factors are often cited as potential causes (the use of birth control pills or an IUD, for example, or a genital herpes infection), none of these are known to produce severe enough changes in cervical cells to lead to cancer. They may accelerate cancerous changes once these have started, however. It is always a good idea, if possible, to change your method of birth control if a Pap smear shows an abnormality (see below), just to see if it makes a difference. At the very least, it gives you the feeling that you are doing something for yourself.

There is also no proof that vaginal infections cause cancerous changes in the cervix.

Pap Smears

The test for cervical cancer is known as a Pap test, which is named after the Greek physician, Papanicolaou, who devised the test. (Wisely, someone shortened the name of the test, because we would have a great deal of trouble convincing women to come in and have a yearly Papanicolaou test.) Pap smears are taken by inserting a spatula into the opening of the cervix and rotating the spatula around the periphery. The surface cells of the cervix are thus scraped onto the spatula and are then transferred onto a glass slide.

Pap smear results are generally divided into four classes. Class I means that all is well, and the test should be repeated in one year for most women. I will come back to class II in a moment. A class III Pap smear indicates a change in the cells of the cervix that correlates with a very high likelihood that the cells will develop into frank cancer if left untreated. This cell pattern is called carcinoma in situ or precancer. But remember that a class III Pap does not mean that you have cancer yet. Class IV indicates a very likely cervical malignancy. (Some Pap smear classification systems include a class V, which is a definite cervical malignancy.)

Now what about that elusive class II? Class II includes all the disordered changes of growth, called dysplasia, in cervical cells that indicate that something unusual is occurring in those cells but not enough to qualify as precancer. The level of dysplasia can be further subdivided into mild, moderate, and severe.

In some parts of North America, the CIN classification of Pap smears is also used. CIN I corresponds to mild dysplasia; CIN II, to moderate dysplasia; and CIN III, to severe dysplasia and carcinoma in situ.

Why this plethora of possibilities, if all we are looking for is cancer? Cervical cancer develops gradually, and we are able to monitor the changes from the earliest stages of inflammation. But in looking for cancer, we pick up a lot of other minor inflammations that will not progress to precancerous changes, although all inflammations need to be monitored because we simply can't tell which will self-correct and which will progress. What is important to remember about Pap smears is that the smears are only as good as the smearer, so to speak, and the lab that reads the slide (the slider?). It's an easy test to do, but all doctors miss the appropriate cells from time to time by not taking the smear from deep enough in the cervix, for example, or by not making a complete rotation of the cervix when taking the smear.

Why aren't Pap smears done more frequently? Luckily, dysplastic changes generally take a long time to become frankly cancerous. Although with the spread of the human papilloma virus (see chapter

13), which seems to strongly accelerate cancerous change, the statistics may change somewhat; it is currently believed that it takes several years on average to change from a noncancerous state to carcinoma in situ.

Depending on the severity and the location of the abnormalities in the cervical cells, further treatment can consist of laser therapy, freezing therapy, or surgery. Although a number of medical treatments have been proposed for the treatment of abnormal Pap smears, especially vitamin A, none of them seem to be greatly effective.

A last warning. Very few women with an abnormal Pap smear have any symptoms, so it is important to have a regular Pap smear whether you have any gynecological problems or not.

MENSTRUAL IRREGULARITIES AND COMPLAINTS (BLEEDING AND ALL THAT)

PMS (As Opposed to AMS, I Suppose)

Premenstrual syndrome (PMS) is a set of symptoms waiting for a definition. There are no universal criteria for diagnosis of this condition. It is best to say that if you experience uncomfortable symptoms in a routine premenstrual pattern, you can be considered to be suffering from PMS. And contrary to what some men think, not every woman suffers from PMS. At least 15 percent of women, and probably many more, feel *better* before menstruation.

It is normal to have some breast fullness, some bloating, some mood changes before a period. But if these normal symptoms become exaggerated, especially if they are accompanied by significant mood swings, then you can consider yourself to have PMS. There are no tests or X rays to confirm your suspicions. If you think you got it, you got it.

The various treatments that have been proposed have all been less than excellent. In fact, in many studies a placebo has been at least as effective as the other treatment studied.

Vitamin B_6 in high doses is still a frequently self-prescribed treatment. If it works, by all means use it. But remember that high doses of B$_6$ can be toxic, so you should be careful even with this "natural therapy." (How come everyone thinks that natural necessarily means healthy?) Some women have gotten relief with antidepressant medications, and some with NSAIDs. Some doctors use progesterone, but there is much dispute about its efficacy. Curiously, some women who are deprived of sleep claim that their PMS symptoms improve. (I am not sure if this means that if you have PMS, you should arrange for your partner to kick you awake three or four times a night.) Ingesting primrose oil is also promoted by some women as an effective (and expensive) treatment.

Probably the best therapy is to maintain normal weight and to exercise regularly. This is not a facetious comment. In all studies, this therapy is at least as effective as any other, and it has many other health benefits as well. Besides, it's cheap.

Pain with Periods

Period cramps are extremely common. They can be minor and barely noticeable. Or they can be so severe that they limit a woman's capacity to function.

As with so many gynecological complaints, there are a host of nonmedical therapies that may work. These include exercise, relaxation techniques, yoga, hot-water bottles, and anything else that Aunt Alice may suggest. You will likely find, however, that these are only helpful for mild, occasional cramps.

For more severe cramps, medication is often required. Since most period cramps are caused by the release of prostaglandins, antiprostaglandin therapy should work to suppress the pain. And it does. The antiprostaglandins (also known as anti-inflammatory medications) most commonly used for menstrual cramps include mefenamic acid (Ponstan) and naproxen sodium (Anaprox, and its cheaper cousin Naprosyn).

In some women, period cramps are due to pelvic disease such as endometriosis or a fibroid. Depending on how severe the condition is, it may be appropriate to try to find such a potentially correctable condition.

Heavy Periods

Heavy periods are normal for some women. But any blood loss over 100 cubic centimeters should be considered abnormal because it can lead to anemia. The interesting point comes up, of course, as to how you can tell if you are losing too much blood. After all, one woman's soaked tampon may be another woman's normal tampon. The best measure of blood loss is your hemoglobin count (which you undoubtedly recall from chapter 3). If you are getting anemic from your periods, that constitutes excessive blood loss. Simple replacement of iron by diet or pills is all that is required in most cases.

The only common obvious cause of abnormally heavy periods in the under-forty-year-old is the use of an IUD. If you don't have an IUD, sudden onset of heavy periods is often due to dysfunctional uterine bleeding (see below).

A fibroid can also produce heavy periods. Fibroids are much more common in aged uteri. In fact, although fibroids are rare in a thirty-year-old, 15 to 20 percent of women over thirty-five have them. Fibroids can either be left alone, waiting for the inevitability of menopause (the real Godot), or they can be surgically removed. If fibroids are very large, the entire uterus must be removed. Fibroids very rarely become malignant, and any woman advised to have a hysterectomy to prevent a future malignancy in a fibroid ought to seriously consider the motivation behind the recommendation. ("What did the patient have?" "Three hundred dollars.") She should get a second opinion.

Irregular Periods

Irregular periods can be too frequent or too far apart; they can be too heavy; they can be too short or too long; or there may be bleeding between periods. In all cases where no other disease is found, we say that a woman with any of these patterns to her periods is suffering from dysfunctional uterine bleeding (DUB). DUB is thought to be due to an imbalance between the estrogen and progesterone concentrations, although blood levels of these hormones in women suffering from this problem are usually within normal limits (another of those "'splain that if you can, Lucy" phenomena). DUB is also often associated with cycles in which no egg is released, or anovulatory cycles.

DUB is frequently self-correcting, lasting only several cycles. If it is not, depending on your age and the circumstances, you should have some hormonal investigations. These investigations prove to be normal in the vast majority of cases. For women over forty, a dilatation and curettage, better know as a D & C, is pretty much mandatory to rule out a (rare) uterine malignancy. A D & C is a procedure in which the cervix is dilated and the uterus is scraped out, or curetted. The cells from the inside of the uterus are then analyzed for any abnormalities. A D & C often improves DUB of recent onset, but it is usually a temporary improvement because whatever produced the DUB in the first place is likely to produce it again in the not-too-distant future. (This procedure was so commonly done in the past that it was virtually a rite of passage for women approaching middle age, which is why, no doubt, the women in Montreal used to call it a dusting and cleaning.)

Besides patience or a D & C, DUB can also be treated with hormones. In the younger woman, birth control pills are frequently used. In the somewhat older woman, progesterone pills taken for the last twelve to fourteen days of the cycle may also produce more normal cycles.

Missed Periods (Amenorrhea)

Women can skip periods for any conceivable reason. (No groans, please. Just thank God that I have resisted the urge this long.) The most common reason, of course, is conception. So any missed period should be followed by a pregnancy test, no matter how remote a possibility a pregnancy might seem. (Every doctor lies and says that as an intern, he or she diagnosed a nun — not the same one, I'm sure — to be pregnant. To be perfectly honest, I have never examined a nun — none nuns, as it were. Nor have I ever seen a rabbi undressed.)

We often blame stress for a missed period. In these cases stress doesn't necessarily mean stress. (Isn't that just like a doctor?) It is better to say that any change in lifestyle can produce amenorrhea.

Women who lose a lot of weight often suffer missed periods as a consequence. Do not send search parties for these missing periods. Just gain some weight. Women who train very hard at endurance events also miss periods, probably because of the weight loss and strange diets that most competitive athletes suffer as much as the training. (Yes, suffer a diet. Everyone knows you suffer with any diet.)

On the low-dose birth control pill, it is common to skip a period. In fact, many women stop menstruating entirely. This does not decrease your future ability to conceive. So we usually just tell you to ignore the amenorrhea while you're on the pill. This is easier said than done. It is always easy for a physician to tell a woman not to worry about her missed periods. The woman, however, frequently has fears about an undiagnosed conception and very much wants to bleed (only a little bit, in fact three drops would do nicely for most women), every month, just for reassurance that she is not with child and that her body is functioning normally.

A lot of women who discontinue the pill may not menstruate for a while, often up to several months. Very rarely, someone may never resume menstruating again. This is called postpill amenorrhea. Although there is no real agreement as to when these women should be investigated for other hormonal irregularities, I think that if a woman is still not menstruating six months after discontinuing the pill, she should at least have some blood tests done.

Another reason for amenorrhea in many women is breast-feeding. Indeed, it is not unheard of to proceed from one pregnancy to another with no intervening periods. (I can get some people mad by calling this papal birth control, but I won't.)

Menopause (discussed later in this chapter) is the ultimate loss of periods that looms in every woman's future. Often menopause starts with periods that are intermittent before they disappear altogether.

Other, less common reasons for amenorrhea include other hormonal and ovarian problems, pituitary tumors, and the use of certain medications, most notably anabolic steroids. (Presumably Ben Johnson didn't worry about this side effect.)

Always remember that just because you are not having regular periods does not mean that you cannot conceive. An egg can free itself from the ovary at any time, so you should still use some method of birth control, preferably one of the barriers.

Cycles with No Eggs (Anovulatory Cycles)

Anovulatory cycles are monthly cycles in which ovulation does not occur. The reason is that very little estrogen and absolutely no progesterone is released. Although there is usually a menstrual period associated with this cycle, the period can be abnormal in length or appear at an unusual time in the cycle. According to some experts, the best indication that ovulation has occurred is the appearance of breast swelling and tenderness before the period. If these signs don't occur, then it is quite possible you are not ovulating, especially if you have abnormal cycles.

Anovulatory cycles, which are common just after periods first start and in the years leading up to menopause, are only important in that they mean that you cannot conceive without medical intervention.

Bleeding between Cycles (Intermenstrual Bleeding)

Intermenstrual bleeding on the pill is known as breakthrough bleeding. This bleeding usually disappears after a few cycles on your new pill. If heavy, the best way to eliminate it is to change the pill, usually by going up to a stronger dose.

In those women not on the pill, intermenstrual bleeding is usually due to some local cause (like someone getting a petition together to save a neighborhood day care). Common local causes of intermenstrual bleeding include cervical erosions and cervical polyps (benign growths on the cervix).

In the older woman (are you getting tired of my saying this?), this symptom needs to be investigated to exclude possible tumors.

Ectopic Pregnancies

An ectopic pregnancy is a pregnancy that implants outside the uterus, most often in one of the fallopian tubes.

Because there are no special symptoms that are specific for an ectopic pregnancy, any woman who is at high risk for one and who has an abnormal period or abnormal pelvic pain (especially following a period) should be suspected of having an ectopic pregnancy until proven otherwise. High-risk women include those using an IUD, those who have had a Dalkon Shield at any time, those who have had a previous ectopic pregnancy, those who have had surgery on a fallopian tube, those with a history of PID, and those who practice high-risk sex by having unprotected intercourse with more than one partner.

An ectopic pregnancy must be evacuated from the fallopian tube because the tube cannot expand with the pregnancy like the uterus does. Eventually, between about the eighth and the tenth week, the tube will rupture, resulting in torn blood vessels running along the tube, which will continue to spurt blood until they are manually (or womanually) tied off. This is a medical emergency. Ectopic pregnancies are the second leading cause of maternal mortality in North America.

If an ectopic pregnancy is picked up early enough, it may be possible to "milk" it out of the end of the tube, and the tube can be saved. But frequently the pregnancy is either too advanced or too adherent to the tube, and the tube has to be sacrificed.

Miscarriages (Spontaneous Abortions)

Spontaneous abortions are better known as miscarriages. As we have become better able to diagnose very early pregnancies, we have realized that miscarriages are very common, probably occurring in between 33 and 40 percent of all pregnancies.

The most prominent symptom of a spontaneous abortion is bright red spotting or bleeding coming through the cervix, often accompanied by abdominal cramps.

It is believed that most spontaneous abortions occur because the embryo was seriously malformed. In theory, a miscarriage is part of the biological imperative of the human race to keep itself more healthy overall (although as a friend of mine points out, when we look at some of the samples around us that have survived, we sometimes have to wonder about this theory). Miscarriages increase with the age of the mother, with uterine abnormalities such as fibroids, and with endometriosis.

One spontaneous abortion, then, is pretty much par for the course for many women. It is worth getting a work-up to exclude genetic problems when you have had three miscarriages, although it is unlikely that a cause will be found and even less likely that anything can be done should a cause be identified.

There is one cause of recurrent spontaneous abortions that is surgically correctable. In some women the cervix opens too easily as the pregnancy progresses, often as a result of a cone biopsy in which too much tissue was removed. Multiple pregnancies and repeated therapeutic abortions can also weaken the cervix. In such cases, the cervix can be surgically tightened with some stitching.

If you bleed in the first or second trimester of pregnancy, you are said to be having a threatened abortion. Sadly, there is no effective treatment for this condition. You should take it easy as much as possible, but there is not much proof that this advice makes a difference to the outcome, except in selected cases.

The bleeding from a miscarriage should stop within a couple of weeks as the products of conception, including the tiny placenta, completely pass out of the uterus and the uterus returns to a normal, nonpregnant state. If the bleeding continues, you have to suspect an incomplete abortion, in which some piece of tissue is still adherent to the inside of the uterus. This piece of tissue must eventually be evacuated with a D & C, or continued bleeding or infection will result.

Toxic Shock Syndrome

Toxic shock syndrome (TSS) is an overwhelming reaction that occurs in response to a toxin released by an infection with a strain of the *Staphylococcus* bacteria. TSS usually occurs in a menstruating woman who has been using tampons, especially the superabsorbent kind, and has been leaving individual tampons in the vagina for many hours at a time (such as overnight). This seems to promote the growth of the type of bacteria that can initiate TSS, although this reaction can also occur in nonmenstruating females, as well as males, most of whom presumably are not using tampons.

Toxic shock manifests itself with the sudden onset of a severe flulike illness, with nausea, vomiting, headache, high fever, and a rash. The toxin can go on to cause a medical crisis called shock, in which the blood pressure drops, and death can result without vigorous treatment.

Any menstruating female who develops a severe flulike illness should be suspected of having TSS until proven otherwise, which means prompt admission to hospital, even though most of the time she will have nothing more serious than the flu.

MENOPAUSE

Menopause happens to every human female who lives long enough (although who ever thought it would happen to our generation?). Generally it occurs in the late forties or early fifties, but it can happen much sooner.

Contrary to much of the early literature on the subject, menopause does not have to be a time of great difficulty. In fact, several studies show that most women welcome this passage in their lives, and it's small wonder. No more periods or cramps, no more tampons, no worries about contraception or conception, no more monthly mood swings.

Menopause usually announces its presence with the famous hot flashes (I prefer "hot flashes" to "hot flushes," which always makes me think of a bidet with the wrong hose attached, something a plumber friend of mine actually installed for an unsuspecting family) and a change in periods. Hot flashes are intense sensations of warmth accompanied by sweating and often followed by chills. They can occur at any time and can be uncomfortable, but for most women they are quite manageable. When the flashes are particularly disturbing, they can be treated with clonidine (Dixarit). These flashes and the gradually lengthening time between periods can go on for several years. Eventually, the periods and flashes stop altogether.

It is now well established that giving estrogen to women going through the menopause, what is known as estrogen replacement therapy, or ERT, not only relieves many of the nuisance symptoms (such as dryness of the vagina and hot flashes) associated with menopause but also lowers the rates of both cardiovascular disease and osteoporosis in the later years.

That, as they say, is the good news. The bad news, or at least the indeterminate news, is that ERT increases the rate of cancer of the uterus (which is of course of no concern to anyone who has had a hysterectomy).

So how do you balance these risks and benefits? Overall, most doctors agree that since coronary heart disease is so prevalent, the benefits of ERT in reducing this risk far outweigh any small potential increase in the number of malignancies.

Besides, it seems possible to modify the tumor-promoting effect of estrogen by taking progesterone at the same time. Progesterone, however, causes mood swings and breast tenderness in many of the women who take it. Even more disturbing, when progesterone is stopped, a period results. This raises the interesting (and not too welcome) possibility of seventy-year-old women still having periods, something that at least one author (male) insisted was worth the price. Currently, the consensus is that progesterone should be given to all women on ERT despite these drawbacks, but it is safe to say that there is still much dispute about this issue.

ERT is not for everybody. Women who should *not* take ERT under any circumstances include those who have had problems with blood clots, such as strokes or phlebitis, and women who have had breast cancer or very high blood pressure.

One last word. Estrogen is now available in patches that can be applied to the skin, which seems to be an improved method of delivery for most women.

MISCELLANEOUS PROBLEMS

Idiopathic Edema

Idiopathic edema is swelling for which we don't know the cause. A surprising number of women — some estimates being as high as 10 percent of all females — swell and gain weight as their monthly cycle progresses. The swelling is most evident in the feet, fingers, and breasts and around the eyes. It is often accompanied by a need to urinate more, and the swelling is often worse after lying down, making it most evident in the morning.

If the swelling is excessive, a short course of diuretics will relieve it. But this treatment should be reserved for very uncomfortable swelling because the body has a habit of accommodating itself to the diuretic when it is used too frequently. Indeed, many women are "addicted" to their monthly dose of diuretic.

Burning with Urination (Dysuria)

BLADDER INFECTIONS — ACUTE CYSTITIS

God must have made a mistake. How else can you explain why the bladder is so close to the vagina and why the female urethra is only about one and one-half inches long? (The male urethra is about eight inches long. That's urethra, guys, not penis.) Why did God not put the female bladder under the armpit, or at least make the urethra much longer.

It is the short urethra and the location of the bladder that causes women to have so many more bladder infections than men. The bacteria that is most commonly responsible for a bladder infection, known as cystitis, is *E. coli,* the common bacteria that inhabit every person's rectum. During intercourse, in a substantial number of women, *E. coli* transfer from the rectum to the vagina and then to the opening of the urethra, where it's a short hop into the bladder. Many women develop their first bladder infection the first time they have intercourse (hence the name honeymoon cystitis). Other contributing factors can be bike riding and irritants like bubble baths. There is no proof that wiping improperly (back to front) has any contributing role (but that doesn't mean that you should do it that way, heaven forbid).

Besides a burning sensation with urination (dysuria), the symptoms of a bladder infection can include blood in the urine, pus in the urine, pain in the lower abdomen, and especially the urgent need to urinate frequently, especially at night.

An important part of the treatment consists of drinking plenty of fluids, which dilutes the urine and lessens the burning sensation. But you should not drink so much that your bladder is constantly full. A full bladder that is not emptied frequently will aggravate the condition rather than ameliorate it. Remember to drink, pee, drink, pee, drink, pee . . .

Folklore promotes cranberry juice as a treatment for cystitis, although "scientific" medical studies have failed to confirm that it works.

Drinking plenty of fluids often improves the symptoms enough that you may think the infection is gone. You may be right, but it's best to get a urine culture test done to confirm that the infection is really gone.

The first few episodes of cystitis usually respond quickly to one of several antibiotics, including the sulfa group (which sounds like a bunch of corporate raiders looking for a takeover candidate), macrodantin, amoxicillin, and ampicillin.

OTHER CAUSES OF DYSURIA

Although most cases of dysuria are due to bladder infections, several other problems can produce the same symptom. About 10 to 20 percent of dysuria is produced by a urethral inflammation (see chapter 13), usually caused by a chlamydia infection. A vaginal infection, especially one caused by *Candida*, can also produce dysuria, as can trauma to the urethra, usually caused by vigorous intercourse. (It is always a source of interest to me that some men, often the same ones who wince at the very thought of anyone's even touching their genitals, not infrequently subject their partner's vulva, and all the parts in its vicinity, to the kind of roughhousing that only Hulk Hogan could enjoy.) Chemical irritants such as bubble baths, feminine hygienic sprays (which are not hygienic or feminine), and even contraceptive foam can also produce urethral burning.

The frequency-dysuria syndrome occurs in those women who have pain with urination and who need to urinate a lot but who do not have bacteria in their urine. You should drink plenty of liquids, and you should be followed carefully to make sure that you do not develop an actual infection. You do not require antibiotics in the absence of an infection, however.

BREAST DISEASE

Want to hear an awful description? "The human mammary gland is actually a cluster of 5 to 9 individual glands closely associated in a fibro-adipose stroma but independent of one another." That, dear readers, is what you and I politely call the breast. Although this description is technically correct, most of us tend to think of a breast in somewhat more romantic terms than that. Until something goes awry, that is.

Fibrocystic Breast Disease

The easiest way to understand benign breast disease (which is usually called fibrocystic disease but which is not really a disease at all) is to think of the breast as being made up of three kinds of tissue: fatty tissue, glandular tissue, and supporting or fibrous tissue. The fatty tissue is the tissue that gives the breast its shape (it really is the first place you gain weight and the first place you lose it too), and unless there is trauma to the fatty cells, which can result in permanent hard lumps, the fatty tissue in the breast is usually nice and smooth and unlumpy. But when the glandular tissue and the fibrous tissue react to hormonal stimulation, the breast texture can become more swollen and tender, often resulting in distinct, tender lumps. Both these effects become more pronounced as the normal monthly cycle gets closer to the next period. The breast pain and swelling can be so severe that a woman cannot sleep on her stomach or do any exercise without pain.

This is what we call benign breast disease (BBD). BBD is very common, with over 70 percent of women complaining of it at some time. It tends to occur mostly in the thirties and gradually dies down the closer a woman gets to menopause. Like so many other problems in this chapter, BBD is most likely the result of an imbalance between estrogen and progesterone. Although caffeine has always been said to aggravate BBD, it is much more probable that caffeine only does this in some women. If you suffer from BBD, always cut back on your caffeine consumption to see if it makes any difference. If it doesn't, then you can safely start back on your coffee habit.

Generally, BBD need not be treated unless it is very severe. The best thing to do is just put up with the symptoms until your period comes, when the pain and swelling will disappear. Occasionally, in the more severe cases, the use of a mild diuretic for a few days may decrease the general fluid load in the body enough to ease some of the symptoms. Vitamin E capsules and iodine preparations may also be useful for mild cases.

When BBD is more severe, it requires more heavy-duty medications. These include bromocriptine (Parlodel) and danazol (Cyclomen). Both these drugs should be reserved for very severe cases because they have a number of potential complications, and they cost a lot.

When a separate, distinct lump persists, it is important to rule out breast cancer, even with a negative mammogram report. The least traumatic way to do this is to put a needle into the lump (often using ultrasound to localize the swelling) and to extract some fluid from the belly of the mass, which is then analyzed for the presence of tumor cells. If the pathology report is not completely reassuring, or if there is any doubt about the benign nature of the lump, it should be completely removed.

Breast Cancer

The sad fact is that breast cancer is *not* decreasing in North America, despite our best efforts. The reason is simple. We just don't know what causes it. We do, however, know who is at special risk for this tumor. A woman who has a mother or sister who had breast cancer is much more at risk herself, especially if the cancer in the relative was present in both breasts or if the relative developed her disease while still premenopausal. The chances that a woman who has had a malignancy in one breast will develop a second malignancy in the other breast are greater than the chances that a woman will develop a first malignancy. Diet seems to play a role, since the rate of breast cancer goes up in direct proportion to the ingestion of animal fats. Early pregnancies (before the age of thirty) associated with breast-feeding have a protective effect, as does vigorous lifelong exercise. The risk of breast cancer goes up with early onset of first menstruation and later onset of menopause (in other words, it may be related to the total number of menstrual cycles), and with higher socioeconomic status. We also know that there is no connection between breast cancer and BBD, nor between alcohol intake and breast cancer.

Although we repeat the statistic that roughly one in eleven North American women will develop breast cancer, it is still, luckily, rare in young women, although every doctor knows of at least one or two patients who developed this tumor in their twenties or thirties. And the rate obviously goes up with age, so that as my generation approaches menopause (far too soon), we will all know more and more women who get this disease.

A malignant lump usually appears as a hard, immobile, often painless swelling that gradually increases in size and that is often accompanied by palpable lymph glands in the armpit on the same side. The skin over the lump may be retracted as the cancer attaches to the surrounding tissue.

Any lump that feels hard, especially if it is fixed to the underlying tissue, should be quickly analyzed with a biopsy. The best way of doing this is by removing the entire lump. With their usual flare, doctors have called this procedure a lumpectomy. Even if the lump proves to be cancerous, this procedure, if done properly at the time of the biopsy, often means that no further surgery will be required. We are luckily beyond the times when all breast malignancies were treated with that disfiguring surgery known as a radical mastectomy, in which the entire breast and some of the muscle tissue of the chest wall were removed. These days, a lumpectomy combined with radiation therapy, hormonal therapy, or chemotherapy is the preferred method of treatment for most breast cancers.

No discussion of breast cancer can be complete without engaging in the debate that surrounds mammograms. Mammograms are breast X rays. There is no argument about the benefit of mammograms in patients over the age of fifty. All studies done in the last few years, as these X rays and the skills of the people who do them have become more refined, provide excellent evidence that mammograms in women over fifty can pick up many tumors before they have spread and consequently lead to better and earlier treatment. The result is that the death rate from breast cancer goes down in elderly women who have regular mammograms.

The controversy about mammograms stems from the recommendation by many authoritative health organizations that all women between the ages of forty and fifty have annual mammograms as *routine* screening procedures. Just as many equally authoritative bodies argue that this policy is a waste of ever-scarcer health dollars because there is no proof that mammograms done for screening in the entire population of young women actually save lives (now I'm calling those under fifty young). They recommend reserving this X ray for high-risk women, at least until the age of fifty.

So what is poor confused you to do, with all these health authorities screaming advice at you, arguing over your breasts, as it were? What's my opinion? (That's why you're reading this book, after all.) My belief is that you should have a yearly mammogram from the age of forty on (although I promise we can still be friends even if you don't follow my advice). If you are at high risk for a breast tumor, you should start having annual mammograms at an earlier age, perhaps as early as thirty-five.

I also believe that it's vital that you get your mammogram done in a center that is experienced at this sort of X ray. Just as a cholesterol count may vary from lab to lab, so too can a mammogram report.

All younger women experience a bit of discomfort when the breasts are squished together when a mammogram is done. (As one of my patients said to me, "How would you like it if some technician came and squeezed your balls in a vise?" I wouldn't like it even if it weren't a technician, I told her.) The thought of pain should not dissuade you from having the X ray, however.

Another frequent concern is the amount of radiation in these X rays. The dose of radiation in an average mammogram is about two to five times the amount you receive as normal background radiation from daily living, which is not a whole lot, you must admit.

One final word. There are no studies that I know of that show that breast self-examination, or BSE, saves lives. When we study large groups of women, some of whom do BSE and some of whom don't, there seems to be no difference in mortality between the two groups.

So why do I stress that all women should do it anyway? Because it is extremely important that patients feel that they are doing something for themselves and because for at least a few women it can make a difference. It is an easy technique to learn if taught properly, and perhaps if all women started doing self-examination from an early age and were at the same time taught about all the other risk factors that we know of, we could make a bigger dent in the death rate from this cancer.

Nipple Discharge

The first patient who ever complained to me of a nipple discharge was a young woman who told me that she had a dark, almost black liquid coming out of both her nipples. I was young. What did I know? I tried to appear nonchalant, but the look that appeared on my face and the way I explained the investigations to her immediately convinced her that she was going to have both her breasts amputated. I looked so scared because I had been taught that a nipple discharge indicated a tumor until proven otherwise. But the truth, as I have relearned many times over the years, is that in a young, premenopausal woman a nipple discharge, even a very black one, is usually (luckily) benign, most often caused by a benign growth in a duct or excess hormonal stimulation.

Having said that, every nipple discharge, especially if it comes from one breast only, should be discussed with a doctor and analyzed to rule out the possibility of a breast tumor or a pituitary tumor. (Remember the pituitary? It secretes a hormone, prolactin, an excess of which can produce nipple discharge.) The dark color, by the way, usually is from old blood.

CHAPTER 12

The Male

*In which the good doctor forever gives up hope of joining a
men-only club, but who would want to anyway?*

I have never done a formal survey, but I am willing to bet that 50
percent of the men who visit our office come in with a story that
begins, "Look, Art, I didn't think this was important, but my wife (or
girlfriend or sister or mother) felt that I should see you about this.
Sorry to waste your time, but you know how much they worry."
(Women have several significant others; men have several significant
mothers.) This declaration of dependence is often followed by a
disingenuous grin or wink, implying that we, the male doctor and the
male patient, understand how nervous women are, and we must
humor them, nudge, nudge, wink, wink.

It is much more likely, however, that the patient himself is secretly
worried about the symptom that brought him to the office. He probably drove his wife batty with his frequent references to his "minor"
problem. You know the syndrome. "Do you think this mole has
changed, Nancy? How can you be so sure? It's my life, after all. Why
are you looking at me like that? You haven't examined it since this
morning. You know how quickly melanomas spread. In twenty-four
hours I could be dead. I suppose you want me to die. I'm not worried,
you know, but I can't really check myself, can I?"

Finally, Nancy, in self-defense, probably said something like,
"Look, Harold" (I once promised myself that if I wrote a book, I'd
have at least one Harold in it, so here he is), "if you're so worried,
why don't you go visit Art? Go, before I kill you." To which Harold
probably replied, "I'm not really worried, but I'll keep you happy and
go so that you can stop worrying. I'll report back to you right away."
I am frequently the court of last report.

Men are different. Outwardly, they're nonchalant about their health. Inwardly, they seethe with doomsday scenarios. Men don't come down with a simple cold; each cough is a probable bronchitis or pneumonia. Men don't get vague joint aches; they automatically have arthritis. When men have rectal bleeding, it can never be due to hemorrhoids but is always the result of an undiagnosed bowel cancer, UPO — until proven otherwise. (Unidentified UPO problems afflict men far more than women; men always think that the symptom they have is due to the worst possible disorder until the diagnosis has been proven otherwise.)

But men usually resist visiting the doctor. They much prefer to pester their mate with their problem. At the same time, men feel that all women, especially their mates, should have annual, if not more frequent, pelvic examinations, because it's the right thing to do if you want to stay healthy. But can you think of a single male who doesn't resist even an occasional rectal exam? "You're not really going to do that to me, Art." "Of course I am. Last time I looked there was no one else in this room to do it to, was there?" Men don't see anything wrong with me, a man, examining their wives and mothers in the most intimate manner. But it's always interesting to see how quickly testicular pain disappears when a man is told that one of my female partners will be seeing him that day.

I know all this because (you will have guessed this, I am sure) I am a typical male. I don't know how often I've convinced my wife that I had pneumonia, for several hours at least. You know how many of my lymph node swellings have been the first stirrings of malignancy? So many that I am no longer allowed to present a new lymph node to any of my family members for inspection. (For a while I was able to get my wife's attention by having one of my sons present my complaints to her. He has just applied for medical school at the age of ten. He knows enough to get in.) I do many pelvic exams each day, but I am extremely reluctant to have anybody, male or female, do a rectal exam on me.

I have a distinct advantage over many of my brothers because (contrary to the rumors you may hear) I actually possess some medical knowledge. So my overreaction to symptoms can usually be justified with a few fancy references, preferably from an obscure journal not available in English, and if available in English, then not mailed outside of Asia. My wife doesn't buy my act any longer, though. Any new cough produces prompt and vigorous advice to go visit one of my partners and bother her instead. This advice usually flies out at me even before I have taken my hand away from my mouth and long before I can develop that "poor me" look that all men are so adept at. My partners, those cruel women, usually refer me back to my wife, often without even examining me. (Is this what is known as having women fight over you?)

Why are men so resistant to publicly admitting any apprehension about their bodies while privately, to their chosen other, men are so prone to overreaction? As usual, I have a theory. Men are brought up from early childhood to deny and suppress their anxieties and hurts. From a very impressionable age, boys are taught to hide their feelings if they are hurt in play, or if they are made fun of. I don't know how often I've seen a coach tell a crying ten-year-old soccer player that he should stop his tears, shake off the injury, and "get back out there," wherever out there happens to be, no matter how reluctant the youngster is to venture into that territory because he's in pain. Eventually, the boys stop crying altogether when they're hurt because the sympathy just won't come and is often replaced with derision. (The very worst thing you can tell a ten-year-old boy is that he's a wimp.)

HOW THE SYSTEM WORKS

It is always a source of amazement to me how little men seem to know about their bodies. (This doesn't mean small men know much about their bodies.) Men are often afraid to say that they don't know where the prostate is, for example (many can't even pronounce it, calling it a "prostrate" gland instead, perhaps because we examine the prostate while the man is lying down), or what a vas deferens is. So when I am doing a rectal on a fifty-year-old patient, he often asks why I am feeling for the prostate through that orifice. (By fifty, most men have lost their reluctance to ask.) My reply is that I have little choice of orifices. Much like a good offense that takes what the defense will give, I just take what I am given.

Men also tend to make jokes about their anatomical parts, probably because they are embarrassed about "body things." Indeed, in writing this, I have thought of several anatomical puns on the sperm of the moment, some of which I have left in, most of which were thankfully deleted by my (female) editor.

The Testicle (Home to Testosterone and Spermatozoa)

The testicles, those organs associated with so much of the male "essence," are, as any child knows, nothing more than two oval balls that hang in the scrotum.

The testicles produce testosterone, the major male hormone, which is released into the bloodstream through blood vessels that connect to the testicles. Testosterone has many effects on the body but is particularly important in the development of secondary male sex characteristics, such as hair distribution, physical stature, deepening of the voice, and so on. If the source of testosterone is destroyed before puberty — by castration, for example — these secondary sexual characteristics never develop, which means that the boy (and later the man) can sing like Michael Jackson for the rest of his life.

You only need one testicle to produce enough testosterone for normal functioning. If one testicle has to be sacrificed for some reason, the other will produce a sufficient amount of testosterone on its own.

The testicles also produce spermatozoa aka sperm. Spermatozoa are little guys, always swimming, furiously doing a modified backstroke in an attempt to be the one sperm that fertilizes the egg. Semen is the fluid in which the sperm live and the fluid that helps deliver the sperm to their target.

You often hear that it takes only one sperm to fertilize an egg. This is true so far as it goes. But one sperm would surely be destroyed on that hazardous journey up the vagina, through the cervix, up the uterus, and along the fallopian tube, where it meets the egg. Radisson and Groseilliers surely never had a harder time in opening up the West.

Sperm get around this difficulty by being plentiful and working as a team. An average normal sperm count is over *sixty million sperm per cubic centimeter of semen*. Think about how many sperm that is. Less than twenty million sperm per cc is considered a low sperm

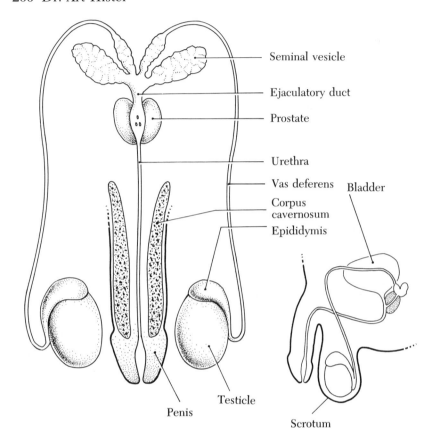

Seminal vesicle

Ejaculatory duct

Prostate

Urethra

Vas deferens Bladder

Corpus
cavernosum

Epididymis

Testicle

Penis

Scrotum

THE MALE REPRODUCTIVE SYSTEM

count, although as we always stress, any sperm count over one can theoretically result in a pregnancy.

The Epididymis, the Vas Deferens, and the Penis

A sperm (I shall forever think of spermatozoa as tiny Woody Allens from *Everything You Always Wanted to Know about Sex*) starts its trip from the testicle to the outside world — although frequently not to daylight — by entering a tube called an epididymis. The epididymis empties into the ductus or vas deferens. The vasa deferentia on both sides meet and enter the base of the penis through the ejaculatory duct. Semen, that protective bath that harbors the sperm, is composed of fluid from several sources, including glands near the urethra called the seminal vesicles, which store the sperm before ejaculation; the prostate gland; and glands in the urethra itself. The bladder also sends a tube to enter the penis.

There are many misconceptions about how the penis functions, but it is actually a very straight forward organ. Basically, the penis is composed of two spongey muscle chambers surrounding a duct. When a male becomes aroused, the nervous system sends stimuli to blood vessels in these chambers, which are called the corpora cavernosa. This stimulation draws blood into these chambers and also restricts the outflow of blood, allowing the chambers to harden and the penis to stiffen. When the blood is drained, the organ returns to its flaccid resting state, which most men claim is about a foot long.

How can one duct, the penis, deliver urine and sperm, yet not mix up the two? Because urination and sperm delivery are under the control of different nerve pathways. And luckily, when either system is in use, it automatically shuts the other one off. Thus, it is virtually impossible to ejaculate when urinating, and vice versa, although I have no doubt that there are many men who claim that they can and do. (See any issue of *Penthouse*, "Letters" section, which I never read, of course, but have heard much about.)

The Prostate (Why Women Do Not Really Envy Men)

Where, oh where, does the prostate come in? In the end, of course. The prostate is a gland that lies just below the bladder and surrounds the urethra. It is best felt through the rectum (although men would say it is never best felt). Its job is to add fluid to the ejaculate, presumably to help in the transport and the nourishment of the nervous sperm about to be sent into the cruel world. (Think of the sperm as Benjamin in *The Graduate*: "Go into plastics," which many, of course, do.)

LUMPS AND SWELLINGS

All men should learn to do testicular self-examination because it's easy to do and it is the simplest way to detect a testicular malignancy before it spreads.

Testicular self-examination is as simple as it sounds. Just like a homemade smoke, you roll your own.

Cysts and Cancers

Small, soft round growths are not uncommon on the testicle, the epididymis, or the vas deferens. Frequently, these lumps are detected by the patient himself or by his sexual partner. Most of these growths are benign fluid-filled cysts and require no treatment unless they enlarge to an uncomfortable size.

A common side effect of vasectomies is the formation of a hard little lump on the cut vas. This is called a sperm granuloma and is completely benign.

Cancers of the testicle are rare. Unlike most other cancers, however, they are more common in younger males. They usually feel harder and firmer and more uneven than the cysts described above. Luckily, the usual type of testicle cancer, called a seminoma, has an excellent prognosis.

Varicocoeles

A varicocoele is an uneven lump in the tubes above the testicle, and it is due to the overgrowth of veins in this area. For some reason, most varicocoeles occur on the left side. A varicocoele is much easier to feel when you are upright and may even disappear when you lie down. Some textbooks have stated that a varicocoele feels like a bag of worms, an impossible statement to verify. How many people do you think have ever felt a bag of worms? Who would want to?

A varicocoele is easy to feel, but it often comes as a revelation to a man that he has one, simply because most men have never compared their spermatic channels with those of another male.

About half of all men who have a varicocoele also have a low sperm count. In those men, the varicocoele is presumed to contribute to the lowering of the sperm count by increasing the temperature around the epididymis and vas deferens. The higher the temperature, the lower the sperm count.

So in a male with a low sperm count and a varicocoele, we usually operate to remove the excess tissue. I have not seen very many successful cases, but it's a simple procedure and is usually worth doing, if only for the psychological satisfaction that you are doing something that may correct the problem.

Recent reports show that if a varicocoele is removed when a man is still young, in his teens or early twenties, there is a better prognosis for fertility in later life.

Fluid around the Testicle (Hydrocele)

A hydrocele is a collection of excess fluid around the testicle. Occasionally it occurs on both sides. The testicle, much like a fetus, is normally surrounded by a small amount of fluid, which cushions it from any excess shock, especially those bumps that occur every day to the hanging scrotal sac. This fluid is constantly turning over, but an infection or injury to the area may result in increased production or decreased reabsorption of this fluid, which results in a swelling around the testicle.

A hydrocele need only be treated when it is large enough to cause problems by its sheer weight. There are two basic forms of treatment. The first is to remove the fluid through a needle (doesn't the thought just give you the creeps?) and then inject some chemical, such as tetracycline, that will cause scarring and prevent the fluid from reaccumulating. This treatment is successful in about three quarters of all hydroceles but occasionally needs to be repeated. The second form of treatment is an operation to remove the sac that contained the fluid.

Lymph Node Swellings

Lymph node swellings in the groin are extremely common. They are produced by infections that drained into those nodes from anywhere south of the umbilicus. Just as throat infections lead to swollen "glands" in the neck, so does any inflammation in the lower parts of the torso lead to swollen glands in the groin, in the creases where your legs meet your torso. Once swollen, the node will often stay somewhat larger and can be easily felt for many months, even years. Swollen glands from old infections should *not* hurt. If a node is tender, you should try to find the source of infection. If a node is gradually enlarging, it is imperative to find the cause.

Hernias (Why Men Should Only Lift Pianos with Their Legs)

The testicles are formed in the abdomen and slide into the scrotum several weeks before birth. To do this, they must penetrate through that muscle layer at the base of the abdomen that prevents your guts from spilling out of the abdomen and into the scrotum. The hole through which the testicles have slid (or as Dizzy Dean used to say, slud) then tightens up, closing the opening. But subsequent physical stress can weaken that channel, allowing the opening to "rupture." This is what is known as an inguinal hernia. Although most hernias happen to people born with a preexisting weakness in that area, hernias are particularly common among people who work at hard physical labor that involves lifting or straining. The increased effort puts more pressure on that weak spot.

Hernias can cause pain, but it is usually minimal. The patient often first notices the hernia when a silent swelling appears in the groin or in the low pelvis. (It was a dark and stormy night. Silently, the hernia descended.) Many if not most hernias are discovered in that famous male rite of passage that starts with "Turn your head and cough." Why turn your head, you may ask. Because I don't want you coughing in my face when I examine you, that's why. When you turn your head, I take the opportunity (opportunity?) of grasping the tube that leads from the testicle into the abdomen and feeling the muscle wall at the point at which the tube disappears into the abdomen. You then cough, increasing the pressure in your abdomen, so if there is a hernial opening, I can more easily feel the tissue sliding down. This is best done with the male standing (the male patient, not the male doctor).

Most hernias should be closed by surgery because they will never go away, and the longer they exist, the more likely you are to develop a complication. The most dreaded complication is called an incarcerated, strangulated hernia. This does not mean that your hernia gets thrown in jail and executed. Rather, an incarcerated hernia is one in which some tissue gets caught outside the abdominal cavity and cannot return. If the blood flow to that tissue gets cut off, much like blood flow to a finger gets cut off if a ring is too tight, then the hernia is said to have strangulated. The tissue below the stricture dies and becomes gangrenous. This is a life-threatening emergency.

How common are incarcerated, strangulated hernias? Well, in eighteen years of practice, I have never seen one. But because a hernia will never disappear, I still believe it should be corrected surgically because it's just not worth the risk and because the hernia is likely to get bigger with time. Unfortunately, exercises do not tighten the opening, and many exercise regimes actually make it worse. The hernia is a hole and will only get wider if the muscles get strained. Corsets do not correct the underlying problem; they merely hide it. Besides, they're ugly.

Surgery, however, is not uniformly successful for hernias and in a significant percentage of cases has to be repeated.

Oh yes. If you have one hernia, there is a good chance that you will have another one on the other side.

DISCHARGE FROM THE URETHRA

Discharge from the urethra is due to some type of infection, usually in the urethra, sometimes in the prostate. The discharge should be cultured for *Neisseria gonorrhea*, *Chlamydia*, and other organisms (see chapter 13).

Frequently the discharge lessens or disappears entirely even if you do nothing. But you should never assume that the infection is gone just because the discharge is gone. You are still a potential carrier of a sexually transmitted disease, and you should still be treated, as should your partner.

PAIN IN THE GROIN AREA

The Testicles

The most common reason for the testicles to ache is from trauma. This discussion always brings a queasy feeling to the pit of my ample stomach.

Trauma to the testicles is not rare, especially in contact sports. You can't say it often enough to young boys: "I know you hate them, but jocks and protective cups were invented for a good reason, which is that your parents should end up being grandparents. Wear them!"

Testicles can become infected and hurt. It is odd what a scary prospect mumps are for even the most rational man. That is because we have read somewhere that mumps in an adult leads to a testicular infection, which is likely to leave us sterile. It is true that about 25 percent of males who get mumps also develop a testicular inflammation called orchitis. But only a very small proportion of those males end up sterile. All the rest recover completely, after a good scare.

There are other organisms that can infect the testicles, but these infections are rare.

Although it's not common in adults, you can still get the dreaded "blue balls" that most of us suffered from occasionally as adolescents. They occur when the male has become aroused and the testicles have swollen with blood but sexual release is not forthcoming. The veins in the testicles then become engorged and cause pain. Until all the swelling does go down, read a book, preferably not an erotic one.

The Epididymis

An infection in the epididymis is a common problem in young men. Generally, the symptoms are sudden onset of pain and swelling. This infection is usually caused by *Chlamydia*, but it may also be caused by other bacteria. The pain can be intense, so pain relief, such as bathing the area or using strong analgesics, is essential.

It is important to differentiate epididymitis from torsion of the testicle, a condition in which the testicle has twisted on its pedicle, or stalk. This problem occurs suddenly in young men as an intense pain just above the testicle. This condition must be diagnosed quickly because when the testicle twists, the blood supply is cut off. If the testicle does not untwist itself, it must be untwisted with surgery, or else it will die of gangrene. Of course you only need one testicle to function adequately, but it does something to your self-image if one of them is removed. (A male nightmare is a picture of a testicle twisting slowly in the desert wind.) If a testicle has twisted once, the problem is likely to recur, so much so that some urologists believe in a prophylactic procedure to prevent this recurrence. (They tie it down — broncobusting, sort of.)

The Urethra

Pain in the tip of the urethra is usually described as a "burning" type of pain. Most of the time it is due to an infection in the urethra, usually caused by *Chlamydia*. It can also be caused by cuts in the urethra, warts, herpes, and other local lesions.

Many men, after a successful treatment for a chlamydial infection, complain of a persistent, mild discomfort in the urethra. More often, the patient complains that all is "just not right down there." This vague discomfort is known as posturethral syndrome and is presumably due to a persistent mild inflammation. It requires no active treatment, except you should probably avoid alcohol and caffeine while the pain persists. It can last for many months, but it usually disappears on its own.

The Prostate

The prostate can become infected with *Chlamydia* and other bacteria. The symptoms that accompany a prostatic infection, or prostatitis, can include a discharge from the penis, blood in the semen, discomfort with urination, and pain. This pain usually occurs in the low abdomen, but it may also appear in the perineum (yes, men have perineums, too) the area between the scrotum and the anus, and in the lower back. The pain of prostatitis is occasionally described as "exquisite," meaning intense, not pleasingly beautiful or delicate. Often this is a difficult diagnosis to make, unless an effort is made to culture prostatic fluid, because the symptoms are not usually dramatic.

In some men, the symptoms of prostatitis can be worsened by alcohol and caffeine.

Opinion is divided on the effect of intercourse on prostatitis. Some people believe that prostatitis is less likely to occur when the prostate is allowed to rest often, which means infrequent masturbation or intercourse (and no, I don't know the definition of infrequent). Others believe that to minimize the risk of prostatitis, the prostate ought to be emptied regularly. Me, I like the second school.

The antibiotics that are used for this infection must be specific to the infecting organism because prostatitis has a great tendency to recur and become chronic. In recurrent cases, there is some evidence that the patient should be treated for up to three months with the appropriate antibiotic.

The prostate can continue to ache for many weeks after an infection has cleared because presumably there is still some mild inflammation left over. These cases all improve eventually.

Chronic prostatitis also usually causes a persistent ache, which improves only when the chronic problem clears.

There is an interesting condition called prostadynia, in which the person complains of prostate pain but no abnormality can be detected. Now I realize that no reader of this book is neurotic (you are all obviously paragons of normal mental health, as you have shown by buying this book), but you must believe me that there are occasional persons who have a tendency to develop what I would call "neurotic" symptoms, especially in areas that involve the reproductive organs. Presumably, that's what many cases of prostadynia are about.

(This gives me the opportunity to yell at those psychiatrists who are members of the renaming police and who want to do away with the term "neurotic." It is a perfectly wonderful term that everybody, doctor and layperson alike, interprets in his or her own way, which is probably what bothers the renaming police. They're all neurotic.)

INFERTILITY

It is commonly said that 50 percent of infertility in couples stems from the male partner. Although this figure may have been accurate in the past, it is no longer true now that sexually transmitted diseases (STDs) have multiplied so quickly. STDs have been much more unfair to women than to men, in that women more often suffer sterility as a complication of an STD.

It is still true, however, that even if the male member of the twosome has sired dozens of inheritors in the past, he should be investigated with a sperm count and analysis if a couple is having trouble conceiving.

The most common, easily changed reason for male infertility (besides lack of biological knowledge) is an increased temperature in the scrotum. (I'm afraid to ask how you measure scrotal temperature.) Anything that raises scrotal temperature, such as frequent saunas, very hot, prolonged baths, or extra underwear in the winter, should be avoided by the infertile man. All men with low sperm counts should also be checked for varicocoeles and hormonal abnormalities.

IMPOTENCE

Impotence is very common. We do not have very good statistics to tell us how prevalent it is, mainly because a lot of impotent men do not complain about it. Even so, it is estimated that over twenty million North American men are impotent. Impotence increases with age. It is not a common problem for thirty-year-olds, but it is quite common for sixty-year-olds.

Many factors can contribute to impotence. If you smoke, guess what? Quitting smoking is the single most important thing you can do for yourself to correct impotence. Cutting down on cigarette intake generally doesn't help, because the nicotine, which decreases blood flow to the penis, from even a single cigarette can linger in your system for a long time. Alcohol is an important factor. When drunk, most men cannot get it up, although their verbal prowess is not diminished. But chronic alcoholism also leads to diminished sexual capacity, presumably through nerve destruction. Psychological impotence is very common. This is one problem that is very hard to self-correct because the more you think about it, the worse it usually gets. Although some sexual clinics brag about their ability to help men with this problem, the truth is that psychological impotence is hard to cure.

Impotence increases with atherosclerotic disease, probably because cholesterol plugs up the small arteries to the penis. Other diseases that can contribute include diabetes and high blood pressure. Curiously, some medications, especially the beta blockers that are prescribed for high blood pressure, make the problem even worse. The medications rarely cause the condition alone. But remember the straw and the camel, and think about beta blockers and impotence that way (although you don't have to compare the penis to a straw, necessarily).

Although there are many counterculture remedies for impotence (including eating the testicles or brains of various huge beasts), there are no accepted medications that can be taken to enhance performance, except a drug called yohimbine, which only works in very mild cases.

One should always try a psychological therapeutic approach because no matter what the original cause, there is always some psychological overlay.

The newest medical therapy is the injection of various compounds, including papaverine and others, into the penis. (This is not for the faint-hearted.) These injections can cause the penis to harden for two hours. If the injections don't work, the only treatments left are penile implants or prostheses.

PROBLEMS OF THE PROSTATE

You will hear more and more about the prostate gland in the coming years. As we baby boomers age, the problems of middle and old age seem to make more of an impact on the media, and the prostate will soon be a problem for more of us.

The prostate tends to enlarge with age, a phenomenon known as benign prostatic hypertrophy, or BPH. Sooner or later, BPH will get you in the end.

I will never forget the time I took my son to a Vancouver Canucks game, and there we were, the two of us, standing at the communal urinal with dozens of other males, all of us blissfully emptying our bladders. In a beautiful soprano voice that could be heard blocks away, my son inspected my trickle, compared it with his river, and asked, "Why does it take you so long to pee, Dad?" I couldn't get another drop out.

An enlarged prostate leads to several symptoms that all of us middle-aged men will appreciate. It may be harder to start urinating, the stream is not as strong, it is harder to unload the entire contents of the bladder, you have to get up at night more often to urinate, and there is more dribbling.

There is no medical treatment for BPH. When the prostate is too large and the symptoms no longer tolerable, there are various surgical techniques to open up the channel. Newer techniques such as balloon dilatation ("Why are you blowing that balloon up there, Daddy?") of the prostate show some initial promise but are still considered experimental.

Prostate cancer is very common in older men but rare in men under the age of fifty. Most prostate tumors cause no symptoms. We pick many up on routine physical examination by feeling a hard nodule on the surface of the prostate. Unfortunately, at least 30 percent of prostate tumors have spread by the time they can be palpated rectally, so the prognosis for palpable prostate tumors is not very good.

That is why so much effort has gone into finding alternate methods of diagnosis. Ultrasound of the prostate is being used more and more for diagnostic purposes, but its use remains controversial. Ultrasound can pick up some prostate tumors before they've spread, but this is a mixed blessing at best. Many of the tumors that we find on ultrasound, especially in older men, would never have bothered the patient. Some are benign growths and others may very well have grown at such a slow rate that the patient, an elderly gent, would have died from some unrelated cause long before the prostate tumor would have caused him any problem. Picking up these kinds of tumors can result in needless surgery with all the potential complications associated with these procedures. Clearly, what we need is much better evidence to tell us which tumors found on ultrasound will cause problems, and in which patients.

COSMETICS

No discussion of the male reproductive tract can be complete without measuring the mystique of the penis. So many men seem to be wrapped up in the mythology of "size of organ."

Size matters only if you let it matter. And you can't do anything about it anyway. Remember, it's the gunner, not the gun, the singer, not the song, the men, not the semen.

You're welcome.

CHAPTER 13

Sexually Transmitted Diseases

*In which the author navigates his way through
the slippery, often odorous minefield populated
by warts and other organisms*

I've told you several times that I'm getting old.

I'm so old I can still remember when most of society was embarrassed at even the thought, let alone the discussion, of venereal disease. I remember when there was only one or two of "those problems." We all knew about gonorrhea and syphilis, but you would have been hard-pressed to name a third.

Now look how far we've come, my babies. The term "venereal disease" has been replaced by the more direct but less romantic term "sexually transmitted disease," or STD for short. At least fifty diseases are now included in this category, frightening news for anyone who is not monogamous. But there is some comfort in the fact that only a few are common.

Luckily, society's attitude towards STDs has changed considerably over the years. Whereas in the past, the patients, and occasionally the doctors as well, whispered their fears about VD, or perhaps snickered at the thought, STDs are now generally treated as routine problems that must be approached in an honest and a forthright manner.

How do you avoid STDs? Always practice safe sex. This means you should stick with one partner whom you know to be monogamous. Don't have sexual intercourse, even oral intercourse, with people you are not sure about until you know them and their sexual history much better. (Read a book together first and talk — think of talking as oral intercourse.) Don't be shy. Ask questions about whom they have been with, what diseases they may have had, what symptoms they may be ignoring. This is one situation where a little bit of knowledge may be vital.

If you do have intercourse with someone you don't know very well, the male partner should wear a condom, preferably a latex one ("natural" condoms can allow passage of some viruses, including the virus that causes AIDS). A condom should also be worn for fellatio. And if you don't insist on a condom, at least make sure that you don't swallow semen. (A good friend of mine uses the excuse that it has too many calories. Just say you're on a diet.)

Gay sex presents unique problems because of the devastating effect that STDs have had among gay males. The best investment a gay man can make is to buy a gross of condoms. He should use them freely, either on himself or by distributing them to his sexual partners.

Gay women are the only group of sexually active adults that up to now has been relatively protected from STDs. However, in the last several years, even gay women have begun to suffer in increasing numbers from these infections.

No matter what your sexual preference, there are only three ways to maximize sexual safety.

1. Have no sex at all (something few of us are able to stick to).
2. Have intercourse only with one other person who has been similarly monogamous his or her entire life. (Such a person is of course at a premium.)
3. Always use a condom for both genital and oral intercourse, until you choose a partner for life, having made yourself as certain as you can that that person has similarly practiced safe sex until you came along. To maintain this safety, you must both of course continue to stay monogamous or use condoms if you don't. It is unfortunately true that when you have intercourse with a new partner who hasn't practiced safe sex in the past, you are in effect sleeping with all the people your partner slept with (a pretty ugly bunch, you'll agree).

What do you do if you think you have an STD? Here are some general rules everyone should know about STDs:

1. You often can't rely on symptoms alone to tell you if you have an STD, because often the symptoms are nonexistent or fleeting.
2. Most STDs require follow-up to see if the problem has cleared, even if you have taken all the prescribed medication, because symptoms are such an unreliable guide to the presence of disease.
3. With most STDs, you have to treat your sexual partner(s) as well, even if he or she has no symptoms. Your partner is very probably carrying the infecting organisms if you have not used condoms for protection.
4. It is important to culture all areas to which the STD may have been transmitted. For example, if you have had oral intercourse, tell the doctor. Otherwise, it's a bit hard for her or him to guess just what it is you do with your partner.

The information in the rest of this chapter describes symptoms mostly as they occur in women because to a great extent women have more complicated histories with STDs than men.

One last thing. Because of the rapidly proliferating and changeable information in this area, if you are in any way concerned about one of these problems, it is imperative that you see a physician who is especially interested in and knowledgeable about STDs. Improper information can have disastrous consequences for your future health.

ORGANISMS THAT CAUSE PID OR NGU

Chlamydia

Chlamydia is the primary organism that causes PID and NGU (see the section on NGU, or NSU later in this chapter).

Unfortunately, *Chlamydia* does not always produce symptoms in an infected person. What is most frustrating about this organism (and what makes it so hard to diagnose) is that in both women and men, a chlamydia infection can vary in intensity, ranging from no symptoms at all to mild, hardly noticeable discomfort to severe pain. The symptoms also vary in location because *Chlamydia* likes to travel, and as it does so, it infects each area it enters. So the general picture in an untreated case in men might start with a discharge from the urethra, associated with pain in the penis, be followed by pain in the abdomen, and end with pain in the scrotum.

In women, the organism tends to follow a similar biological route, starting in the cervix, ascending into the uterus, and ending in the fallopian tubes. This route correlates with a host of symptoms that include cervical discharge, bleeding with intercourse, burning with urination, period cramps, heavier periods, and various types of pain in the low pelvis. In short, *Chlamydia* can cause practically any symptom in the reproductive area. The most discouraging aspect of chlamydial infections is that the infecting organisms cause absolutely no symptoms in most people. Yet they still continue to produce an inflammatory fluid in the area that they are infecting. This fluid is sticky, and if it is present in narrow areas like the fallopian tubes, it tends to glue the sides of the tubes together, leading to narrowed tubes. Once inflammation is present in the tubes for a prolonged period, scarring sets in. Thus, the long-term effect of chlamydial infections is to cause infertility because of tortuous, blocked tubes. Chlamydial infections are the most common cause of mechanical infertility in women, or infertility that results from a mechanical barrier between the ovum and the sperm. If the tubes are only partially blocked, they eventually become more tortuous or somewhat twisted, greatly increasing the chance of having an ectopic pregnancy (see chapter 11).

Chlamydial infections have also been implicated in a higher rate of miscarriages. They also cause a host of infections in the newborn, including infections of the eye (conjunctivitis) and of the lungs (pneumonia). For this reason, all pregnant women should be tested for *Chlamydia* before delivery.

How can you tell if you have picked up *Chlamydia*? There are several tests available, but most of them are as yet not too reliable. I always stress that in the person who may have been exposed to *Chlamydia*, or in the person who has symptoms that are compatible with the diagnosis of a chlamydial infection — for example, in a woman, a pelvic infection or a raw, bleeding cervix, and in a man, urethral discharge — it is advisable to be treated for this infection, even if the results of the tests are negative. And always remember that all your sexual partners should be treated at the same time as you are. Otherwise, if you have sex with the partner who infected you, and you have not synchronized your treatments, you may become reinfected. (As yet, synchronized treatments are not a demonstration sport at the Olympics.)

People at particularly high risk are those who have had multiple sexual partners and those who are diagnosed to have another STD. The term "multiple" doesn't mean "many." Two or more sexual partners should be considered multiple. Also remember that if your partner has had one other partner, that makes you a contact of multiple sexual partners, and you consequently become a high-risk person, even though you are only sleeping with one other person.

Treatment regimes for a chlamydia infection are likely to change as newer and better antibiotics become available. At the time of the writing of this book, the recommended treatment for adults is some type of tetracycline in high doses.

When in doubt, test. If still in doubt, get treated. No matter what the tests say. And don't forget to have your partner(s) treated at the same time. And if he or she or they refuse, consider a career of abstention (which should persuade him or her or them to get treated).

Neisseria gonorrhoeae

Every time I speak to a group about STDs, I am invariably asked, "What ever happened to gonorrhea? Did it just go away?"

'Fraid not, folks. Gonorrhea, caused by the bacterium *Neisseria gonorrhoeae* ain't gone. It has changed somewhat, however, and in its newer guises it poses a distinct public health problem, although not yet on the scale of some of the other STDs. But give it time, and it might.

Women frequently have few symptoms with gonorrheal infections of the reproductive tract. There may be a thicker cervical discharge or burning with urination. But often there are no symptoms, and the organism is first suspected when the patient develops PID (see below). Like untreated chlamydia, untreated gonorrhea can lead to blocked fallopian tubes and infertility.

Classically, men with gonorrhea in the urethra develop a thick, yellow discharge that leads to a burning sensation in the penis with urination. These symptoms usually appear two days to two weeks after exposure. But many men develop only minimal discharge or often none at all. Yet they are still able to transmit the infection in the absence of symptoms.

Gonorrhea can also infect the oral cavity and the rectum. Although gonorrhea can produce an obvious throat infection that mimics any other infection in that area, it is often "silent" in its oral form (think about the concept of a silent oral infection). In the rectum, gonorrhea produces a thick discharge and rectal irritation.

Gonorrhea that's left untreated can spread to any other organ (especially the joints) and result in infections that are very difficult to diagnose and treat.

The tests for gonorrhea are also less than completely reliable. If you have been told that your partner has gonorrhea, you should be treated for this infection, whether your tests are positive or not (in the world of STDs, a positive test, unlike a positive comment, is not a good thing).

Whereas in the sixties practically all gonorrheal infections responded to ordinary penicillin in large doses, now some infections require newer, very sophisticated antibiotics. All proven gonorrhea infections should be closely monitored for response to the antibiotic that is chosen. This is particularly crucial if you happen to pick up gonorrhea in the third world, where resistant strains are much more endemic.

Never rely on homemade remedies for treatment of gonorrhea. The symptoms can often disappear, and you will wake up one day with a pelvic infection, or to a phone call from a partner, informing you that he or she has symptoms and you were his or her only contact. Gonorrhea, like taxes, does not go away just because you want it to.

PELVIC PAIN — PID (PELVIC INFLAMMATORY DISEASE)

PID is the acronym for pelvic inflammatory disease. In PID, there is an infection of the fallopian tubes (and usually the cervix, the uterus, and the ovaries as well), often caused by *Chlamydia*, but also produced by *Neisseria gonorrhoeae* and other organisms (see previous sections). The infection results in the release of a sticky, inflammatory fluid that tends to make the sides of the tubes stick together, eventually resulting in narrowed, tortuous tubes. PID can be acute, subacute, or chronic.

When you get acute PID, you are usually quite sick, with pain in the abdomen being the major symptom. The pain can be on either side of the pelvis or, more often, on both sides, and the pain is often worsened by most physical activities, especially intercourse. As well, you may have heavier and crampier periods. There is often a new sexual partner involved, and you may or may not notice a changed cervical discharge. If you have an IUD in place and you happen to be exposed to *Chlamydia* or *Neisseria gonorrhoeae*, you are more likely to develop PID than a woman without an IUD who is exposed to the same organisms.

On examination, you may or may not have other symptoms of infection, such as a fever. Most important, the cervix is usually exquisitely tender to touch, especially when it is manipulated. (How do you manipulate a cervix? Promise it riches and fame?) The lower pelvic cavity is exquisitely tender as well, often with a palpable swelling.

Unfortunately, though, some women who have PID are just not that sick, and it takes a high index of suspicion to diagnose such subacute cases. Many doctors do not diagnose this condition unless there are changes in blood tests consistent with an acute infection, but I believe that the history and the examination are the most important clues to diagnosis, and hang the blood tests. (Call me a Hanglophile.) A lot of women will be overdiagnosed for this problem by my simple criteria, but I believe that overdiagnosis is preferable to missing some of the milder or subacute cases, which occurs when we use only very strict criteria such as blood tests.

Cultures should always be done to try to isolate the responsible organism, although the tests frequently do not yield the culprit. Treatment consists of the appropriate antibiotics, often given intravenously, and strict rest, preferably in bed, to allow the inflammation to die down. Acute PID may require prolonged therapy, even with the most aggressive treatment, the most difficult part of which is always convincing the acute PID sufferer to rest in bed.

In some women acute PID turns into a problem of chronic abdominal pain. It is probable that once the tubes have been damaged, they will inflame more easily in the future when exposed to the organisms that can cause this infection. More commonly, the original infection often leaves damaged tubes behind, ones that are somewhat twisted and narrowed and that have many adhesions, or areas that are stuck together. Inflammation around these adhesions frequently results in a pelvis that feels exactly like one with an acute case of PID, even though no acute infection is present. As a result, a woman with this kind of pelvis may be overtreated with antibiotics because the physician tends to overdiagnose a flare-up of acute PID.

Chronic PID has several unhappy sequelae. There is the already-mentioned chronic inflammation, in which the pelvis hurts and the patient is sick, sometimes for weeks or even months at a time. Chronic PID can also result in twisted, scarred tubes that greatly increase the chance of an ectopic pregnancy. If the tubes are sufficiently scarred, the patient is left sterile.

There is no good treatment for chronic PID. The only way to correct some of the damage is through pelvic surgery, but surgery that merely attempts to correct some of the problems (like the cutting of adhesions) is usually just a temporizing move, and the pain often soon returns. In very intractable cases, radical surgery to remove the uterus and tubes (and the ovaries, if they are also inflamed) is occasionally necessary, but again, depending on the source of the problem, there is no guarantee of success with this operation either.

URETHRAL DISCHARGE — NGU, OR NSU

Nongonococcal urethritis, or nonspecific urethritis, is an infection of the urethra resulting in urethral discharge and burning with urination in which *Neisseria gonorrhoeae* is not the offending organism. Now that we have better testing media, we know that most such infections are caused by *Chlamydia*, but other organisms can also cause this problem.

NGU is always treated as if it were due to *Chlamydia*, with the same treatment schedule.

VAGINAL DISCHARGE

A vaginal discharge is not usually caused by an STD, although both *Chlamydia* and *Neisseria gonorrhoeae* can produce changes in the discharge. Certainly, any woman who has a change in discharge that she can't readily explain, especially if she has recently had a new sexual partner with whom she has had unprotected intercourse, should have appropriate tests done. (For a fuller discussion of vaginal discharge and vaginal infections, see chapter 11.)

GENITAL ULCERS OR SORES

Herpes

Although herpes infections have been present since biblical times, this virus didn't achieve its present notoriety until the last two decades. *Time* magazine anointed the era of the herpes epidemic when it featured a cover story about herpes with a huge red letter *H* on the cover (which, contrary to popular local opinion, did not stand for Hister). This official media acknowledgment merely confirmed what most health workers had noticed for several years — the number of cases of herpes had been increasing dramatically since the dawn of the so-called sexual revolution, and the infection had begun to spread rapidly through the sexually active population.

A herpes infection is caused by the herpes simplex virus (HSV). Although there are several types of herpes virus, there are only two types of herpes simplex virus, which are imaginatively named herpes virus type 1 and herpes virus type 2 (people who name viruses do not write creative books for children). Herpes 1 primarily causes cold sores on the lips or around the mouth. Herpes 2 primarily causes genital sores. But when herpes 1 is transmitted to the genital area by oral-genital sex, it can cause exactly the same problems in the pelvis as herpes 2.

The incubation period of a herpes infection generally varies from two days to two weeks. The infection makes its appearance with a superficial ulcer, or a group of tiny, wet sores. The first time a herpes sore appears, it may hurt a lot and last for several weeks. But for most people, the first herpetic infection may produce only a very transient, mild skin irritation that is easy to dismiss as meaningless. Or the most noticeable symptom may be a burning sensation with urination, or a vaginal discharge. The sores, in fact, may not even be noticed at all, and you many not find out you have the infection until someone tells you that you passed an infection on to her or him. So, no matter how innocuous a sore in the pelvic area may seem, even if your partner has handed you an affidavit of a clean bill of health from a list of previous contacts ("Read this! Now are you satisfied? So now can we go to bed?"), you should still get tested for herpes, especially if the sores come back for a few days every so often.

Unfortunately, when the sores clear, the herpes virus has not left. The virus has sort of gone into hiding, living in nerve cells in your body. From time to time it may reappear, even as long as years later.

For a great many people, herpes comes on once or twice and never bothers them again. In other folks, however, herpes does recur. When it does, it generally comes back for several days and disappears without any treatment. In some people, however, genital herpes recurs frequently and may require the use of suppressive medication for relief from outbreaks.

For those people with recurrent herpetic sores, the recurrence often announces its impending arrival by causing a tingling sensation or an itch in the area where it will break out. This phenomenon is known as a prodrome.

Stress is usually put down as the number-one cause for a herpes recurrence. A simple question: do you know anybody who lives a stress-free existence? Outside of an institution, I mean. My case rests. Certainly, stress can lead to a recurrence, but always look for factors that are easier to control. For example, there are theories that excessive exposure to sun reactivates all types of viral lesions in your body, including herpes lesions around the genital area if you expose your genitals to the sun (a strange rite of summer that many people seem to practice, especially here on the west coast). So if you get frequent summer recurrences of herpes, keep your precious parts out of the sun.

Intercourse can precipitate a recurrence of herpes both through the direct physical trauma to the area and through the anxiety associated with the possibility of a flare-up. The solution is simple. Make sure that you do not traumatize the area unnecessarily, and RELAX.

Unfortunately, the only way to be certain that you won't pass a herpetic infection on to your sexual partner is to have intercourse only with a condom on at all times. Although it is easier to pass the virus on when there are evident symptoms, which includes anything from the prodrome to the healed sores, it is still possible to transmit the virus even when no symptoms are present. Most health authorities counsel that it is best to practice safe sex (read *condoms*) until you have chosen a lifelong partner, who may then decide for himself or herself if he or she wants to take the risk of contracting this infection.

Many home remedies have been proposed for the treatment of herpes outbreaks. The most common in the counterculture segment of my practice is the amino acid lysine (not Lysol). There is absolutely no objective medical evidence that lysine works better than a placebo. But never discount the placebo effect. If lysine works for you, then by all means continue to take it. (By the way, if you want to buy a bridge, contact my office. I have several bridges in the Vancouver area that I am trying to sell to a nice owner. The deeds are included, of course.)

The prescription drug acyclovir (Zovirax), available both as a pill and as an ointment, can decrease both the severity and the length of a new case of genital herpes. The pill is definitely more effective and when possible should be started as soon as your first episode of herpes is suspected.

Acyclovir ointment is absolutely ineffective in recurrent herpes (although it is frequently prescribed for this condition). Oral acyclovir, however, drives the virus underground a day or two more quickly than would happen if you took no treatment at all. So unless you get very frequent recurrences, this treatment is not worth the high cost. For frequent recurrent bouts of herpes, oral acyclovir can reduce the frequency of recurrence and the length of each attack.

Like most STDs, herpes is much more problematic for women than men. In men, the only complications of herpes are the discomfort of the sores, the emotional consequences of the infection, and the knowledge that it can be passed on. It causes no long-term health problems in otherwise healthy heterosexual men, although it can cause severe rectal infections, which are much more common in gay men.

For women, the road is more tortuous. Although there is a good deal of controversy about whether the following "fact" is quite as true as it used to be, HSV infections have been linked to a higher rate of cervical cancer (the controversy stems from the recent conjecture that this higher rate of cervical cancer is not caused by the HSV but by the human papilloma virus (HPV), as both viruses tend to infect the same people). Nonetheless, it is very important that women with herpes get regular Pap smears.

Equally important to every woman is that herpes infections can be devastating in a newborn infant, causing a high rate of blindness or brain damage and even death. To avoid this rare consequence, any pregnant woman with a genital herpes infection that is active at the time of delivery should have a cesarean section, which prevents the fetus from coming in contact with the herpes virus in the vagina. The most important thing to stress here, though, is that most people with herpes do not know they have it. So if there is any chance that you have come in contact with the HSV, you must tell the doctor helping with the delivery. If an examination for herpes at the time of delivery shows no active infection, a vaginal delivery is safe.

Any wet sore in the genital area should be cultured for the presence of herpes virus. A negative test never means that you don't have herpes. But a positive test does confirm your suspicions and alerts you to future consequences.

Remember, for most people an HSV infection is an inconvenience, a bother, a problem that must be monitored, but not a cause for alarm.

Syphilis

Syphilis is making a comeback. Most people thought that syphilis was like Gordie Howe — it had hung in there seemingly forever but had finally retired in the last few decades. But instead, like Guy Lafleur, syphilis has flowered again, and new cases are on the rise once more.

Syphilis is caused by an organism called *Treponema pallidum.* In a new case, the treponeme causes a sore, or chancre, at the site of infection, which is usually the penis in men and the vulva or vagina in women. The chancre lasts for several weeks and then disappears, leaving no sign behind (such as Syphilis Slept Here).

Two to twelve weeks later, syphilis enters the second stage, in which it causes a flulike syndrome accompanied by a transient skin rash. This stage too fades without treatment. It is in the third stage that syphilis is devastating. It lurks in the body as a hidden menace for many years. It can invade any body system and destroy it. It particularly tends to affect the cardiovascular and nervous systems.

The diagnosis of syphilis depends on a high index of suspicion. Any individual at high risk, such as a person who has not been practicing safe sex, should be tested with routine blood tests. If sores are evident, these can be tested directly for the presence of the syphilitic organisms.

As usual, practicing safe sex ought to keep you away from this infection.

Treatment is high doses of injectable penicillin.

Other Causes of Venereal Ulcers

There are several other causes of ulcers or sores in the pelvic area, but these are much less common. They include STDs such as lymphogranuloma venereum and chancroid, and non-STD causes such as yeast infections, reactions to drugs, trauma, and tumors, which are very rare.

WARTS

Human Papilloma Virus (HPV)

Human papilloma virus (HPV) is the virus that causes warts in the genital area. There are many subtypes of HPV, and they can cause several types of genital warts. Those ugly, large grapelike clusters that all of us have had a peek at in venereal disease textbooks are called condyloma accuminata. But HPV also produces a flatter type of wart that is considerably more difficult to diagnose because it can hide itself very well for years before producing its damaging effects. Why should we worry about HPV? After all, warts are just warts, True, they're yucky, but so what? Treat them with eye of newt and brain of toad and they'll disappear.

We worry about these infections because we now have very good proof that a few types of HPV can cause cancers (although most types do not). The areas that can definitely develop HPV cancers include the cervix in women, the penis in men, and the anus and rectum in both women and men. The HPV can act very quickly at instituting changes in your cells. Although rare, it is thought that in some women, an HPV infection can change a normal (class I) Pap smear to a precancerous (class III) Pap smear in less than a year.

HPV warts can grow in your body for many years before they become visible to the naked eye (as opposed, I suppose, to the fully dressed eye, which can see them earlier). In fact, many warts require sophisticated equipment like a colposcope (a magnifier of cervical cells) to be properly seen. You may be told for many years that your Pap smears are normal, yet you may be incubating HPV; it cannot be easily detected with currently available tests. If you do have warts, it's important that your partner be carefully checked for warts as well. In addition, any visible warts make it important to look hard at all other potentially infected areas, such as deep in the vagina.

What do you do with warts caused by HPV? First, always practice safe sex so that you don't pass them on. Second, you must treat them. Like warts in other areas of the body, some venereal warts disappear spontaneously. But you should never rely on that eventuality.

Condylomata are usually treated with a solution of a substance called podophyllin, which is painted onto each wart. Other solutions, like trichloroacetic acid, can also be used. If these solutions don't do the trick, venereal warts can be burned with lasers, frozen by cryotherapy, or removed surgically. Another treatment, which is generally not readily available, is to inject interferon (an antiviral drug) into the wart. But no matter what treatment is used, warts tend to recur.

If you have warts, or indeed if you ever did, you must be checked frequently for the emergence of new warts that were incubating at the time you were last treated. This warning (wartning?) applies particularly for areas that are difficult for you to see yourself, such as around the anus or in the vagina. (Of course if you can see these areas easily, I have a job opportunity I'd like to discuss with you.) In addition, you should be carefully monitored for a long time (preferably by somebody particularly knowledgeable about this problem) for the first symptoms of premalignant change.

Molluscum Contagiosum

Molluscum are those tiny, round, pearly warts that usually show up in bunches around the genitals. They can, however, occur anywhere on the body. They are transmitted by close person-to-person contact, often through intercourse.

Unlike other types of warts, these are not produced by the HPV. And also in contrast to other venereal warts, most molluscum will disappear if you wait long enough. So all you really need to do is not transmit them to a partner. If you want to treat them, liquid nitrogen freezing is very effective.

PELVIC ITCHING — PARASITE INFECTIONS

An itch in the pubic area can be caused by yeast infections and skin problems such as the various types of dermatitis (see chapter 10), but it is also commonly caused by parasites.

Crabs

Can you think of an uglier thing than a crab? I mean crabs are *ugly*. What's more, they move. Freddie Krueger in miniature!

Crabs are little critters that you generally only get from sexual transmission, although I have heard an incredible assortment of alternate explanations from people, usually in front of their partners, as to how they came to possess these bugs. You can get them from toilet seats, but this is not very common, especially for men, who are blessed with paraphernalia that allows less sedentary use of the toilet.

The major symptom that crabs produce is itching. Most people seem to assume that if they have crabs, they will see the little bugs dart about frantically (sort of a pubic Japanese bullet train or a pubic antelope, I suppose). In fact, a large percentage of crab owners refuse to believe they have the infection unless the physician confirms this movement, which can only be done by staring at the pubis for a long time. (I'd rather see *Guys and Dolls* again.) But crabs don't really move much. Why should they? After biting your skin, they bloat and become contented, sort of like me after a huge dinner. They will then just sit there in your pubic area.

Crabs can climb out of the pubic area. They have been spotted in eyebrows and armpits, although they are not thought to infect the scalp. It is important to check all hairy areas for crabs if you are infected. It is also very important to treat your partner(s) simultaneously. And to have a good explanation ready.

Crabs are treated with lindane (Kwellada). Usually one application is effective.

Other Parasites

Scabies (see chapter 10) often infects the pubic area, especially in men. All other superficial parasites, such as body lice, can also infect the pelvic area, but they generally prefer other haunts.

OTHER STDs

AIDS

A meaningful discussion of AIDS (aquired immune deficiency syndrome) is beyond the scope of this book for one simple reason — the information about this disease is changing at such a rapid rate that something written today may be out of date by the time this information is published. Thus, I will only mention several facts that everyone should know.

AIDS is caused by a slow-growing virus called the human immunodeficiency virus (HIV). Currently, the virus cannot be cultured directly from a blood sample, so what we test for instead are antibodies to the virus. If your blood tests positively for these antibodies, it means that you have been exposed to the HIV. We do not know how many people who have been exposed to the virus will develop full-blown AIDS, although we know that at least 50 percent do, and this number will probably prove much higher eventually.

It is generally agreed that after exposure to the virus, most people who are tested will show antibodies in under eight weeks, but some people have not tested positive for more than a year (and a rare few, even longer) after exposure to the virus. Newer, more sensitive tests will soon be available that should greatly improve our ability to find the virus in all its hidden forms and probably at an earlier stage.

In Canada, AIDS is still mostly a problem only for groups who practice high-risk behavior. This high-risk behavior includes unprotected vaginal or anal intercourse with unknown or infected partners, and intravenous drug use. There is absolutely no proof that you can get AIDS from sharing towels or cups, or from any other type of direct physical contact, except those covered in the high-risk categories. If those high-risk patterns are not part of your lifestyle, you probably have more of a chance of being struck by lightning than you have of contracting AIDS.

At this time there is no evidence that AIDS is transmitted through oral sex. But a good friend of mine, who sees a lot of AIDS patients, says that you really should never exchange bodily fluids if you want to be completely safe. Why take the risk?

An active HIV infection attacks the lymphocytes, those cells that fight off infection. Thus, the AIDS patient is prone to opportunistic infections (like disseminated herpes and candida infections) that the normal person can fight off.

There are no universally effective treatments that prevent an HIV-positive patient from developing an active infection. There are similarly no medications that kill the AIDS virus, although AZT (Retrovir) seems to retard the progression of the illness in most people, especially if given early, before the patient is very ill. Work is currently being done on several other medications that may prove to be of benefit, as well as on immunizations that could perhaps be used on people who practice high-risk behavior.

Even Other STDs

Several other problems such as giardiasis (see chapter 8) and hepatitis B (see chapter 4) are also often sexually transmitted, but these are all dealt with in other parts of this book.

CHAPTER 14

Contraception

In which you finally find out why your IUD may only be tuned to a country and western station

There are two important things to remember about birth control. One, there is no perfect method of contraception. Since reproduction is biologically necessary for the continuation of the species, anything that interferes with it is bound to produce unwanted side effects, just as any interference with other biologic functions such as eating or sleeping produces such effects. Two, when contraception fails, the woman suffers much more severe consequences than the man. For this reason, it is the woman who should choose the method of contraception that a couple will use. In doing so she must carefully consider the pros and cons of each method, recognizing that these change throughout life — what was appropriate at twenty does not necessarily make sense at forty. In fact, it is a very rare woman who at forty is still using the same method she used at twenty.

What, then, are the most important factors that you should take into account in choosing your method of birth control?

1. The frequency of intercourse in your life. If you are only having sex once a month, you are likely to choose a different method than if you are having intercourse every night (an exhausting prospect at my advanced age).
2. The possible reasons for failure of each method. If you are not a very disciplined person, you may not demand that your partner put on a condom each time you make love, especially if he is the typically reluctant male. (Quickly now, can you name a single male who shouts "hurrah" and gleefully claps his hands at the

297

thought of putting on a condom?) Or you may be very forgetful and consequently fail to take a pill every day.

3. Your fear of pregnancy. If it is absolutely essential that you do not get pregnant, then you must obviously choose the method that can come closest to guaranteeing no possible failure (and the answer is not abstention, which tends to be abandoned rather precipitously).

4. Your partner's views. Sex is often a political as well as an emotional and a biological act. By this I mean that sex is often more than simply coupling. There are many more emotions involved than simple biologic urges. You should talk to your partner about his preferences and give them some weight in your decision. If a man says that he loathes condoms, it is likely that he will be quite reluctant, at inopportune moments, to put one on, which is one hell of a time to start an argument, especially one that you might lose. I have found over the years that methods that interfere with normal sexual routines tend to be abandoned. The alternative for many couples is not to have intercourse as often, and this generally leads to other problems in the relationship if any resentment develops.

5. The side effects of the method. All methods of contraception have some manner of side effect, and some can have serious complications as well.

6. Your medical history. Certain methods of contraception cannot be used by some women because they may produce serious if not life-threatening complications. Thus, if you have ever had a blood clot, for example, you should avoid the pill at all cost because the pill can lead to clots. If you only have periods every three months, you may not be able to tolerate the uncertainty of a diaphragm, because you would constantly be concerned about a possible pregnancy.

7. Your fear of certain eventualities. I have heard many women say that no matter how reassuring the medical profession is about the pill, they still cannot relax and use that method comfortably. This is an important consideration. If you are unsure about the safety of a particular method, you are much less likely to use it properly, a factor doctors call a lack of compliance. Lack of compliance can lead to all sorts of problems, not the least of which is an unhappy

patient who runs a higher risk of getting pregnant. It's very important that you discuss these anxieties with your physician and settle them to your satisfaction.

You negotiate your way through this confusing and constantly evolving maze by thoroughly informing yourself about the various choices, how they work, what their potential problems are, how often they fail and why, and what factors we are still in doubt about. This is not as difficult as it sounds. Most of the information you need is available in various publications, including this book. Stay up to date by asking your doctor every time you visit if there is something new or different you should know. Although often somewhat dramatic, the popular press is an excellent source of new information that you can often read even before your doctor has had a chance to find it out. (I am always surprised by the obscure articles patients bring into the office, which they have read in God knows what magazine, but which often, surprisingly, give useful advice.)

Talk to friends. I have frequently prescribed a new method of birth control that the patient asked for, instead of my original recommendation, because a friend of hers had recommended that this other method might suit her better ("no matter what your doctor says"). This kind of recommendation is often quite appropriate.

And don't be afraid to argue with your doctor or to change your mind. Living situations change, fears change, relationships evolve and dissolve. (One woman's diaphragm is another woman's IUD — an old Welsh proverb.)

THE BIRTH CONTROL PILL

The pill is the most-studied drug in history. For the first time ever, a medication has been given to millions of humans not to correct an unhealthy state but, in most cases, to provide convenience.

The medical profession has been holding its collective breath (picture thousands of blue-faced physicians) to see if women on the pill will develop any unexpected complications, especially cancer. Mostly, the news is good. Many women who have taken the pill have received health benefits from using it, some of which continue even after they have come off the pill (see the discussion of advantages, below). Recently, however, there have been several reports that the rate of breast cancer increases in some women who take the pill, seemingly those who are quite young when they first start and who take the pill for a long time. These findings are in dispute, but if they are confirmed in more studies, we will have to be much more cautious about who takes the pill and for how long.

How It Works

The birth control pill is a combination of two types of female hormone, estrogen and progestin, which is a close relative to the normal female hormone progesterone. The different types of pill merely use different types of estrogen and progestin and in different doses.

The main contraceptive effect of the pill is to prevent the ovary from releasing an egg: no egg; no fertilization; no fetus. (The pill also causes changes in the cervical mucus and creates a less hospitable environment on the inside of the uterus for an egg.) The ovary doesn't release an egg because the progestin fools the pituitary gland (remember the gofer?) into believing that the woman taking the pill is pregnant. The pituitary gland then does not release its hormones, preventing the ovaries from releasing an egg.

There has been a trend to use lower dosages of estrogen in the pill over the last two decades. The lower dosages have helped cut down on many side effects and complications that stemmed from the higher doses that were formerly used. It is rarely necessary for a woman to take a pill with more than thirty-five micrograms of estrogen in it. (I really don't know, and you don't have to either, how big a microgram is. Just take my word for this.) Progestins too have gradually come down in dose.

Advantages

In the charts showing the effectiveness of different methods of birth control, there are usually two columns — one showing the theoretical effectiveness in a perfect world (one in which we stay young forever and in which the Dodgers and Les Canadiens never lose a game), the other showing the actual effectiveness in a world that depends on imperfect humans (Dan Quayle?). The second column reflects the user failure rate, and it is important to keep this figure in mind when you weigh the advantages and disadvantages of any method of birth control.

Here are the main advantages of the birth control pill:

1. The pill virtually guarantees that you won't get pregnant. The pill is close to 100 percent effective. For most women, it *is* 100 per cent effective. Certainly you can get pregnant if you don't take the pill properly. But in eighteen years of practice, I can recall only two women who became pregnant while on the pill. And both of them may have missed at least one pill, if not more. So although it's possible to become pregnant on the pill, it's highly unlikely to happen.
2. The pill is easy to use. It is certainly easier to swallow a pill than to insert a diaphragm or pressure a partner to use a condom.
3. The pill seems to protect against PID (see chapter 13).
4. The pill regulates menstrual cycles.
5. Periods are lighter on the pill. This means there is less chance of becoming anemic through blood loss.
6. Women on the pill have much fewer period cramps than women who are not on the pill. In some reports, pill users even complain less of premenstrual tension (although this is not common).
7. Lighter and less crampy periods mean an improved lifestyle for many women, with less time lost from work and recreation.
8. Pill users have less endometriosis (see chapter 11) than other women.
9. Women on the pill have a lower rate of ectopic pregnancies than other women.
10. Pill users are much less prone to develop cysts on the ovary.
11. They have fewer benign breast lumps.
12. Acne clears on the pill.

There are other gains as well.

A much-quoted study that compared a group of 100,000 women who took the pill with a group of 100,000 who didn't showed that the pill users had 235 fewer biopsies for benign breast lumps, 320 fewer cases of iron-deficiency anemia, 117 fewer cases of ectopic pregnancies, 600 fewer admissions to hospital for pelvic inflammatory disease, 50 percent less ovarian cancer, 50 percent less uterine cancer, less frequent first attacks of rheumatoid arthritis, and 35 fewer operations for benign ovarian cysts.

Disadvantages

For the most part, the side effects of the pill are a nuisance that can usually be tolerated or adjusted to with little cost to your comfort. Following are the main disadvantages of the pill:

1. The most common complaint is breakthrough bleeding, or spotting during the month. The reason for spotting is that the pill only gives you a small amount of hormone, and some women simply require more hormone to control the lining of their uterus. Spotting is minimized if you take the pill at the same time every day (which doesn't mean at the same exact minute but roughly at the same hour).

    Most of the time spotting is minimal and usually disappears after a month or two on the pill. In some women, however, spotting can be very heavy and even mimic a regular period that just goes on and on. Occasionally, breakthrough bleeding can be lessened by changing pills, but sometimes the only way to get rid of this symptom is to increase the strength of the pill. You should accept this solution only reluctantly because when you increase the dose, you increase the risk of other side effects and complications.

2. A fair number of women lose their periods while on the pill, a problem called amenorrhea. Amenorrhea occurs because the estrogen content of the low-dose pills is not sufficient to allow the buildup of a thick enough lining on the uterus. Thus, there is little lining to shed at the time the period should come. The first time that you get amenorrhea on the pill, you should have

a pregnancy test. Once pregnancy has been ruled out, you can safely go back to using that pill. There is no proof whatsoever that if you don't have periods while taking the pill, you will have more trouble getting pregnant when you discontinue its use. Amenorrhea can usually be corrected by increasing the dose of estrogen. But as for breakthrough bleeding, be very careful about making this adjustment.

3. A very common complaint on the pill is weight gain. I have heard women complain that the pill caused them to gain twenty-five pounds, but it's commonly agreed that anything more than a five-to-seven-pound weight gain is probably not due to the pill. Instead, check the frequency with which you open the fridge.

4. The pill can increase blood pressure, and for this reason every woman who is using the pill should have a yearly blood pressure check. Any increase in blood pressure should be carefully monitored. If it is above 140/90 on more than two occasions, you should discontinue using the pill, and your blood pressure should then return to normal. There is no proof that the pill increases blood pressure permanently.

5. The pill can increase both the severity and the frequency of headaches, especially migraines, but this is not true for everyone. I also know of women whose headaches have been mitigated by using the pill, probably because they stopped worrying about becoming pregnant.

6. There is no doubt that the pill lessens libido in some women, but libido seems to be increased in just as many women.

7. The pill is commonly accused of increasing vaginal yeast infections, but this is not nearly as common with the lower doses of pills currently in use.

8. Nausea, which is not unusual on the pill, generally disappears after one or two cycles.

9. For many women, breasts swell and become more tender, but both these symptoms generally also disappear with continued use.

10. For a small proportion of women who stop using the pill, it takes a while for periods to restart. It is not uncommon to have one or two cycles that are irregular, but some women take several

months to return to normal; a few take more than a year. This problem is called postpill amenorrhea. It is significantly more prevalent in those women who had abnormal cycles before they started the pill. Fertility is not affected; in the long term, you are just as capable of conceiving as women who have used other methods of birth control.

11. The pill increases the blood's ability to clot and also leads to higher cholesterol levels in the bloodstream, thus increasing the risk of strokes and heart attacks. This risk is minimal for most women under thirty-five but increases steadily as they pass that age, especially if they smoke or have diabetes. This has led many doctors to tell all women over thirty-five to choose an alternate method of birth control. But judging by current evidence, I believe that a woman over thirty-five or even over forty who doesn't smoke and who has never smoked, and who doesn't have other risk factors such as very high cholesterol or diabetes, can probably safely take the pill.

12. The pill can sometimes lead to depression, but just as many women have told me that their mood improved on the pill.

13. The pill can cause liver damage, and it can also stimulate certain hormone-dependent tumors (such as those in the female reproductive organs). Both of these are rare complications.

Occasionally the fear is raised that the pill may damage subsequent offspring, especially if you discontinue using the pill just before becoming pregnant. In fact, there are studies of women who took the pill *while* pregnant, some who even took the pill for the full nine months of their pregnancy. (I know there are always rationalizations, but somewhere, somehow, that bulge in the lower half should have been the source of at least an odd question or two.) Children of such women do not have a higher rate of tumors (although I think that the children of those women who took the pill while pregnant should definitely get their sex education at school and not at home).

Precautions

Before starting on the pill, you should talk to your doctor about your medical history and your family history. ("My Uncle Syd is a nut, my brother is a loser with foul breath, but I'm perfect.") You should then have a thorough physical examination to include at the very least a blood pressure reading, breast examination, liver evaluation ("you have a great liver there"), and thorough pelvic exam. This type of examination should be done every year. You should also have a Pap smear, a blood count for hemoglobin, a urinalysis, and, if you have been sexually active, tests for the various STDs. Although not everyone agrees with this, I also test every woman starting the pill for cholesterol.

The pill is certainly not for everyone.

Among the problems that should absolutely disqualify use of the pill are a history of previous problems with blood clots, a history of phlebitis (an inflammation in a vein, which leads to higher rates of blood clots), a history of stroke or heart attack, any liver tumor, a suspected breast malignancy, any currently active liver disease, and any problem with undiagnosed, abnormal vaginal bleeding. A woman with high blood pressure should probably not be on the pill either. In addition, in the last few years, many doctors have started advising women with high cholesterol not to take the pill.

There are some conditions that don't automatically disqualify you from using the pill, but if you do happen to have any of these risk factors, then the pill should probably not be your first choice for contraception. But if you weigh all these risks carefully (how exactly do you weigh a risk — in kilorisks?), you may still decide that it is worth your while to take the pill. These relative contraindications include a history of diabetes, gestational diabetes (diabetes while you were pregnant), gallbladder disease, epilepsy, lupus erythematosis, and fibroids.

Certain drugs, such as Dilantin and Phenobarbital, can occasionally lower the effectiveness of the pill. There has also been some concern that sometimes the commonly used antibiotics ampicillin and tetracycline can also interfere with the pill, although it is extremely unlikely that using these antibiotics for an acute infection for seven to ten days can produce enough interference for you to become pregnant. As with all medication, you should take the lowest dose of pill that works. Unfortunately, far too many women were put on higher doses a few years ago, and they have renewed the prescription year after year. Each time a prescription for the pill is renewed, you should ask if there is a lower dose you can take.

One other very important reminder. If you are on the pill, any time you develop a symptom that you can't easily explain, check it with your doctor. Certain symptoms should be checked immediately. These include coughing up blood, significant and sudden pain or swelling in the legs, sudden severe headache, and sudden visual disturbance. Although most of the time these symptoms are not caused by a major problem, they should nonetheless never be ignored.

And finally, there is no proof that you ever have to take a break from taking the pill. You can take it for many years in a row without requiring a switch to another method of contraception.

THE MORNING-AFTER PILL (MAP)

The morning-after pill (MAP) is a misnomer because it is rarely *one* pill that is used, and you can even take them the same night. Today the most popular form of MAP consists of two Ovral birth control pills followed by two or more such pills twelve hours later. These should be taken as soon as possible after the main event, but definitely within seventy-two hours. The success of this approach is said to be about 97 percent, but it is clearly more successful the sooner the pills are taken. The main side effect is nausea.

You will not know until your period is due whether or not this method has worked for you, because the only sign of success is a period at the normally expected time.

THE DIAPHRAGM

A lot of people, especially men, who come asking about a diaphragm have never actually seen one, and the ideas that they have about size and shape are truly astounding. Even some women express amazement at the size when they first see a diaphragm. A typical reaction might be, "You're not going to get that into me." But we usually manage with little discomfort. As a matter of fact, the next reaction is usually, "It's not really in, is it?"

How It Works

A diaphragm is a rubber dome that is inserted into the vagina before intercourse. The part of the diaphragm that goes closest to the cervix should be filled with spermicidal cream or jelly (before insertion, of course). The amount of spermicide that is recommended varies according to what you read. A good rule is that if you squeeze a diaphragm, it will develop two or three grooves in its dome. If you fill the grooves with spermicide, that is usually a sufficient amount. You can also apply a bit of spermicide around the rim of the diaphragm as a first line of defense against all those invasive sperm. It is the spermicide, rather than the diaphragm, by the way, that is probably the most effective part of this method of contraception.

The diaphragm is inserted so that it covers the cervix and is anchored behind the pubic bone in front. It *must* cover the cervix; otherwise nothing prevents the sperm from swimming up their favorite swimming hole.

Although there is some dispute about this, it is commonly recommended that you not insert the diaphragm more than two hours before having sex. Some people say you can safely insert it up to six hours before the Big Bang. It must be left in place for at least six hours after intercourse. If you happen to have intercourse again during that time, you should inject some more spermicide into the vagina (this advice too is questioned by some people), but do not take the diaphragm out.

Diaphragms come in various sizes. When a diaphragm fits well, you generally can't feel it in place, except for a bit of pressure on the walls of the vagina.

It is always difficult to measure the effectiveness of the diaphragm because there is so much "user failure." It is generally accepted that when used perfectly, the diaphragm has an effectiveness rate of over 90 percent. The actual rate of protection, when user failure is taken into account, is more like 75 to 80 percent. But if you are a reliable user, you should get fairly good protection from this method.

Advantages

1. The diaphragm is a temporary method of birth control. Thus, unlike the IUD, which is continuously irritating the uterus, or

the pill, which you must take every single day whether you want to sleep with someone else or not, the diaphragm sits in your purse or your drawer when you don't need it.

2. The diaphragm is composed of inert rubber. As a result, no chemicals enter your bloodstream. The side effects are restricted to the vagina.

3. The diaphragm is relatively cheap, usually costing under twenty dollars. It can last for several years, and the only cost besides the original outlay is the cost of the spermicide.

4. The diaphragm is under the control of the woman. It is therefore harder for a woman to be talked out of using it in those situations where the man tends to be more obstinate.

Disadvantages

1. There is some fuss and muss involved with the use of a diaphragm. Because a diaphragm must be left in place for several hours after intercourse, it can be messy, especially for women who have had intercourse in the morning. They must walk around with the diaphragm inside them for much of that day.

2. The diaphragm interferes with sexual spontaneity. A diaphragm makes intercourse a more calculated activity, something that seems to bother men more than women. Many women say that they would use a diaphragm, but the man in their life doesn't or wouldn't like it. So they choose something else, which is generally a wise decision because, as mentioned before, any method that interferes with one's sexual relationship is likely to be soon abandoned.

3. A subtle disadvantage is that the man can always feel the diaphragm during the act of making love. And although the rubber dome is exceedingly thin and soft, intercourse being intercourse and men being men, they will occasionally complain that they do not like the feel of the rubber.

4. Because of the way it sits in the vagina, a diaphragm increases a woman's risk of developing a bladder infection. The diaphragm pushes up on the urethra and interferes with proper urination,

making those little bacteria that are always lurking around the urethra much more likely to push into the bladder and infect it. Someone has recently developed a diaphragm with a U-shaped nick in the rim, which presumably will put less pressure on the urethra.

Precautions

The most important precaution to remember about a diaphragm is to use it. Be realistic about your ability to be disciplined, your partner's discipline, the frequency of intercourse in your life, and your anxiety about a method that is about 90 percent effective. If you can honestly decide that you will use this method without fail, you will probably be very happy with it.

When using a diaphragm, do not use foam as a spermicide rather than cream or gel, since the foam can apparently interact with the rubber in the diaphragm.

Because the rubber thins over time, a diaphragm should be periodically checked for leaks (not leeks). This is done either by holding it up to the light or by seeing if it leaks when filled with water.

Do not use a diaphragm to help you with excess bleeding during your period. There have been a few (rare) reports of toxic shock syndrome (see chapter 11) associated with diaphragm use.

Also, according to some people, the diaphragm works best in that position favored by the missionaries. All other positions slightly increase the risk of dislodging it.

THE CONDOM

Condoms are excellent contraceptive devices. However, I have yet to meet a man who likes them. Many women dislike them as much as men do. This general lack of affection for the condom leads to a high user failure rate.

It is generally accepted that when used properly, and when the quality of the condom can be assured, the effective rate of contraception with condoms is 95 to 99 percent.

Condoms fail for several reasons. First, they fail because of lack of quality control in the manufacturing process. Condoms are like microwave ovens. They can leak and they can break, although this is less likely to occur with the quality, brand-name condoms.

Condoms also break if they are improperly stored, especially in warm, moist areas. There are men, and some women, who have been carrying the same condom around in their back pocket for years, in case they "get lucky" and score, which hasn't happened since the Cubs last won the pennant, several decades ago. It is much more likely that that particular stored condom will break in a pinch.

How It Works

Although every male likes to believe that he was born with the knowledge of how to use a condom (after all, where else can it go, huh?), many men err when confronted with the actuality of using one. Here, then, are Art Hister's simple rules for condom use:

1. The woman should make sure that the condom is put on before there is any attempt at penetration. In fact, it should be put on as soon as you start thinking about what is going to happen (about dinnertime for most men).
2. You have to leave room at the tip to collect ejaculate, or the condom can literally explode like a balloon. Just think of the force behind that biological urge.
3. When putting on a condom, you have to roll it up to the top of the shaft of the penis so that it cannot come off easily inside the vagina.
4. When withdrawing from the vagina, you must pinch the top of the condom so that it won't go for a solo swim in the vagina.
5. Condoms are not recyclable. Use once and discard.

It's monkey see, monkey do. But monkey must see first. And then monkey should practice.

Advantages

1. The major advantage of a condom is the lack of side effects, especially for the woman. Aside from occasional rashes in response to the lubrication or lack of it, it is exceedingly rare to see other side effects in either the man or the woman.
2. Condoms, like diaphragms, can safely be stored until they are needed, although as mentioned above I would not advise storing a condom for too long without replacing it.
3. When you rely on condoms as your method of birth control, you have nothing going through your body while you are celibate.
4. The latex condom is a major armament in the battle against the spread of AIDS. Natural condoms made from sheep intestine (what's natural about using a sheep intestine to cover your penis?) do *not* protect against the virus that causes AIDS.
5. Condoms can also protect against gonorrhea, herpes, chlamydial infections, trichomonas infections, warts, hepatitis B, and other STDs.

Disadvantages

1. The major disadvantage of the condom is that it is not under the direct control of the woman. Unfortunately, the consequences of failure of contraception are much more severe for the woman. Or to put it another way, many men don't care as much as they should about what happens when birth control fails. When the man is the one responsible for contraception, it doesn't take the brain of an Einstein to see that it is more likely that this method will occasionally (frequently?) be abandoned.
2. Condoms interfere with the mechanics of the sexual act. Unlike the diaphragm, which can be put in before you go to bed on the assumption that something important is going to happen soon (sleep for most of us), condoms can only be put on at the time the need arises. This necessitates an interruption that is difficult for many couples to incorporate comfortably into their sexual relationship.

3. Depending on the frequency of intercourse, this may be a some-
    what expensive method of birth control.

Precautions

There is only one important precaution. If you decide to use condoms, make sure you always have two around, make sure you know
how to use them, and *use them*.

The only other precaution is that if lubrication is a problem, either
buy only lubricated condoms or use water or spermicide. Do not use
petroleum jelly or mineral oil, because they can damage the condom.

THE CERVICAL CAP

Apparently the cervical cap was very popular in the early years of
this century and then faded in popularity for unknown reasons. Like
Neil Sedaka and the Rolling Stones, however, it has made a comeback.
But its comeback is considerably more successful than Sedaka's (thank
God). (Apparently the Stones are now promoting their own label of
sportswear. Given their ages, do you think that their next project will
be Rolling Stones Old Age Homes? Complete with the large-tongue
logo, of course.)

How It Works

The cervical cap looks like a hard, pliable thimble. It should be
filled with spermicide before being inserted. It is then pinched onto
the cervix and sticks to it by suction. You remove the cap by flicking
it, which breaks the suction seal.

The cervical cap is about as successful as the diaphragm in preventing pregnancy.

Advantages

Most of the advantages that were listed for the diaphragm are applicable to the cervical cap as well:

1. A cervical cap is cheap.
2. A cervical cap is inert.
3. A cervical cap provides temporary birth control.
4. A cervical cap is under the control of the woman.

A cervical cap, however, does have significant advantages over the diaphragm for the appropriate patient:

1. A cap is less messy than a diaphragm, since it often requires less spermicide.
2. A cap can be left on the cervix for longer than the diaphragm can be left in the vagina, up to several days. But remember that the longer that it's left in place, the worse the smell (it is, after all, a foreign body) and the greater the likelihood of a vaginal infection.
3. Because a cervical cap is small and placed far back in the vagina, the man may not be able to feel it, unlike a diaphragm, which he can always feel.

Disadvantages

1. The cervical cap often takes a bit of practice before you know how to use it properly. At first it may feel as if you'll never be able to do it. But as with the violin, if you practice, you can be a virtuoso (although I doubt if you will be paid to play your instrument at Carnegie Hall).
2. A cervical cap does not fit every cervix. Because there is some room for error, you should always have your cap fitted by someone who has some experience fitting these devices.
3. Cervical caps are made of thicker rubber than diaphragms. If the man happens to be able to feel it, ouch. The thick rubber can hurt his delicate parts, depending on how directly he hits the cap (and depending on how delicate his parts are).

4. The fact that the man can hit the cap is a real problem to the woman as well because the force of the thrusts during intercourse can dislodge a cervical cap. It may come as a rude surprise to you the next morning when you go fishing for the cap and you find it floating freely in the vagina. Thus, with every new partner, a woman with a cervical cap is well advised to use another method of birth control (usually condoms) as well for the first few weeks. During that time her homework is to experiment with intercourse in various positions to see if the cap can be dislodged, not a tough assignment for most.
5. As with diaphragms, there have been occasional reports of toxic shock syndrome with use of the cap. It is worth stressing that the cap is not meant to be used as an alternative to menstrual pads or tampons.

There is no proof that a cervical cap can worsen a cervical inflammation. Thus, it can be used safely even by women with abnormal Pap smears.

Precautions

The only precaution is to say that if you want to use a cap, practice. End of story.

THE SPONGE (FROM OUTER SPACE)

A new barrier method of contraception has recently been loosed on the women of Canada, although it's been available in the United States for several years. It's called a contraceptive sponge.

How It Works

The sponge is (surprisingly) a spongelike device loaded with spermicide that is inserted into the vagina before intercourse. The sponge is merely a more attractive material than rubber in which to load the spermicide.

Advantages

The spongey material is quite soft and is apparently well tolerated by most men and women. The safety profile, effectiveness rate, and pattern of use are similar to those of other barrier methods. (Speaking of barriers, the least effective barrier method of birth control is a father who doesn't let his daughter date.)

Disadvantages

Do not be fooled by ads. Although the manufacturer may advertise the effectiveness rate as approaching 100 percent, objective evidence shows that this method is no better at preventing pregnancy than other barrier methods.

THE INTRAUTERINE DEVICE (IUD)

The IUD is an instrument loved by lawyers. It is surrounded by controversy and lack of adequate information (as well as by the uterus, of course). Thus, women will come into the office and say that they don't want an IUD because it's only for women over forty. Or others will refuse an IUD because they have a girlfriend who ended up with a pelvic infection, and they have heard that all women who have an IUD are at high risk for pelvic infection. I even had one woman tell me that she had never considered an IUD for herself because she had heard that only fat women could tolerate them. All of these fears are groundless.

How It Works

We still do not know exactly how the IUD works. It's always fashionable to bring up the fact that nomadic Arabs put stones into the uteri of camels on those long treks across the desert. (I move in strange circles, where people know stuff like this.) Apparently, the intrauterine stones worked well to prevent pregnancies in the camels. But we really have never known exactly how the stones worked. My own theory is that male camels don't choose to have intercourse with female camels who have stones in their uteri. It's not a completely appealing prospect, you must admit, even to a horny camel. Besides, it must be so noisy when they finally do mate.

For the longest of times it was thought that an IUD works by aborting a conceived fetus. That is, the egg and sperm get together and do their thing, but the product, a new embryo, has nowhere to go because the IUD irritates the lining of the uterus too much, turning the usual home for the fetus into an inhospitable environment.

We now know that this is not its only (or main) mode of action. An IUD certainly does irritate the inside of the uterus at the points at which they are in contact. In fact, this irritation is what produces the heavier, longer, and crampier periods that women with IUDs suffer. But the IUD also alters the sperm in a way that prevents the little guys from fertilizing the ovum. The IUD also seems to alter the way the fallopian tubes move (what is known as tubal motility) in a fashion that may protect against pregnancy.

The IUD is fairly efficient at doing what it is meant to do. Statistics vary, but the IUD seems to be about 97 percent effective. What this means is that if 100 women use an IUD for one year, 97 will not get pregnant. More to the point, especially to those others, is that 3 women *will* get pregnant. The pregnancy rate for the IUDs that we insert in our office is lower than that. Perhaps we are more selective in our patients, or perhaps our patients do not have intercourse as frequently (something I very much doubt); there are many variables.

Advantages

1. The IUD is cheap. Depending on where you buy it, it costs about thirty to forty dollars, which is not too much money if you amortize

it over the several years you may keep it. The original cost of the IUD is your only expense (except for more tampons from heavier periods).

2. Once it's in place, you no longer have to think about contraception until the IUD must be replaced. Intercourse can then be as spontaneous as human beings can make it (which means that you can "do it" as soon as the male of the species stops flipping channels at night).

3. The IUD is effective instantly. (Once after I'd inserted a woman's IUD, she ran up to me in the hall while I was chatting with several other patients and asked me breathlessly, "When can we make love, Art?" "I have to do rounds first," I replied.)

Many doctors, and the companies that manufacture IUDs, recommend removing all IUDs after two years or thirty months. But in many clinics, including my own office, the doctors leave most IUDs in place up to four or five years (except for the Progestasert, which must be replaced every year), and the pregnancy rate does not seem to increase from one year to the next. I don't think that IUDs should be left in place longer than five years, because there are some reports that the rate of infections begins to go up after that amount of time.

Disadvantages

1. For the longest time, doctors were concerned that the IUD seemed to be prominently implicated as a cause of PID (see chapter 13). It is now clear that the IUD by itself does not cause PID. However, if you happen to be exposed to the organisms that cause PID, an IUD will accelerate the passage of these organisms into the uterus and fallopian tubes, allowing the infection to occur more quickly and probably more severely.

    That is why before having an IUD inserted, it is extremely important that you evaluate your risk of being exposed to these organisms. If you are a young teenager who has never had children and who has multiple sexual partners, you are definitely a poor risk for having an IUD. If, however, you are a thirty-year-old woman who has had all the children you want and have only one sexual partner, who can be trusted not to have multiple partners on his own, you are a good candidate for an IUD. (Did you know that you could be a candidate for an IUD? "C'mon down Susie, you're our next contestant on 'One Size Fits All.'")

2. A controversial point is whether or not someone who has had a previous pelvic infection, should ever use an IUD. Most doctors counsel patients who have previously had PID to never even think of having an IUD because the risk of future infections and sterility is too high.

    I am more ambivalent. In the selected, highly motivated, vigilant patient, I think it's worth a try if there are no good alternatives. But at the first hint of possible pelvic inflammation, the IUD should be removed and the woman should be treated with the appropriate antibiotics.

3. If you become pregnant with an IUD in place, you have a greater chance of having an ectopic pregnancy (see chapter 11). If you have an abnormal period, and most particularly if you miss a period and you have an IUD, it is imperative that you check with your doctor.

4. IUDs cause heavier and crampier periods. For most women, this is not too severe a problem. For some women, however, it may mean abandoning the IUD as their preferred choice. This is especially true for women who have uterine fibroids, who should probably never have an IUD at all. If you have heavy periods, you should be checked periodically for iron-deficiency anemia.

5. The IUD has a string that projects out of the cervix into the vagina. Occasionally men can feel this string during intercourse, and it may irritate the penis. I have always felt that some men complain too much about the sensitivity of their penises. If you tell these men that there is a dime in the vagina, they will feel obligated to tell you if it's heads or tails that they can feel. Suffice it to say that most IUD strings are so thin and so covered with mucus that even if the man can feel it, the string shouldn't bother him excessively. If it continues to be an irritant, it can be shortened (the IUD string, not the penis). But it cannot be cut too short, or else there will not be enough string left to tug on when the IUD must be withdrawn.

Precautions

It is preferable to insert an IUD towards the end of menstruation. First, a period ensures that you are not pregnant. Second, at the end of the period the cervix is also slightly more open, making it easier to insert an IUD. And third, since there is always a bit of bleeding with an insertion, you will not notice it as much if you are menstruating.

Some doctors put IUDs in immediately after delivery of a baby. I prefer to wait until the uterus has returned to normal, about two months after the delivery. Immediately after a therapeutic abortion, however, it is relatively simple to insert an IUD.

Some doctors routinely inject a local anesthetic into the cervix to relax the cervix before inserting an IUD. I believe that most women can relax enough to permit easy insertion if the doctor spends some time helping them relax. In the excessively tense person, a small dose of tranquilizer can help (the patient, not the doctor).

An IUD should always be rechecked after a few days or weeks have passed to see if it has moved or been expelled. I usually advise returning after the next period, when enough time has elapsed for any events to occur that might dislodge the IUD.

You should periodically check the IUD string by inserting a finger into the vagina and feeling the string at the end of the cervix. If you ever feel that the IUD string has lengthened, you should be examined by a doctor. The IUD may have moved and may need to be replaced.

If you can feel any hard plastic tip at the opening of the cervix, the IUD has moved into the cervix, having left its permanent residence in the uterus. It is then no longer as effective for contraception and must be removed.

If you miss a period, or even if your period is somewhat different (if it's much lighter or it comes much sooner, for example), it is important to check for an ectopic pregnancy.

If you have an IUD and you experience a new, unexplained pain in the pelvis or lower abdomen or an unexplained vaginal discharge, you should always get checked for a pelvic infection.

If you have an IUD, it is quite important that you get a yearly pelvic examination. At that visit, you should reevaluate your need for that particular method of contraception; you should be checked to see if the IUD is still in place; you should have a Pap test; and you may require screening for possible STDs.

If you happen to become pregnant while you still have your IUD in place, you should have it removed as soon as the pregnancy is diagnosed. Even though removing the IUD leads to a higher rate of miscarriage, leaving it in place during the rest of the pregnancy leads to a higher rate of complications, including miscarriages later in the pregnancy, infections, and bleeding problems. If you insist, however, the IUD can be left in place until delivery, in which case you are likely to hear, "Congratulations, Mrs. Gumby, you have a copper T."

VASECTOMY

How It Works

To sterilize a man, all you have to do is to interrupt the flow of semen to the waiting outside world. Under local anesthetic, a small cut is made in the scrotum on each side. Each spermatic cord is found and cut. The patient is then stitched and sent on his way, slowly.

Advantages

1. Vasectomies are simple procedures.
2. They are virtually 100 percent effective.
3. Vasectomies are cheap. The medical plan generally pays for them.

The overwhelming proportion of men will tell you it's the best thing they ever did. And so will their partners.

Disadvantages

1. Complications are rare but include infection and bleeding, which is usually minimal.
2. A small percentage of men become temporarily impotent, usually

for several weeks, There is no physical reason for this problem. It is probably due to the fact that the male's "essence" is somewhat wounded by this procedure, at least at an emotional level. When the man realizes in his soul that he is really unneutered by this surgery, his prowess quickly returns.

3. Many men who are sterilized have a small rise in their cholesterol levels, and for a long time there was concern that these men would have a higher rate of heart attacks and strokes. This does not occur. In fact, in some studies men who have undergone vasectomies have fewer cardiac problems than their unaltered brothers, although the difference is minimal. (They probably worry less.)

Precautions

Never have a vasectomy done assuming that you will want to reverse the procedure. Even though vasectomies can be reversed with a success rate of 60 to 70 percent, you should always go into the procedure waving a permanent good-bye to your spermatic cords. (A bon voyage party is not a bad idea.)

I generally put it this way to my patients: "If Brooke Shields were to walk in here, Harold, and she were to tell you that she must have your baby, would you still be happy that you had had the vasectomy? If the answer is "Regretably, yes," then go ahead with the procedure. But if Ms. Shields could seriously tempt you with that type of offer, don't do it.

Circumstances change. "Forever" sometimes turns out to be six more months, and the person in your life now may not be the main person in your life a year from now. Your new partner may desperately want a child, and your operation may be a serious hindrance to a happy new relationship. Before you have it done, be honest with yourself about what you would do if your circumstances were to change.

An important precaution is not to trust the results of the vasectomy until three months have passed, because the procedure fails in a small number of men, some of whom have an extra spermatic cord lingering in there. You should "beware the lurking sperm" and use another method of birth control for three months postcut, at which point you should have a final sperm count done. The number of sperm seen at that time should be zero.

TUBAL LIGATION

How It Works

Unlike a vasectomy, a tubal ligation is not a minor procedure. To interrupt the fallopian tubes, whether by cutting them or burning them or using some other method, requires entry into the abdominal cavity. This was done in the past by making an incision, called a bikini cut, at the bottom of the abdomen — a major procedure. Now a much smaller cut, called a laparoscopy incision, is made in the area of umbilicus and results in a quicker recuperation.

Advantages

1. Tubal ligations rarely fail. It appears that failure is more likely to occur when the tubal ligation is done at the time of a cesarean section, or in the postpartum period.
2. The other important advantage is that the woman does not have to worry about contraception in any new partnership.
3. Tubal ligations are cheap (free, actually).

Disadvantages

1. Tubal ligations require more anesthetic and longer recovery times and produce more complications, such as bleeding and infections, than vasectomies.
2. It is also necessary to spend a small amount of time in hospital.
3. A small but significant number of women complain of heavier and crampier periods after having tubal ligations.

Precautions

If Robert Redford insisted that he wanted you to be the mother of his next child, would you regret your decision to tie your tubes? A tubal ligation is much more difficult to reverse than a vasectomy, with successful reversals averaging, at best, 30 percent of attempts.

Mr. Redford may not wait around to assess the results of your attempts at reversal. If you have hesitations about whether or not you might want to become pregnant in the future, do not have your tubes tied.

NATURAL BIRTH CONTROL

Natural birth control is a general term to cover all methods of contraception that attempt to predict when a woman will ovulate. These methods include the rhythm method, measuring basal body temperatures, the cervical mucus method, "astral" birth control, and others. What they all have in common is that the proponents of each method believe that they have developed a good predictive tool for ovulation, and to avoid pregnancy all you have to do is avoid intercourse at unsafe times. What all these methods also seem to have in common is that they don't work very well for most women.

How It Works

As described in chapter 11, ovulation generally occurs fourteen days *before* the next period. That means that you have to be psychic to make ovulation methods of birth control successful. You have to know how long the *next* cycle is going to be to predict when that egg that is just dying to be fertilized will emerge.

This inexactitude is made even more complicated by the fact that ovulation does not always occur exactly fourteen days before a period. It may occasionally occur twelve days before, or even ten days. Add to that the fact that sperm can live for up to seventy-two hours in the female reproductive tract, and you know why there are so many little offspring of devout Catholics running around. Rhythm is at best an inexact method of contraception. And it merely has to fail once a year to ensure a continuing population increase.

For those who do not want to rely only on inexact numbers to predict when ovulation will occur, there are physical changes that appear in some women that correlate with ovulation. In most women, mucus from the cervix becomes much thinner at ovulation. This happens so that sperm can more easily pass through on the way to do their job. In addition, the body temperature rises about a degree in many women when they ovulate.

Many women tell you that they "just know" when they are about to ovulate or when they just have ovulated. They usually experience subtle, nonmeasurable changes that correlate to the time the egg emerges from its nest, and they are usually correct.

Advantages

The obvious advantage of a natural method of birth control is that if it works, there are no possible side effects, and you can't beat the price.

Disadvantages

Unfortunately, many women just don't go through the same distinct changes every month. So even though you may be able to tell on some months that ovulation is about to occur or has already happened, on other months the same changes don't take place. Which means that you must have another method of birth control handy, just in case (sort of like going on a two-week vacation to somewhere in Asia and packing clothes "in case it rains, in case it snows, in case the regime is overthrown, etc."). More of an irritant is the fact that some changes, like the one in the cervical mucus, can occur even though you haven't ovulated. These false positives lead to many days (nights, really) when you must avoid intercourse even though you are in no danger of conceiving.

But the major problem with ovulation-predicting methods of birth control is that sperm live so long. Predicting fertile periods is only useful if you can avoid intercourse for at least three days before you ovulate.

SPERMICIDES AND FOAM

Spermicides are chemicals that immobilize or kill sperm. Foam disperses better than cream or gel, so when a spermicide is used alone, use only foam. And remember that it needs to be put into the vagina thirty minutes before intercourse.

When used without any other concurrent method, spermicides have a poor track record in preventing pregnancy. They should be used only as occasional alternatives to another, more reliable method.

WITHDRAWAL

A word about the withdrawal method of birth control. I have read that in certain cultures, coitus interruptus, or the withdrawal method, is a very successful method of contraception. (In my house, coitus interruptus means that the phone always rings at the wrong moment. And yes, I always answer it, even though I know it's usually for the kids.) And many couples will tell you that they practice this method, with a good result, which presumably means that no pregnancy occurs until they want it to. However, in objective studies of typical North American couples, withdrawal has not proven to be a very effective method of contraception. Males, like old pipes, leak. And it takes only one sperm to fertilize an egg. Add to that the fact that many men delay withdrawal until the last split (spilt?) second, and there is an even greater likelihood that extra sperm will spill into the vagina.

CHAPTER 15

Designer Diseases

*In which the good doctor loses some of the friends
he has made over the years*

This will come as no surprise to anyone over the age of three, but life can be tough. I realize that one or two people may have said this before me, but it bears repeating. Life is often difficult. Three-year-olds understand this better, and can handle it better, than some adults.

In our sometimes-difficult and often-frustrating struggle with the many details of our daily existence, we often end up fatigued or depressed or run-down. Or we develop chronic headaches, sleeping difficulties, or itchy, persistent skin rashes or a host of other troublesome symptoms. These symptoms are usually mild and transitory. But sometimes they can be overbearing and completely consume the sufferer. Likewise, the symptoms can last for an evening and be relieved by a good night's sleep, a glass of wine, meditation, or a pleasant meal with friends. Or they can be so severe as to require a significant change in lifestyle.

Most of these symptoms are primarily produced by our physical and emotional situation at the time. My question to most patients who come to me with these complaints is this: "If you were living on Maui, having just won a ten-million-dollar lottery, and you were being fed grapes and macadamia nuts by a loving partner on a white-sand beach, would you still have these symptoms?" Most patients can smile and say, "I doubt it."

We have developed the unfortunate tendency of saying that these symptoms are due to "stress." This is true only in the very general sense that all of us are all of the time subject to some type of stress.

It is impossible to conceive of a stressless environment. But most people who complain of undue fatigue deny any extra or excessive stress in their lives at that time. Indeed, most responsible adults are capable of dealing with particularly stressful situations simply because they know they have no alternative. At such times they rarely develop fatigue, probably because they cannot afford to.

I believe that it's more accurate to say that these symptoms are due to our inability to adapt well to the normal stresses that are part and parcel of daily life, to our unhappiness with our situations and our lifestyles. Stress will never disappear from our lives (even living on the beach on Maui with unlimited funds can be stressful — will it be too sunny, are the mangoes overripe, is the surf really up, will someone take it all away from us?), but we can adapt to our particular lifestyle in a more wholesome and healthful way, and this change in adaptation generally relieves the symptoms. At least for a while.

Most patients who suffer from chronic fatigue are willing to accept this explanation. In fact, most of them arrive at the office saying, "I know there is probably nothing really wrong with me. I'm just feeling very tired and I want a checkup to know that I'm all right."

These are the easy ones to deal with. They rarely require expensive and fruitless tests (such as a blood mango level) to confirm their suspicions. Reassurance is usually sufficient, often curative.

There are, however, a substantial number of people who demand a physical explanation for their symptoms. These people invariably complain that they know that everybody feels somewhat tired, but they are more tired than the others. Or they have spent the last five months with a daily headache, and there must be a physical cause for this problem because they know they are not really tense individuals. What is often hard to ignore, but impossible to verify, is the accompanying assertion that there was a time when they did not feel this way. So something physical must be amiss.

Invariably, all the tests that our unsophisticated science can offer these people produce normal results. Traditionally trained doctors are seldom able to find a physical cause for these patients' symptoms. Such patients often make tours of dozens of doctors' offices searching for what is essentially an unobtainable solution to their problem. They are a very frustrated and often a very angry group of people.

These patients are particularly susceptible to what I call designer diseases. A designer disease is a disease or syndrome that purports to explain some, if not all, of the vague and ill-defined symptoms that plague most of us from time to time.

Every few years a new designer disease appears in the public domain, usually accompanied by a cover story in one of the mass-market magazines. The earliest one I remember was hypoglycemia. Today there are two main contestants for the all-symptom crown. In the near corner we have chronic mononucleosis (more recently named myalgic encephalomyelitis), and in the far corner, the yeast syndrome. They seem to have appeared on the scene concurrently, and they are by no means mutually exclusive. Recently, SAD and fibrositis have appeared as new "contendahs" but for the middle-weight, not the heavy-weight, crown (they don't try to explain as many symptoms). And food allergies always lurk in the background as possibilities.

I imagine that currently somebody, probably somewhere in California, is busily working on a new syndrome to be loosed on the world as soon as yeast books fall from the best-seller lists. Designing a new disease is not as hard to do as you might think. If you have a minimal amount of medical information, you can probably design your own. You must simply remember the features that all designer diseases have in common and include as many as you can.

Designer diseases should always deal with vague, ill-defined, hard-to-verify symptoms. If your hair turns green every time you eat a certain food, for example, that's a very exact symptom. That means that we can easily define an experiment to prove whether or not that food causes your hair to glow green. However, if you pick headaches or fatigue as the symptoms to explain, defining a reproducible experiment becomes considerably more difficult. How do we measure fatigue? How can we compare your fatigue with the fatigue of someone else? ("Hey, man, I'm more tired than you." "Oh yeah? Prove it!") One person's weariness is often another person's normal state (an old Irish proverb).

It is vitally important that designer diseases be very difficult to diagnose. The most effective way to do this is to say that everybody seems to suffer from the syndrome to a certain degree. There can therefore be no good test to separate nonsufferers from the afflicted.

It is also important that believers in designer diseases claim a conspiracy against the disease. This conspiracy should include especially all doctors who don't believe the problem exists. The charge must be made that doctors either are incapable of diagnosing the problem or do not want to diagnose it. Often it is both. To counter this conspiracy, there is always a host of "alternate" practitioners, including many classically trained doctors, available to cater to those suffering from these new afflictions. These alternate healers often use tests and treatments that scientifically trained doctors do not recognize as valid.

It is easy to focus on doctors as unenlightened conspirators because even at the best of times, the medical establishment can be a slow-moving, conservative, show-me dinosaur. For many reasons, which are beyond the scope of this book, traditional doctors are often unwilling to entertain new concepts that question established medical protocol. Doctors are conservative healers, making them as a body an excellent target for conspiracy theorists.

There is one other aspect that these syndromes share — a willing public ready to accept these explanations for their symptoms. This aspect is more of a factor than it was fifty years ago. We are more affluent, are better educated, and have more time to spend analyzing our aches and ills than did our grandparents and parents. They were too busy surviving two world wars and the depression to worry about any fatigue they may have had. They were either too hungry or too busy to wonder why they were tired at night. Or perhaps it was just obvious to them.

We seem to have more time to worry about these things. We are also a generation that demands explanations. And there is always someone available to explain the unexplainable. (Take the stock market, for example. Have you ever met a broker who couldn't tell you after the fact why a stock fell in price? Where was she before the price sagged?)

Now for the million-dollar question. (Actually, if I could answer this, I would earn considerably more than a million.) Do these designer diseases actually exist?

The Jewish answer is mostly no and somewhat yes. I realize that this answer will leave no one satisfied, but as with much else in life, you have to learn to live with it (an old Jewish proverb).

There are undoubtedly some people who suffer from each of these problems. There is no doubt that there are people who absorb a knockout blow from a viral infection, for example. They stay sick with fatigue and other viral symptoms for a long time after the virus has gone. But a large number of people who claim they are affected by such symptoms are not suffering from a viral haymaker. Many are suffering instead from a psychiatric problem, usually depression. Unfortunately, this diagnosis often makes both the patient and the doctor quite uncomfortable, so both parties are often reluctant to even mention that possibility. It is considerably more difficult to tell people you think they are depressed than it is to tell them that they have some vague medical syndrome that we cannot adequately diagnose. ("Well, Mr. Smith, you seem to have a chronic case of Who-Knows Disease, a rare disorder found only in men of your age and background, but that means, you'll be extremely happy to know, that you are psychologically as sound as the yen. By the way, I must tell you that there's nothing we can do for sufferers of Who-Knows, except to see them once a month. See you next month.") In our culture, physical disease is much more acceptable, spiritually, emotionally, even financially than is psychiatric disease. (It's generally easier to get an insurance or disability claim in your favor if you have a physical problem than if you have a psychological problem.)

A lawyer friend once said to me, "I'm getting close to burning out on this job, and I feel very much like those people you described with chronic fatigue syndrome." (Lawyers listen to my show because they think they're going to get everything I describe and they want to hear of new diseases they can sue someone for.) "Too bad I can't afford to get it. My boss just wouldn't buy it."

This cynical observation is, unfortunately, accurate in many situations. The assembly-line worker rarely suffers from chronic fatigue syndrome or burnout. He or she can rarely afford to.

CHRONIC FATIGUE SYNDROME

Chronic fatigue syndrome has gone through several name changes in its brief existence. It has been called yuppie flu, postinfectious neurasthenia, chronic mononucleosis, chronic Epstein-Barr virus (EBV) syndrome, myalgic encephalomyelitis (ME), and chronic fatigue syndrome (CFS). The latter is probably the best name because it doesn't pretend to name the cause or define the pathology.

CFS is a problem in search of a name. It is, as well, a problem in search of an explanation.

To understand the most accepted explanation for CFS and the reason for this plethora of names, it is important to understand what happens to us when we get any acute viral illness. Most people who get the flu (or any other viral illness) suffer from fatigue and depression (why me, O Lord?) for a few days (or a few weeks with acute mononucleosis). These symptoms are real and are probably nature's way of telling us that all the work we are doing is not really so terribly necessary and that we should rest a while and take care of ourselves. Chicken soup, juices, sympathy, and some soaps on the tube are pretty good treatments for most viruses. Mothers treat flus and other viruses at least as well as physicians (although a mother's bill is often in different currency from a doctor's). And mothers have been at it a lot longer.

CFS is diagnosed in patients who complain of excessive and prolonged fatigue following any viral illness. This fatigue is often associated with feelings of depression, sleeping difficulties, and lack of libido. People with these symptoms also often complain of frequent exacerbations of their symptoms if they have to exert themselves physically. Another common complaint is that they get sick much more often than their neighbors and that they are unable to fight off any type of virus making its rounds in the community.

The typical patient is most likely to be female (perhaps because women visit doctors more for this kind of symptom than do men), generally young to middle-aged, a professional or middle-class person, a high achiever (hence the perjorative term "yuppie flu," although rumor has it that you don't need to own a BMW or a cappuccino machine to qualify).

We do not really understand why people develop this prolonged tiredness. The favorite medical explanation has been that these people are simply depressed and that their depression manifests itself with the symptom of fatigue. The patients respond by saying, "Of course we're depressed. Wouldn't you be if you were tired all the time? Our problem is not depression. Something else is going on."

CFS is a disease that the patients themselves tell us they have.

Because there are no tests to separate the sufferer from the healthy, you can label yourself as suffering from CFS as soon as you consider your fatigue excessive or prolonged. (The Epstein-Barr antibody tests that are done by a lot of doctors are in no way connected to an accurate diagnosis of this condition.) The only way a doctor might help you is by ruling out other causes of fatigue, such as anemias and other metabolic abnormalities.

There is no known drug treatment for CFS. We cannot treat most viruses anyway, but we certainly cannot treat what we can't diagnose. Medical treatment, therefore, consists of the euphemistic support, rest, and reassurance. This means living a healthy lifestyle, resting as much as possible, and — the hardest part of the treatment — waiting.

Most people eventually recover from CFS, although symptoms can last for many years. I have no doubt that as time goes on and more and more patients are labeled as having CFS, we will discover that some people suffer from this condition for life.

So far, CFS seems to be a syndrome without major medical complications. We have not detected an increased mortality rate in the people who say they have this condition. If this is really an immune system problem, we should be able to detect other immune system defects eventually, such as a rise in the rates of some kinds of tumors. So far, this has not been measured. But on this point the jury is still out, mainly because we have just not been aware of the syndrome for long enough.

CFS is a frustrating problem for both the doctors and (mainly) for the patients. What we urgently need is some kind of test to confirm the presence of this illness in those who really have it. This would relieve the pressure on the patients, who have no way of proving they are sick, and on the doctors, who cannot treat what they can't diagnose.

HYPOGLYCEMIA

The first time that I heard of a medical conspiracy was from a patient who told me that his reflexologist had diagnosed him to be suffering from hypoglycemia after he had visited several doctors who had not been able to identify his condition. He had had numerous medical tests, all of which were negative, even for hypoglycemia. The reflexologist had told him, however, that doctors' tests are unreliable for this problem and that he was still suffering from hypoglycemia even in the face of negative results. By the time he came to see me, the patient had been given a hypoglycemic diet by the therapist, and all his symptoms were now gone. Why hadn't the doctors told him, he demanded to know? What were we afraid of? Needless to say, I was stumped. (Why did this 130-pound bespectacled male strike fear into the hearts of all the doctors he came in contact with? I still haven't figured it out.) Fortunately for me, he had his problem under control by the time he visited me, so I was not covered by this blanket condemnation of the medical profession. We have continued a pleasant doctor-patient relationship over the last fifteen years. I have never repeated the tests. (He does continue to consult his reflexologist when he doesn't completely buy my medical explanations.)

Hypoglycemia is a condition in which the glucose in your blood is too low. Glucose is generally called sugar, although blood glucose is not simply a reflection of sugar intake. More accurately, blood glucose is a reading of how much carbohydrate you have ingested and how your body's insulin is clearing this glucose from your bloodstream.

To understand the theory behind hypoglycemia, you have to understand what happens when you eat. When you ingest any food, it is broken down in the stomach into simpler components that are then reabsorbed in the intestines. These components are then either used by the body for its various functions or else they are stored for future use. What is not needed passes out.

Carbohydrates are reabsorbed as glucose, which is essential for normal body functioning.

Too much glucose in the blood is unhealthy. If the blood glucose level is too high, you have diabetes.

The way your body deals with the glucose load is to call in a type of glucose cleanser, the Zamboni (all true Canadians know what a Zamboni is) of the carbohydrate system. This glucose cleanser is called insulin. Insulin is released as soon as food is ingested. It makes sure that all excess glucose is absorbed into your body's cells and that glucose doesn't continue to circulate and damage your arteries.

With hypoglycemia, the insulin acts like an overprotective parent. It does too good a job, and the blood glucose level continues to drop.

Eventually, the insulin either runs out or tires out, permitting the blood glucose to return to normal levels.

What happens if your blood sugar drops too low? For most people who claim they suffer from hypoglycemia, the symptoms are usually that vague constellation that includes lack of energy, mood swings, inability to concentrate, headache, weakness, and so on. This problem is quickly corrected by eating a food that restores blood sugar to normal.

The glucose level in the bloodstream can hit its trough at anywhere from two hours to six hours after a meal. That is why the definitive test for hypoglycemia is a six-hour glucose tolerance test. A blood sample is taken after a fast of at least eight hours to establish the baseline for blood glucose. A defined amount of glucose in the form of a sugary drink is then ingested, and blood samples are taken every hour for six hours afterwards. And you wonder why most people become extremely fatigued while having this test?

The medical profession defines a low level of blood glucose in a very strict way. The endocrine experts claim that you do not suffer from hypoglycemia until your blood sugar drops below 60 mg/dl, and only if you develop definite symptoms at that time. By these criteria, hypoglycemia is a very rare problem (except in diabetics who accidentally inject too much insulin).

The not-so-traditional experts have much less strict criteria. Although they often attempt to explain this problem biochemically, when they can't, many of these "experts" say that hypoglycemia is really, after all, a self-diagnosed illness. This means that if you say that you feel weak every afternoon at four, and if you feel better after you have an appropriate snack at that time, then you indeed suffer from hypoglycemia no matter what the tests say. You are *when* you eat.

Unlike CFS, hypoglycemia can be treated. The mainstays of therapy are twofold. Avoid excess sugar intake (the sugar gives a prompt relief of symptoms but results in the release of excess insulin, which soon worsens the symptoms) and eat frequent small meals. To be more exact, you should eat some of the chosen foods shortly before you expect the symptoms to occur. So if you get weak four hours after meals, you should have a snack three to three-and-a-half hours after your last meal.

Hypoglycemia seems to be a problem without serious medical consequences. People diagnosed to have hypoglycemia do not have a higher rate of frank diabetes later in life, for example.

FIBROSITIS

Like chronic fatigue syndrome, fibrositis is a new problem with many names. It has been called fibromyalgia, fibromyalgia pain syndrome, and myofascial pain syndrome.

Fibrositis is a problem in which the soft tissues — the muscles, cartilage, and ligaments — of the body are thought to become inflamed, resulting in pain in various parts of the body. Inflammation cannot be easily measured. When an organ or tissue in the body becomes inflamed, white cells rush into that area to help fight some perceived insult. That body part then swells, often to a barely perceptible degree. The inflammation causes that area to hurt. In significant inflammation, you can also feel the swelling and see some redness and fullness (as with a sprained ankle or a bruise).

In fibrositis, the soft tissues of the body are presumed to become inflamed for unknown reasons. This inflammation is rarely visible and can only be diagnosed because the patient complains of pain and tenderness when that particular body part is touched.

The inflamed areas are called trigger points. Touching a trigger point can lead to varying degrees of pain. Usually the patient has multiple trigger points and consequently is often in some degree of discomfort. The pain can be so severe that the patient may require large doses of heavy-duty analgesics to obtain proper pain relief. Along with the pain, the patient also usually suffers from excessive fatigue, poor sleep, and morning stiffness in various joints.

The typical patient with fibrositis is the same as the typical patient with chronic fatigue syndrome. Usually it's a woman, in middle age, who is described as a high achiever and a perfectionist.

As with all designer diseases, there are no acceptable tests to differentiate the sufferers from the well.

There do not seem to be any severe long-term sequelae to fibrositis. People with fibrositis are no more likely to develop arthritis than is the rest of the population.

Many people with fibrositis can be successfully treated by changing their lifestyle, especially getting more exercise, and by taking antidepressant medication. The commonly used antidepressants seem to dull this type of pain significantly, to the extent that these folks can function with minimal disruption to their lives.

THE YEAST SYNDROME

The diagnosis and treatment of the yeast syndrome is a medical growth industry the likes of which I have rarely seen.

We all have some yeast, or candida, in our bodies, especially in our digestive tracts. Most women have some yeast in their vaginas as well. This has always been felt to be the normal state of affairs. Until recently, that is.

At some point in the last decade, there emerged a theory in some parts of the healing community that some people may have "too much" yeast in their systems. This state of affairs garnered the name of the yeast syndrome, or the candida syndrome.

The people who diagnose yeast infections tell us that the main reason that we have so much yeast in us is that our North American diet emphasizes food that is refined, preserved, and eaten in the wrong combinations (we eat far too much protein, for example). If you combine this diet with the overuse of antibiotics (which kill the organisms that keep yeast in check) in both humans and animals, and you also throw in a stressful lifestyle, you then have the necessary preconditions that lead to the growth of excess yeast.

The usual gang of symptoms results, including fatigue, irritability, mood swings, headaches, and the rest of the Alouettes. Candida infections are also implicated by true believers in all types of bowel complaints, pelvic problems, and immune disorders. You name the symptom, I can name you someone who will swear it is due to candida.

Traditional medicine does not recognize this syndrome. Counter-culture medicine, or alternate medicine, in contrast, not only believes this syndrome exists but also stresses that it is virtually of epidemic proportions. To diagnose it, these practitioners have produced a host of testing possibilities. The most common tests are called challenge tests. These involve putting some candida, usually in the form of a pill or an injection, into some part of the body and then measuring the reaction. Any reaction is deemed to be proof of sensitivity to this organism. I'm sure you won't be surprised to learn that I have never heard of a person who was tested who didn't react somewhat positively. There are three possible explanations I can think of. We all have it (nah, impossible, I say); only people who are truly sick volunteer for the test (another long shot); the test is not all that accurate (eureka!).

Can yeast infections be serious? There are certainly conditions in which a candida infection can be a serious, even life-threatening illness. People with unstable diabetes, people on cancer therapy regimes, and people with AIDS can all have candida spread through the body in brushfire fashion. The candida can seed the heart, the brain, and other body organs, causing untreatable, terminal infections. But these very serious yeast infections are quite different from the milder symptoms associated with the yeast syndrome (although I am certain that no one with this syndrome thinks that his or her own symptoms are mild).

To treat the yeast syndrome, you are often first given antiyeast medication in the form of pills, usually in large amounts for several weeks. In theory, this treatment kills all the yeast in your system. Traditional medicine argues that even if it does eliminate much of the yeast, the yeast instantly regrows; it's normal for it to be there.

Along with the medication, the yeast sufferer is also told to eliminate all yeast-producing foods from the diet. Despite what the yeast gurus may assure you, this diet is very restrictive. It is virtually impossible to function as a normal person in our society and still follow the diet guidelines carefully. Here is just a partial list of foods you should not eat on a yeast-free diet: all sugars (including, of course, honey), all alcohol and vinegar, all cheeses (except cottage and ricotta, but whoever thinks of those things as cheeses anyway?), all fruit, all nuts, all mushrooms, all "regular" breads. You can eat meat (without sauce, of course), vegetables (likewise without sauces), fish, chicken, eggs, and grains. Remember, if you also plan to follow a low-cholesterol diet, there goes much of the red meat and the eggs. Have a nice day.

I remember a woman who had suffered from extremely painful periods and had indeed found some relief with a yeast-free diet. But she tearfully told me that she had stopped following the diet and reverted to painful periods because she had become a "diet cripple" as a result of all the restrictions she had put on herself and her mate. She couldn't go out to eat without cross-examining the servers. She was unable to eat at friends' houses without ruining the meal with all her questions and demands. She spent hours in markets reading labels. Better to put up with the symptoms, she said.

If you want to believe you have yeast syndrome, by all means follow the diet and see if you improve. If you do improve, you must then decide whether your symptoms are sufficiently better to warrant this change in your lifestyle. We have no proof that this diet can harm you physically. I make no promises about your psyche (and dinner at my house is off).

FOOD ALLERGIES

The first patient who told me she had food allergies that the medical profession had not been able to diagnose also informed me that there were a couple of other things about her physical and mental state that I should know. In short, she was a Jewish lesbian celiac (a person who is allergic to gluten, present in wheat, oats, barley, and rye), which I believe is a rather small minority of the population (although probably very well organized). I have never forgotten her, possible because I too am Jewish and a celiac. I also prefer women as my sexual partners, so we had much in common.

Food allergies are the easiest designer disease to define. The name tells you all you need to know. Traditional medicine accepts that food allergies do indeed exist, but there is much difficulty in diagnosing them properly (see chapter 4). Most people who label themselves as having food allergies have never had confirmatory tests done. These people just say that they have certain symptoms when they eat the foods to which they are allergic. These symptoms include all the usual ones as well as multiple bowel problems. The latter include "poor digestion," gas from either end, abdominal cramps, changes in bowel movements, and similar complaints.

The two most common food groups that people claim they are allergic to are wheat and dairy products. In fact, there are many people who cannot tolerate dairy products, or foods that contain lactose. That is because these people lack an enzyme called lactase, which breaks the lactose down. So when they eat dairy products, they only partially digest those foods, and they can suffer from various digestive symptoms as a result. Strictly speaking, this is not an allergy because there is no antigen-antibody reaction (see chapter 4). Interestingly, these folks can tolerate fermented lactose, so they can generally eat cottage cheese and yogurt.

Real allergy to gluten is associated with a small but significant risk of several kinds of bowel tumors (a fact that keeps me up many nights). People who have this condition should be told emphatically to avoid all gluten-containing foods, and they should be carefully monitored for changes in their bowel symptoms as they age (even though we are not certain that sticking to the diet really reduces the risk of tumors, another fact that keeps me up when the first one doesn't).

You would be truly amazed, by the way, at how adept food manufacturers are at putting some type of wheat or barley extract into their products. Thus, if you are a strict celiac, you must avoid most soy sauces, many ice creams, all fast foods, most luncheon meats, beer, and most hard liquors, not to mention all breads, pastas, and pastry. You end up eating lots of cheese (if you are not lactose intolerant as well) and chicken (the interesting thing about chicken is that I have never heard of anyone who is allergic to it).

There are no medications to take to alleviate true food allergies, although lactose-sensitive individuals can drink milk to which a commercial lactase enzyme, Lactaid, has been added. Lactaid can digest up to 90 percent of the lactose in milk. But with real allergies, you must simply avoid those food groups.

SAD

You know how down you get when the days become short and the nights seem to be endless? All of us experience a type of sadness related to short winter days. We call this the winter blues, or blahs, or winter doldrums.

The psychiatrists have now come along to tell us that there are people in whom this sadness is really a sickness. They have named it seasonal affective disorder, or SAD.

I am not sure exactly how you diagnose SAD, but I suppose that if you are more depressed than expected from a simple change in the seasons (especially if you eat more at that time), then you must have SAD. There are no good tests to tell you if this diagnosis is correct.

There is a treatment, however, which consists of shining light on yourself, so that the days feel longer.

Epilogue

In which the good doctor signs off

So there you have it. For $27.95, less if you bought this book on remainder, and nothing if you borrowed it or stole it, you have learned all the important facts that I believe are needed to encourage your health and well-being.

I hope all the material was comprehensible and relevant. (My publisher is praying mostly that it was accurate.) If you are not certain about anything I have written, always check it out with your local expert, who is generally your family doctor. Most family physicians I know are usually only too happy to correct something that you read somewhere else (which sounds pejorative but is not).

The last word is this. Always give yourself credit when dealing with your body and its malfunctions. You know that old bod better than anyone else. (Really, now, who else would want to know it as well?) And always do everything with a sense of moderation, using the common sense you were born with.

That's all, folks.

Glossary

Words can be confusing. Paul Simon says that one man's ceiling is another man's floor. If he had an M.D., he might have said, "One woman's pain is another woman's normal state" (an old German proverb). In medicine, this type of confusion can result in needless distress. Here are just some of the words that I have found over the years may be a ceiling to one, a floor to another.

Abscess   An abscess is a walled-off area of infection. Antibiotics cannot penetrate an abscess, so it must be drained surgically; otherwise it will continue to fester and expand.

Benign   A tumor that is not malignant is benign. Some benign tumors can still be a problem. For example, a benign growth in the brain can be a real hazard if it continues to grow because we often have no good way of getting at it.

Biopsy   A biopsy is a procedure in which tissue is removed from the body for further analysis. Biopsies don't necessarily require anesthetic or stitches.

Cancer   A cancer is a malignant growth.

Carcinoma   A carcinoma is a cancer that grows from the cells lining any particular organ. It is the most common type of cancer.

Hernia   A hernia is a rupture in some body tissue. The most common hernias occur in the groin area in males (inguinal hernias) and in the muscular diaphragm (hiatal hernias).

Infection   An infection is an inflammation due to the presence of a foreign invader such as a bacterium, virus, or parasite.

Inflammation   Inflammation is a reaction of body tissue to an injury. The result is swelling, heat, redness, and pain.

Malignant   A tumor that will kill you if allowed to grow is a malignant tumor. A malignant tumor either spreads or erodes through essential adjacent tissue.

Tumor   A tumor is a swelling. It is not necessarily a malignant growth. A benign swelling is a tumor as well.

Ulcer   An ulcer is a deep erosion in the lining of a tissue or on the skin.

INDEX

abdominal pain, 160–61
Accutane, 207
acetaminophen, 59
Achilles' tendon, 193
acne, 205–208
  and therapy, 206–207
acute abdomen, 165–66
acute mononucleosis, 78
acyclovir (Zovirax), 214, 289
Adalat, 82
addictions, 5–6
additives in food, 24
adenoids, 100–101
adrenalin, 73
Advil, 59
aerobic exercise, 13, 193–94
aerosol sprays, in asthma, 114
AIDS (acquired immune deficiency
  syndrome), 294–95
  test, 47
alcohol:
  benefits of, 8
  effects of, 6–9
  as a factor in heart disease, 128, 141
  and impotence, 275–76
Alcoholics Anonymous, 9
alginic acid compound (Gaviscon), 156
allergens, common, 70
allergic:

conjunctivitis, 72
  dermatitis, 209
allergies, 69–75
allopurinol (Zyloprim), 185
alopecia areata, 223
alveoli, 106
amenorrhea, 248–49
anaerobic exercise, 13
Anakit, 73
anal:
  fissure, 170
  itching, 167
analgesic medications, use in chronic
  pain, 57
anaphylactic reactions, 73
Anaprox, 242, 246
androgen in puberty, 206
anemia, 80–81
angina, 122, 143–44
angiotensin-converting enzyme (ACE),
  137–38
ankylosing spondylitis, 180
anovulatory cycles, 250
antacids, 156
anti-allergic kits (Epipen or Anakit), 73
antihistamines, in treatment of
  allergies, 71
anus, 152, 167–76
anusitis, 170

apnea, 98–99
arthritis, 180, 183–86
arthroscopy, 53
ASA, 59
astemizole (Hismanol), 71
asthma, 111–15
asthmatic attacks and antihistamines, 72
Atarax, 225
atheromas, 121
atherosclerotic heart disease, 121–22
athletes, and anemia, 80
athlete's foot, 212
automated reagin tests (ART), 42
AZT (Retrovir), medication for AIDS, 295

back pain, low, 179–82
back problems, prevention of, 181
bacterial conjunctivitis, 86
bacterial infections of the skin, 216–18
Bactrim, 74
Bactroban, 216
bad breath, 92–93
baldness, 222–23
Bartholin's glands, 231
baseball, 194–95
Benemid, 185
benign breast disease (BBD), 257–58
benign prostatic hypertrophy, 276
Benson, Herbert, 26
beta blockers, 67, 137
Betadine, 239
biopsies, 51
birth control:
    factors in choice, 297–99
    pill, 299–306
bisacodyl (Dulcolax), 172
bites and stings, 227
bladder, 230–31
    infections, 255–56
bleeding between cycles, 250
blepharitis, 87

blood levels of medications, tests for, 42–43
blood pressure:
    acceptable levels, 134
    measurement of, 133
blood tests, 42
blood urea nitrogen (BUN): tests for, 43
boils, 217
Borrelia burgdorferi, 220
bowel cancer, 162–64
    diet concerns, 163–64
bowel movements:
    black, 175
    changes in, 171–72
    narrow, 176
bowels, 160–62
breakthrough bleeding, 250
breast:
    cancer, 250–61
    disease, 257–61
bromocriptine (Parlodel), 258
bronchitis, chronic, 110–111
bronchodilators, 113
burning, with urination, 255–57
burping, 152–53
bursa, definition of, 179
bursitis, 188

caffeine:
    as an addiction, 9–11
    and CHD, 130
    and heart attacks, 11
    and pregnancy, 10
calcaneal spur, 193
calcium:
    and nutrition, 23
    test for, 43
calcium-channel blockers, 138
calluses, 225
cancer:
    of the bowel, 162–64
    breast, 258–61
        and caffeine, 10

cervical, 243–45
of the prostate, 277
of the skin, 221–22
of the testicle, 268
Candida albicans, 234, 237
cankers, 93
carbohydrates and diet, 21
cardiovascular system, 118–46
carpal tunnel syndrome, 81
CAT scans, 51
cellulite, 205
cellulitis, 217
cervical:
   cancer, 243–45
   cap, 312–14
cervicitis, 234–35
cervix, 231
   pain from, 240
checkups, routine, 34–37
chest pain, 58, 116–17, 143
chlamydia, 272–73, 281–87
   and childbirth, 282
chloasma, 226
Chlor-Tripolon, 71
chlorhexidine (Hibitane), 216
chlorpheniramine (Chlor-Tripolon), 71
cholesterol:
   count, 43–44
   definition of, 124–25
cholesterol levels, 118–19, 121
   factors that affect, 127–31
   and heart disease risk, 123, 124
   tests for, 126–27
   treatment to reduce, 131–32
cholestyramine resin (Questran),
   131–32
chronic fatigue syndrome (CFS),
   330–32
chymopapain, for disc problems, 181
cilia, 108
cimetidine (Tagament), 157
Clinoril, 184
clitoris, 232
clonidine (Dixarit), 253

cluster headaches, 67
cocaine, 5
codeine, 59–60, 109
colds, 77
colon, 150–52
colonoscopy, 171
complete blood count (CBC), 44
condom, 280, 309–12
condylomata, 292
conjunctivitis, 85–86
constipation, 172–73
contact dermatitis, 209
contraception, 297–325
corneal abrasions, 88
corneal ulcer, 87
corns, 225
coronary artery disease (CAD), 121–46
coronary heart disease (CHD), 121–46
   rates of, 122–23
   risk factors, 123, 124–31
corpus luteum, 232–33
cough:
   chronic, 110–112
   suppressants, 109
coughing, 108
   blood, 116
   produced by bronchial irritation, 109
   produced by colds, 108–109
crabs, 218, 293–94
creatinine, tests for, 43
cromoglycate (Opticrom), 72
crotamiton (Eurax), 219
CT scans, 51
cultures, 52
cycling, 195
Cyclomen, 241, 258
cystitis, 255
cysts:
   in males, 268
   mucous, 94

Dalkon shield, 251
danazol (Cyclomen), 241, 258

DeBakey, Dr. Michael, 123
dermatitis, 208–210
dermographism, 226
Desenex, 212
desensitization therapy, 72
designer diseases, 326–40
deviated nasal septum, 96
dextromethorphan, 109
diabetes, 45–46
    as a factor in heart disease, 140
diaphragm (birth control device),
    306–309
diarrhea, 173–75
diclofenac (Voltaren), 184
diet, and heart disease, 20–21, 129–30
diet plans, weight-loss, 24–25
dilatation and curettage (D&C), 248
disc problems, 181–82
dislocation injury, 188
Dixarit, 253
doctors:
    how to choose, 28–30
    how to visit, 31–32
drugs, recreational, 4–6
dry hair, 223–24
Dulcolax, 172
dysfunctional uterine bleeding (DUB),
    247–48
dyspareunia, 239
dysplasia, 244
dysuria, 255–56

E. coli, 255
ear:
    description of, 89
    infections of, 91–92
    pressure, 92
    ringing in, 90
    wax, 89–90
early pregnancy test (EPT), 44
echocardiogram, 146
ectopic pregnancies, 233, 250–51
eczema, 208

electrocardiogram (ECG), 52
electrolytes test, 44–45
emphysema, 111
endometriosis, 240–42
endoscopy, 53–54
epididymis, 266–67
    infection in, 272–73
Epipen, 73
erythrocyte sedimentation rate (ESR),
    45
esophagus, 150, 152
estrogen, 232
estrogen replacement therapy (ERT),
    253–54
Eurax, 219
exercise, 11–16
    drawbacks, 16
    as a factor in heart disease, 128,
    141–42
    how to start, 13–16
    target heart rate in, 16
expectorants, 109
eye:
    blood in the white of, 86
    structure of, 84–85
eyelid, inflammation around, 87
eyes, runny, 72

facet impingement syndrome, 180
fallopian tubes, 230, 233, 251
farting, 166–67
fascia, definition of, 193
fatigue, 60
    chronic, 326–27
fats in diet, 20–21
Feldene, 184
female, 229–61
    cycle, 232–34
    reproductive system, 230–32
ferritin test, 45
fever, 60–61
fiber in diet, 24
Fibermed, 172

fibrocystic breast disease, 257–58
fibroids, 242, 247
fibrositis, 335–36
Fibryax, 172
fimbria, 230
Fivent, 113
Flagyl, 236, 239
floaters, in vision, 88
flu, 76–77
follicle-stimulating hormone (FSH)
    test, 45
folliculitis, 217
food:
    allergies, 338–39
    poisoning, 158–60
foot injuries, 193
frequency-dysuria syndrome, 256–57
Friedman, Dr. Meyer, 139
fruits and vegetables, nutritional value
    of, 22
fungal infections, 211–12
furunculosis, 217

gallbladder, 150
    disease, 164–65
gallstones, 164–65
Gantrisin, 74
gardnerella infection, 234–36
Gardnerella vaginalis, 234–36
gastritis, 154–57
    treatment for, 156–57
gastrointestinal system, 148–76
    description of, 149–52
gastroscopy, 53
Gatorade, 173
Gaviscon, 156
gay sex, 280
gemfibrozil (Lopid), 132
genital ulcers, 287–91
Giardia lamblia, 175
giardiasis, 175
glaucoma, 86
glucose tests, 45–46

gonorrhea, 283–84
gout, 185–86
group A beta-hemolytic streptococcus,
    101–103

hair problems, 222–24
halitosis, 92–93
headaches, 58, 62–69
    from trauma, 68
    see also specific types of headaches
hearing, decreased, 90–91
heart, how it works, 119–20
heart attack, definition of, 122
heart disease, 121–46
    and diet, 20–21
    and medications, 142
    symptoms of, 143–46
heart murmurs, 145–46
heartburn, 153–57
heel spur, 193
hemoglobin test, 46
hemorrhoids, 167–68, 169–70
hepatitis, 78–80
    test, 46
herald patch, 215
hernias, 270–71
herpangina, 93–94
herpes, 87–88, 287–90
herpes simplex virus (HSV), 213–14,
    287–90
    and childbirth, 290
herpes zoster, 214
Herplex-D Liquafilm, 213
HI titer test, 46
hiatus hernia, 157–58
Hibitane, 216
hiccups, 152
high blood pressure, 132–38
    medical therapy for, 137–38
    techniques to lower, 134–37
high-density lipoprotein (HDL), 125
hip pain, 193
hirsutism, 224

Hismanol, 71
HIV (human immunodeficiency virus) test, 47
hives, 226
hoarseness, 104
home testing, 37–38
hormones, role in female cycle, 232
hot flashes, 253
human papilloma virus (HPV), 291
humidifiers, and allergic symptoms, 74–75
hydrocele, 269
hydroxyzine (Atarax), 225
hypertension, 132–38
hyperventilation, 115–16
hypnotics, 18
hypoglycemia, 46, 328, 332–35
hypothalamus gland, 232

ibuprofen:
    (Advil), 59
    (Motrin), 184
idiopathic edema, 254–55
idoxuridine (Herplex-D Liquafilm, Stoxil), 213
immunoglobulin (antibody) test, 47
immunotherapy, 72
Imodium, 175
impetigo, 216
impotence, 275–76
incarcerated, strangulated hernia, 271
Inderal, 137
infertility in males, 274–75
influenza, 76–77
insomnia, 17–18
interferon, treatment for warts, 292
intermenstrual bleeding, 250
intestinal tract, 150–52
intrauterine device (IUD), 315–20
iritis, 86
iron in nutrition, 23
irritable bowel syndrome (IBS), 161–62, 176

ischemic, 122
isoniazid, 111
isoretinoin (Accutane), 207
itching skin, 224–25
IUD (intrauterine device), 251

jaundice, 79–80

ketoprofen (Orudis), 184
knee problems, 192, 194, 195
Kwellada, 219, 294

large intestine, 150
laryngitis, 104
lice, 218–19
ligament:
    definition of, 179
    sprains, 193
lindane (Kwellada), 219
    treatment for crabs, 294
lipoprotein, 125
lips, swelling on the, 94
lithotripter, 165
liver function tests, 47
locomotor system (LMS), 177–98
loperamide (Imodium), 175
Lopid, 132
lovastatin (Mevacor), 132
low back pain, 179–82
    prevention of, 181–82
low-density lipoprotein (LDL), 125–26
lumpectomy, 259
lung, 106
luteinizing hormone (LH) test, 45
Lyme disease, 219–20
lymph node swellings, in men, 269
lymphangitis, 217

Maalox, 156

male, 262–78
  infertility, 274–75
male-pattern baldness, 222
malignant melanoma, 221
mammograms, 259–60
marijuana, 5
massage, 190
medical tests; *see* tests, medical
medication:
  and cholesterol levels, 131
  for headaches, 64
  and heart disease, 142
  questions to ask about, 32–34
mefenamic acid (Ponstan), 246
melanin, 200
menopause, 249, 253–54
menstrual:
  cycles with no eggs, 250
  irregularities, 245–53
menstruation:
  heavy, 247
  irregular, 247–48
  missed, 248–50
  pain with, 246
Metamucil, 132
metatarsal bones, 193
metronidazole (Flagyl), 236, 239
migraines, 65–67
  medication for, 67
minerals in diet, 23
minoxidil (Rogaine), 222
miscarriages, 251–52
mitral valve prolapse (MVP), 146
moles, 221–22
molluscum contagiosum, 215–16, 293
mononucleosis (mono), 78
morning-after pill (MAP), 306
Motrin, 184
mouth, 92–94
mumps, and males, 272
mupirocin (Bactroban), 216
murmurs, heart, 145–46
muscle, definition of, 179
musculoskeletal system, 177–98

myocardial infarction, 122

nail abnormalities, 227–28
Naprosyn, 246
naproxen sodium (Anaprox, Naprosyn),
  242, 246
nasal:
  allergy symptoms, 72
  congestion, 95–96
  sprays, use of for colds, 96
natural birth control, 323–25
neck pain, 182–83
Neisseria gonorrhoeae, 283–87
Neomycin, 74
neurodermatitis, 209
niacin, 131–32
nifedipine (Adalat), 82
night leg cramps, 83
night sweats, 82
nipple discharge, 261
nongonococcal urethritis, 286
nonsteroidal anti-inflammatory drugs
  (NSAIDs), 59, 155–56, 184, 190
nose, 94–98
nosebleeds, 96–97
nuclear medicine tests, 54
nutrition, 18–25

obesity, as a factor in heart disease, 141
onychomycosis, 213
Opticrom, 72
orchitis, 272
orthoses, 191
Orudis, 184
osteoarthritis, 185
osteoporosis, 23, 186
otitis:
  externa, 91–92
  media, 91
ova and parasites, tests for, 54
ovarian cysts, 242
ovaries, 230

overuse injury, 188
ovulation, in cycle, 233

pain:
    abdominal, 160–61
    acute, definition of, 57–58
    from the cervix, 240
    chronic, definition of, 56–57
    female, 239–43
    in groin area, 272–75
    during a heart attack, 144
    hip, 193
    low back, 179–82
    neck, 182–83
    pelvic, 242–43
    in pelvis and abdomen, 240
    rectal, 170
    vaginal, 239–40
painkillers, and headaches, 62
palmar warts, 215
palpitations, 145
Pap smears, 234, 243–45
papilloma virus, 244
parasite infections, 218–19, 293–94
parasites and ova, tests for, 54
Parlodel, 258
paroxysmal atrial tachycardia (PAT),
    145
patello-femoral syndrome, 194
patient rights, 30
Pedialyte, 173
pelvic:
    inflammatory disease (PID), 284–86
    itching, 293–94
    pain, 242–43, 284–86
penicillin, and allergic reactions, 73–74
penis, size of, 277–78
peri-oral dermatitis, 218
perianal dermatitis, 167
period cramps, 246
periods:
    heavy, 247
    irregular, 247–48

missed (amenorrhea), 248–50
    pain with, 246
personality types, A and B, 138–40
pesticides, hazards of in foods, 24
pharynx, 106
phosphates, test for, 43
physical examinations, frequency of,
    34–37
pigment changes in the skin, 225–26
pinworms, 168–69
piroxicam (Feldene), 184
pituitary gland, 232
pityriasis rosea, 214–15
placenta, 233
plantar fasciitis, 193–94
plantar warts, 215–16
plaque in the arteries, 121
plastic surgery, 228
platelet test, 48
pleurisy, 116–17
pneumonia, 110
pneumothorax, 116–17
podophyllin, 292
Ponstan, 246
postinflammatory discoloration, 226
potassium in nutrition, 23
povidone-iodine (Betadine), 239
pregnancy:
    and caffeine, 10
    test, 44
premenstrual syndrome (PMS), 245–46
probenecid (Benemid), 185
progesterone, 232–33
projectile vomiting, 158
propranalol (Inderal), 67, 137
prostate, 267
    cancer of, 277
    pain in, 273–74
    problems of, 276–77
prostatitis, 273–74
protein:
    in diet, 21–22
    test for, 43
pruritis, 224–25

psoriasis, 211
psyllium, 132
pterygium, 88

Questran, 131–32

racquet sports, 196
ranitidine (Zantac), 157
rapid heart rate, 145
Raynaud's disease, 81–82
rectal:
    bleeding, 170–71
    itching, 168
    pain, 170
rectum, 152, 167–76
red eye, 85–86
reflux, 153–55
reflux esophagitis, 154–55
    medication for, 156
    treatment for, 155
Relaxation Response, The, 26
respiratory system, 105–117
    how it works, 106–108
Retrovir, medication for AIDS, 295
Reye's syndrome, 61
rheumatoid arthritis, 183–84
rheumatoid factor test, 48
RICE (rest, ice, compression, eleva-
    tion), 189–90
rifampicin (Rifampin), 217
Rifampin, 217
ringworm, 212
Rogaine, 222
running, 191

safe sex, definition of, 279–80
salt in the diet, 24
saturated fats, 125
scabies, 218–19
sciatic nerve, pressure on, 181
sciatica, 178–79

seasonal affective disorder (SAD),
    339–40
sebaceous:
    cysts, 204–205
    glands, 200
seborrheic dermatitis, 209–210
sebum, 200
Seldane, 71
Selsun shampoo, 212
semen, 265–67
Senokot, 172
Septra, 74
sex, as a factor in heart disease, 140
sexual safety, how to maximize, 280
sexually transmitted diseases (STD),
    238–39, 279–96
    about, 280–81
    organisms that cause, 281–84
"shin splints," 188
shingles, 214
shoulder injuries, 197
sigmoidoscopy, 171
silent ischemia, 122, 140
sinus:
    congestion, 99–100
    headaches, 68
sinusitis, 99–100
skiing, 196
skin, 199–228
    cancers, 221–22
    and chemicals, 202
    description of, 200
    how to protect, 201–203
    infections, 211–21
    sun and, 201
    tests for allergies, 54
sleep, 17–18
    apnea, 98–99
    disorders clinic, 99
sleeping pills; see hypnotics
small intestine, 150
smell, sense of, 94–95
smoking:
    as a factor in heart disease, 128, 141

hazards of, 2–4
and impotence, 274–75
and the skin, 202
snoring, 97–98
sodium cromoglycate (Fivent), 113
sore throats, chronic, 103–104
spermatozoa, 265–67
spermicides and foam, 325
spidery veins, 204
spinal column, 178–79
sponge, barrier method of contraception, 314–15
spontaneous abortions, 251–52
sports injuries, 186–98
    medications, 190–91
    prevention, 188–89
spot mono tests, 48
sprain, 188
sprained ankle, 192
stings and bites, 227
stomach, 150, 152
    flu, 77
Stoxil, 213
strep throat, 101–103
stress:
    and headaches, 63–64
    in life, 25–26
    and personality types, 138–40
stress fracture, 188
stroke, 122
styes, 87
subconjunctival hematoma, 86–87
substance abuse, 4–6
sulfa drugs, and allergic reactions, 74
sulfamethoxazole-trimethoprim
    (Bactrim, Septra), 74
sulfisoxazole (Gantrisin), 74
sulindac (Clinoril), 184
sunscreens, 202
Surgam, 184
swallowing, 153
swimmer's ear, 91–92
swimming, 197
syphilis, 290–91

test for, 42

T_4, TSH tests, 48
tachycardia, 145
telangiectasia, 204
temperomandibular joint (TMJ), 69
tendon, definition of, 179
tendonitis, 187–88, 193
tennis elbow, 196
tension headaches, 62–65
terfenadine (Seldane), 71
testicle(s), 265–66
    cancer, 268
    pain in, 272
    self-examination, 268
    torsion of the, 272–73
testosterone, 265
    test, 49
tests, medical, 32, 39–55
    false positives and false negatives, 40
    questions to ask, 40–41
theophylline preparations, 114
thoracic cavity, 106
throat, 100–104
tiaprofenic acid (Surgam), 184
Tinactin, 212
tinea versicolor, 212–13
tinnitus, 90
TMJ syndrome, 69
tolnaftate (Tinactin), 212
tonsillitis, 100–101
tonsils, 100
toxic shock syndrome, 252–53
trace elements and nutrition, 23
trachea, 106
tranquilizers, and headaches, 64
traumatic injury, 188
Treponema pallidum, 290
trichomonas, 238–39
Trichomonas vaginalis, 234
triglycerides, 126
tubal ligation, 322–23
tuberculosis (TB), 111–12

292s, 59
Tylenol, 59–60

ulcers, 155–57
 treatment for, 156–57
ulnar nerve, 196
ultrasound and heart murmurs, 55, 146
undercyclenic acid (Desenex), 212
urethra, 232
 discharge from, 271
 pain in, 273
urethral discharge, 286
uric acid test, 49
urinalysis, 50
uterus, 230

vagina, 231
vaginal:
 discharge, 234–39, 287
 pain, 239–40
varicocoeles, 268–69
varicose veins, 204
vas deferens, 267
vascular headaches, 67–68
vasectomy, 320–22
vasomotor rhinitis, 95–96
vegetables and fruits, nutritional value
 of, 22
vegetarians:
 and anemia, 49, 80–81
 and nutrition, 22–23
venereal:
 disease; see sexually transmitted
  diseases
 ulcers, 291
 warts, 215
  how to remove, 292–93

vertebral column, 178–79
viral:
 conjunctivitis, 85–86
 infections, 75–76
 of the skin, 213–16
vitamin A acid cream for skin, 203
vitamin B_{12} deficiency, 80–81
vitamin B_{12} and folate tests, 49
vitamins and nutrition, 22–23
vitiligo, 225
Voltaren, 184
vomiting, 158
vulva, 231

walking, 198
warts, 215–16, 291–93
wheezing, 112
whiplash, 182
white blood count, 50
Winston Churchill Syndrome, 154
withdrawal method of birth control,
 325
wrinkles, 203

X rays, 51
xanthine family of drugs, 9–10

yeast:
 infections, 237–38
 syndrome, 336–38
yohimbine, 276

Zantac, 157
zits, 205–208
Zovirax, 289
Zyloprim, 185